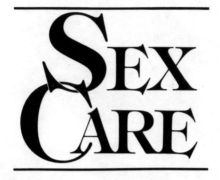

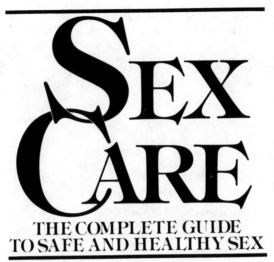

SEX CARE

THE COMPLETE GUIDE TO SAFE AND HEALTHY SEX

Timothy R. Covington, Pharm. D.
Birmingham, Alabama

and J. Frank McClendon
Huntington, West Virginia

PUBLISHED BY POCKET BOOKS NEW YORK

Another *Original* publication of POCKET BOOKS

POCKET BOOKS, a division of Simon & Schuster, Inc.
1230 Avenue of the Americas, New York, N.Y. 10020

ISBN: 0-671-52398-8

First Pocket Books trade paperback printing June, 1987

10 9 8 7 6 5 4 3 2 1

POCKET and colophon are registered trademarks
of Simon & Schuster, Inc.

Printed in the U.S.A.

To Betsy,
my love, my life,
my inspiration.

T.R.C.

Acknowledgments

I wish to acknowledge the many individuals instrumental in the development and production of this book:

Marnie Hagmann for her early advocacy of the prospectus.

Stacy Prince for her encouragement and commitment.

Christine Young for her excellent artwork.

David Lief Anderson for his superior job of copy editing.

Sydny Weinberg Miner and Sally Peters for their patience, loyalty, support, enthusiasm, and commitment to this project.

Drs. James G. Stevenson, Charles D. Ponte, Marie A. Abate, and other professional colleagues who provided invaluable input and/or encouragement.

Betsy, Courtney, and Abby for their constant patience, encouragement, sacrifice, and support that only family members can provide.

T.R.C.

Contents

INTRODUCTION   1

I
CONTRACEPTION

Chapters 1 through 8 emphasize proper use, safety,
effectiveness, adverse effects, precautions, warnings, and
special considerations.

1 Oral contraceptives   15
2 The intrauterine device (IUD)   39
3 Condoms   59
4 Barrier methods: Diaphragm and contraceptive sponge   79
5 Spermicidal gels, creams, and aerosol foams   99
6 Other contraceptive methods   115
7 Voluntary sterilization   136
8 Investigational contraceptives   158

II
SEXUALLY TRANSMITTED INFECTIOUS DISEASES: THEIR PREVENTION AND TREATMENT

Chapters 9 through 16 emphasize cause, symptoms, prevention,
and treatment of each infectious disease.

9 Gonorrhea   183
10 Genital herpes   194
11 Acquired immunodeficiency syndrome (AIDS)   215
12 Syphilis   233
13 Nongonococcal urethritis   246

14 Pelvic inflammatory disease (PID)   *255*
15 Trichomonas vaginalis   *266*
16 Other sexually transmitted diseases   *275*

III
SPECIAL CONSIDERATIONS IN SEXUAL HEALTH

17 Premenstrual syndrome (PMS): A therapeutic enigma   *293*
18 Toxic shock syndrome (TSS)   *307*
19 Drugs and diseases that affect sexual function   *316*
20 Methods of pregnancy detection   *333*
21 Pregnancy termination (abortion)   *347*
22 Rational approach to feminine hygiene   *364*
23 Sexual myths and fallacies   *375*

INDEX   *391*

Preface

Sexual health encompasses (1) effective birth control, (2) avoidance of a host of sexually transmitted viral and bacterial diseases, and (3) recognition of numerous factors that may enhance or detract from the state of sexual well-being. Sexual health is not guaranteed; it does not just happen. Optimal sexual health requires a base of fundamental knowledge and conscientious application of that knowledge.

The author realized the need for a comprehensive guide to sexual health some years ago. Statistics on pregnancy and sexually transmitted disease are alarming. Consider, for example, that despite the change in attitude about sexual education in the United States in the last few decades:

- Of 393 sexually active U.S. college coeds surveyed in 1978, 65% used "high-risk" methods of conception control (withdrawal, rhythm, douche) or no method at all.
- The number of unwanted pregnancies is rising and approximately one in five (17.9%) of all births in the U.S. were to unmarried females in 1985.
- Approximately 1 million 15 to 19 year olds become pregnant each year in the U.S., and 600,000 of them will deliver offspring.
- Over 1.3 million legal abortions secondary to unwanted pregnancies have been conducted in the U.S. each year of the 1980s.
- Of a group of 3,592 U.S. college students surveyed in 1984, 90% expressed a strong desire for more information on methods of contraception prior to marriage.
- Approximately 14 million unplanned pregnancies occur annually in the U.S.

The physical, psychological, moral, ethical, religious, and economic considerations associated with unwanted or unexpected pregnancies cannot be minimized by society.

Furthermore, the serious issue of sexually transmitted disease is only now beginning to receive the attention it deserves. In an editorial in the *Journal of the American Medical Association*, Edward N.

Brandt, Jr., M.D., Assistant U.S. Secretary of Health, stated: "Sexually transmitted diseases are becoming the 'epidemic' of the 1980s and 1990s and a 'human tragedy' resulting in a great deal of unnecessary suffering." This statement is supported by the following public health statistics derived by the U.S. Department of Health and Human Services during the 1980s:

- Approximately 300,000 to 500,000 new cases of genital herpes are diagnosed each year in the U.S. Approximately 20 million Americans currently harbor this incurable virus. Cases of genital herpes increased 1,086% (over tenfold) between 1965 and 1981.
- Approximately 1.3 to 1.8 million new cases of gonorrhea are reported annually in the U.S. Because as many as 50 to 80% of patients may not develop symptoms, over 3.0 million cases exist in the U.S. at any one time. Approximately 200 million new cases of gonorrhea occur throughout the world each year.
- Approximately 100,000 new cases of syphilis are reported annually in the U.S. Approximately 40 million new cases of syphilis occur throughout the world each year.
- Approximately 3.0 million new cases of trichomoniasis occur annually in the U.S.
- A significant portion of the 200,000 new cases of hepatitis B reported annually in the U.S. are sexually transmitted.
- More than 1.0 million annual episodes of pelvic inflammatory disease (PID) in the U.S., which occur secondary to undiagnosed and untreated gonorrhea, result in loss of fertility in approximately 100,000 women annually.
- In the 1980s over 100,000 babies per year had diseases or malformations associated with a sexually transmitted disease of the mother.
- In a 1984 survey of married women in the U.S., 38% reported having had a sexually transmitted disease.

There are well-defined methods for preventing both the spread of sexually transmitted disease and unwanted pregnancies. Effective treatment of sexually transmitted disease is generally available, as are effective birth control methods. And there are many other special considerations essential to sexual health—key topics such as pregnancy termination, pregnancy detection, drugs and diseases that affect sexual function, feminine hygiene, and sexual myths and fallacies—on which helpful information is important. No book on sexual health would be complete without providing detailed information on these topics. Greater appreciation of these somewhat unrelated topics can contribute substantially to your physical, psychological, social, and emotional well-being.

The purpose of SEXCARE: The Complete Guide to Safe and Healthy Sex is to provide a comprehensive manual that will assist you in maximizing sexual health and enjoyment while decreasing the probability that an adverse health event or unwanted pregnancy will occur. This book's 23 chapters cover four major areas: (1) the proper use, safety, effectiveness, adverse effects, precautions, warnings, and special considerations of available birth control methods, (2) a discussion of prevention and treatment of sexually transmitted diseases, (3) a discussion of contemporary topics in sexual health (such as pregnancy termination, drugs and diseases that affect sexual function, toxic shock syndrome, and premenstrual syndrome), and (4) an overview of reproductive physiology (in the Introduction).

The book is designed to be a thorough, but easy-to-understand, guidebook or manual for the general public, one that will help you be an informed consumer of preventive health care and medical services and attain the highest possible degree of sexual health and enjoyment.

T.R.C.

Introduction

The consequences of casual or uninformed sexual practices can do much to compromise the quality of life of individuals—from adults and adolescents to unwanted children and even developing fetuses. Cultural attitudes have contributed to problems of secrecy, taboos, and fears concerning sex. Such societal attitudes are changing for the better, however, and sex is increasingly viewed more appropriately as a natural and fulfilling part of life. Attitudes toward sex are changing in a positive manner, but there is one dimension to healthy sex that is impossible to overstate: The key to sexual health and liberation lies in more effectively educating *ourselves* about how to maximize sexual health and enjoyment while minimizing the chance that an adverse health event or unwanted pregnancy will occur.

There is abundant evidence that many of us require more information about sexual health. A very high percentage of contraceptive failures are due not to a defect in a drug or device, but rather to the fact that the user did not utilize the drug or device properly. Most of the millions of cases of sexually transmitted diseases (STDs) diagnosed each year could have been prevented if appropriate contraceptive measures and hygienic practices had been observed. Even if STDs occur, most can be effectively treated if prompt medical attention is obtained.

Below are tragic examples that further reveal the need for more sexual health information:

- A 15-year-old unwed mother-to-be became visibly distraught in the fifth month of pregnancy. Finally, during the sixth month of pregnancy, and after suffering much mental anguish, the young woman asked a co-worker how the baby was going to be born through her navel.
- Some teens think there is no possibility of pregnancy if

1

you are not married, if the female doesn't have an orgasm, or if you have sex standing up.

- A letter to a syndicated columnist/counselor, which is reprinted from time to time, asks if a female can get pregnant by kissing a male on the lips.
- A student nurse was admitted to a hospital with symptoms of endometrial adenocarcinoma (cancer of the uterus), severe iron deficiency anemia, and excessive menstrual flow. After several days of hospitalization and numerous expensive diagnostic tests, one physician finally asked the woman if she was taking any medication. The patient reported she was taking four oral contraceptive tablets per day for 21 days each month to "guarantee" that she would not become pregnant. When the woman stopped taking the oral contraceptive, her symptoms disappeared. Her overzealous and uninformed approach to self-treatment, however, almost cost her life.
- Approximately 75% of teens surveyed in 1986 think if they develop a sexually transmitted disease and are successfully treated they cannot have the disease again.
- Approximately 91% of teens surveyed in 1986 feel that sexually transmitted diseases aren't really dangerous to one's health.
- Numerous women who failed to seek prompt treatment of gonorrhea have developed pelvic inflammatory disease (PID) and become sterile.

While these are fairly extreme examples, it is clear that many sexually active individuals do not seem to understand or appreciate how to prevent pregnancy or sexually transmitted disease effectively—or in some cases even how a baby is started or born. The social and economic consequences of unplanned pregnancy, sexually transmitted diseases, and other sexual and personal hygiene misadventures can be devastating to the affected individual, spouse, children, family, and friends and perhaps to a developing fetus as well.

THE RESPONSIBILITY OF THE INDIVIDUAL

Consumers bear great responsibility for educating *themselves* about numerous matters of sexual health. Although society is becoming more liberal in matters pertaining to sex and sexual health, there is little opportunity for formal education; in fact, a Surgeon General of the United States has stated that the next great improvement in public health will occur when people undertake *personal* efforts to reduce health risks. Today's society is actively involved in a health improvement renaissance. The consumer is demanding and assuming a larger role in self-care.

In tracing the history of 20th-century medicine, Art Ulene, M.D., has stated that we entered this century in an era of *infectious disease medicine*. Sanitation measures, immunizations, and antibiotics allowed staggering gains in life expectancy. In the 1950s we entered an era of *mechanical medicine* where we fixed or replaced our diseased organs or parts with surgical procedures, new organs, or prostheses. We are now in an era of *life-style medicine,* which deals with health matters over which we have personal control. Information is the greatest resource in an era of life-style medicine.

Episodes of psychological and/or physical suffering due to poor understanding of sexual health matters can involve most adults at some time in their lives. For example:

- Premenstrual syndrome (PMS) was not generally viewed as a legitimate medical condition until a few years ago. Women have been suffering unnecessarily for centuries because of PMS. Numerous approaches to treatment can alleviate many, if not all, discomforting symptoms of PMS in a large percentage of women.
- Toxic shock syndrome (TSS) can be prevented if women are aware of risk factors and avoid them.
- Legal and illicit drugs often have an adverse effect on sexual function.
- Inappropriate approaches to pregnancy termination often expose the female to extreme health risks.
- The public is cheated out of tens of millions of dollars annually for products claimed to have mystical or magical sexual properties.
- Thousands of unwanted pregnancies occur each year because individuals do not use contraceptive drugs or devices, do not select an appropriate contraceptive for their individual needs, or do not use a particular contraceptive properly.

Statistics, such as those listed in the Preface, only tell part of the story. Although we would like to think we are a sexually liberated society and are well educated and informed about how to achieve sexual health, facts reveal that we are not. There is much room for improvement, but improvement is only possible when we are better educated and informed in all matters that pertain to sexual health.

A WORD ABOUT POPULATION TRENDS

About 10,000 years ago (around 8,000 B.C.) when the agricultural revolution began, there were about five million people in the world. As humans began to domesticate animals, stay in one spot, and grow crops, life became more secure; subsequently the birth rate increased and the death rate decreased. At the time of the birth of Christ, the world population stood at 200 to 300 million. That number did not double until approximately 1,650 years after the birth of Christ. The world population reached the one billion mark by 1830. By then, the industrial revolution was in full swing. Fossil fuels were burned, transportation was improved, agriculture became more advanced, sanitation and other public health measures were developed, and population growth began to surge. In only 100 years (1930) the world population had doubled again, to two billion. Growth has been almost a geometric progression since 1930. It only took another 30 years (1960) to reach a world population of three billion. The global population was four billion in 1975, and is over five billion today.

TABLE 1
YEARS REQUIRED TO ADD ONE BILLION PEOPLE TO THE WORLD POPULATION*

Number	Years Required	Year Reached
1 billion	2,000,000 +	1830
2 billion	100	1930
3 billion	30	1960
4 billion	15	1975
5 billion	11	1986
6 billion	9	1995

*1 billion is 1,000 million

A population of six billion is projected by 1995. By 2050, it may well reach 10 billion (see Table 1). Experts predict that the explosive increase in population may not level off for 125 years. The earth currently gains 150 persons per minute—that's 9,000 per hour, 216,000 per day, and 80 million per year. The increase in world population is approximately the equivalent of adding one Bangladesh or Mexico per year. The overall growth in the global population is 1.7% per year, with the highest growth rate in the most undeveloped countries (by 1976, only six countries [East Germany, West Germany, Austria, Belgium, the United Kingdom, and Luxembourg] reported stable or declining populations). Some undeveloped countries have annual growth rates of 4.0%.

Neither futurists, ecologists, demographers, biologists, nor any other group can say what the "carrying capacity" of the earth is. Anyone can understand, however, that economic and population growth cannot continue indefinitely on a finite planet with limits on natural resources, food supplies, and tolerance for pollution.

The French use a riddle to teach children the nature of exponential growth. They say that if a pond contains a single leaf on day one and the number of leaves doubles each day—that is, two leaves the second day, four the third day, eight the fourth day, and so on—the pond is full of leaves on the 30th day. The teacher then asks when the pond is half full. The answer is obviously the 29th day. Using this analogy, the global lily pond on which five billion of us currently live may already be half-full. The next generation could "fill the pond" entirely. If this doubling of the population occurs at a rate beyond our technical ability to cope with it, as is probable, a large number of countries will face economic, ecological, health, energy, nutritional, social, and political stresses that could prove unmanageable.

Signs of stress on the world's principal biological systems and energy resources are already present. The earth's primary biological systems—oceanic fisheries, grasslands, forests, and croplands—are currently stretched to their limits of capacity. Oil production will peak in the early 1990s, and the nuclear dream is fading. The economic system of the future may be designed around a post-petroleum, non-nuclear world employing renewable sources of energy. How we will address the needs of a rapidly expanding world population if growth continues as projected will tax the intellectual capacity of the human mind.

There are excellent short-term approaches to coping with population growth, however. One of the most fundamental approaches is contraception. The only reasonable solution to the problem of unchecked population growth is to conscientiously apply birth control procedures worldwide. The world need not be on a collision course with disaster. The key to solving the problem is education and informed decisions by individuals.

REVIEW OF REPRODUCTIVE PHYSIOLOGY

Many of you have a general picture of the human reproductive system but are unclear on the details. What follows is a review of the basics of normal human reproductive physiology.

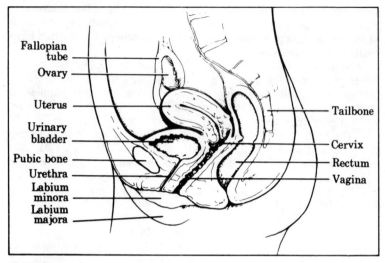

FIGURE 1

Side view of female reproductive system

FEMALE REPRODUCTIVE PHYSIOLOGY

Glands, ducts, and supporting structures comprise the female reproductive system (see Figure 1). The *primary* sex organs of a woman are the two ovaries. Her *secondary* sex organs are two fallopian tubes or oviducts, a vagina, a uterus, a vulva, and two breasts.

Primary Sex Organs

The *ovaries* are two glands resembling almonds in size and shape. They are located on each side of the uterus. The two purposes of the ovaries are to produce an ovum (egg), and to secrete the female sex hormones, estrogen and progesterone (see Table 2). Most women are born with approximately 400,000 ovarian follicles, each containing one immature egg; no new ones develop after birth. Only a few, approximately 400, ever reach full maturity, and the rate at which they mature is usually one per menstrual cycle. All the others degenerate, and few, if any, are present by the time a woman reaches menopause.

Over a period of 30 to 40 years, a woman's body prepares itself for pregnancy with each menstrual cycle. The egg matures in a small sac or follicle of the ovary. When the egg is "ripe," the follicle splits open, releasing the egg. This process occurs near the middle of the

TABLE 2
SELECTED PHYSIOLOGICAL EFFECTS OF THE TWO PRIMARY FEMALE SEX HORMONES

ESTROGEN
- Growth and development of ovaries and ova (eggs)
- Growth and maintenance of healthy muscle and tissue of the vagina, uterus, and fallopian tubes
- Growth and development of breasts
- Growth and development of external genitalia
- Development of typical female body shape, such as narrow shoulders and broad hips
- Maturing of bone growth in adolescence

PROGESTERONE
- Stimulation of normal secretions of healthy uterus
- Decrease in movement of smooth muscles in the fallopian tubes
- Stimulation of breast growth and development
- Stimulation of growth of uterus in pregnancy

menstrual cycle and is known as ovulation. The egg remains viable (fertilizable) for approximately six to 24 hours following ovulation. Once released, the egg travels down one of the two fallopian tubes to the uterus.

Secondary Sex Organs

The *fallopian tubes* are attached to the uterus. The other end of each fallopian tube expands into a funnel-like portion with fringe-like projections that sweep over the ovary toward the fallopian tube. Once "swept" into the three- to six-inch-long fallopian tube during ovulation, the egg begins its trip toward the uterus. Fertilization, the union of egg with sperm, normally occurs in these tubes, and the fertilized egg is then carried to the uterus for implantation. Numerous hormonal and physical changes then take place that allow for normal development of the fetus. If the fertilized egg is not implanted in the uterus, but begins instead to develop in the fallopian tube, this is called a tubal pregnancy. This type of pregnancy is rare, cannot survive, and may result in serious complications for the woman. If fertilization of the egg does not occur, the normal cycle continues on to menstruation.

From an external view, the *vagina* is located above the rectum and below the urethra which drains the bladder. The vagina receives the male organ during intercourse and is the receptacle for sperm before they start making their way toward the egg. The vagina is normally three to four inches deep and is very elastic and capable of expansion. The vagina is largely made up of smooth muscle and is lined with mucous membranes that assist lubrication. The primary functions of the vagina are to (1) receive seminal fluid from the male, (2) act as a channel for elimination of menstrual flow and secretions of the uterus, and (3) serve as the lower portion of the birth canal.

The *uterus* (womb) is a pear-shaped organ approximately three inches long, two inches wide, and one inch thick. The upper portion of the uterus is called the body, and the narrow neck that projects downward into the vagina is called the cervix. When a woman is pregnant, the uterus undergoes remarkable changes in size to accommodate the developing baby.

The uterus is a powerful muscle and has three walls or layers. The *inner lining* is known as the endometrium, and the tissue of this layer sloughs off during the menstrual period. The *middle layer* is composed of layers of muscle that extend in all directions and give the wall of the uterus great strength. This powerful muscle is structurally adapted to facilitate childbirth, as it is thickest near the back of the uterus where the force of a contraction can help push a fetus down and out of the uterus; the lower portion of the uterus (cervix) is

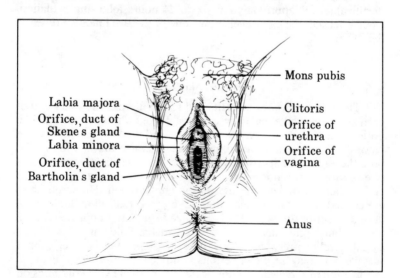

FIGURE 2
External genitalia of female

thinner so it can stretch and allow a fetus to pass into the vaginal canal. The *outer layer* of the uterus consists of a thin membrane covering only the upper portion of the uterus.

The *vulva* is the anatomical term for the *external genitals* of the female, and includes the mons pubis, labia majora, labia minora, clitoris, urethral orifice (opening), vaginal orifice, and Bartholin's and Skene's glands (see Figure 2). The *mons pubis* is a skin-covered pad of fat that lies over the pubic bone. Hair appears in this area at puberty. The *labia majora* are two large folds of tissue surrounding the vaginal opening. They are composed mainly of fat and small glands that lubricate the vaginal canal. The *labia minora* are located within the labia majora. The *clitoris* is a small organ, about one-half inch in length, composed of erectile tissue and lying between the labia, above the urethral opening, and below the mons pubis. The clitoris is the trigger of female sexual excitement and corresponds to the male penis in shape, position, and sensitivity. Involving the clitoris in lovemaking is the key to pleasurable sex for many women.

The *urethral orifice,* which lies between the clitoris and vaginal orifice, is the small opening through which urine flows. The *vaginal orifice* is the opening into the vaginal canal. *Bartholin's glands* are two small bean-shaped glands, one on either side of the vaginal opening. *Skene's glands* are located near the urethral opening. These two sets of glands normally secrete a lubricating fluid. They are frequently infected by sexually transmitted organisms, particularly the organism causing gonorrhea. Gonococcal infections of these glands are very difficult (though not impossible) to treat.

The *breasts* lie over pectoral muscles of the chest. Growth and function of breast tissue is determined largely by the hormones estrogen and progesterone. Breast size is determined more by the amount of fat around this glandular tissue than by the amount of glandular tissue itself. Therefore, size of the breast has little to do with functional ability (for example, secretion of milk for nourishment of newborn infants).

MALE REPRODUCTIVE PHYSIOLOGY

As with the female, the male reproductive system consists of a series of glands, ducts, and supporting structures. The primary function of the male reproductive system is to produce mature sperm, then introduce them into the female reproductive tract so fertilization of an egg may occur (see Figure 3). The male reproductive glands are a pair of testes, a pair of seminal vesicles, a prostate gland, and a pair of bulbourethral (Cowper's) glands. The duct system on each side consists of an epididymis, a vas deferens, and an ejaculatory duct, which connects to the urethra. Other structures include the scrotum and penis.

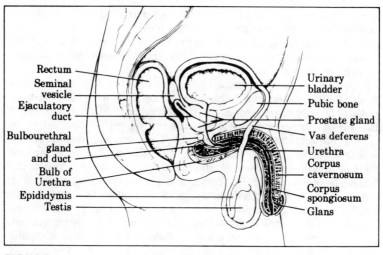

Rectum
Seminal vesicle
Ejaculatory duct
Bulbourethral gland and duct
Bulb of Urethra
Epididymis
Testis

Urinary bladder
Pubic bone
Prostate gland
Vas deferens
Urethra
Corpus cavernosum
Corpus spongiosum
Glans

FIGURE 3

Side view of male reproductive system

The *testes* are small, oval glands that lie in a pouch-like sac (scrotum) behind the base of the penis. Each testicle is about one and one-half inches long. The two primary functions of the testes are to produce sperm (spermatogenesis) and to secrete hormones, primarily the masculinizing hormone, testosterone.

The *epididymis* is a tightly coiled tube of very small diameter, but approximately 20 feet in length. An epididymis lies along the top and side of each testicle and (1) serves as a channel through which sperm travel in their journey to the outside, (2) stores a small quantity of sperm prior to ejaculation, and (3) secretes a small volume of seminal fluid (semen). The secretion of the testes and epididymides comprise less than 5% of the seminal fluid.

The *vas deferens,* which is an extension of the epididymis, passes up into the abdominal cavity, extending over the top and down the back of the urinary bladder, where it joins the duct from a *seminal vesicle* to form an *ejaculatory duct.* The two ejaculatory ducts are short tubes that pass through the prostate gland to the urethra.

The two *seminal vesicles* are pouches that fill with sperm cells and act as a storage area for sperm. The seminal vesicles secrete a thick liquid portion of semen that adds to the swimming ability of sperm. The secretions of the seminal vesicles account for about 30% of seminal fluid volume.

The *prostate gland* lies below the bladder and is shaped somewhat like a doughnut. The urethra passes through a small hole in the prostate. The prostate secretes a thin alkaline substance that constitutes approximately 60% of the seminal fluid volume. This liquid, like that produced by the seminal vesicles, promotes sperm movement, and its alkalinity protects sperm from the acid normally present in the male urethra and female vagina.

Two *bulbourethral (Cowper's) glands* are located below the prostate gland. These two pea-sized glands function like the prostate to release into the urethra an alkaline fluid that represents about 5% of seminal fluid volume.

The *penis* is the organ through which sperm are introduced into the female vagina. The urethra passes through the middle of the penis and is the exit duct for both sperm and urine. Erectile tissue surrounds the urethra. When the man is sexually stimulated, the arteries of the penis flood and stretch the space in the erectile tissue while compressing its veins. Blood enters the penis through wide arteries and leaves through narrow veins so the penis becomes larger and rigid—an erection.

The head of the penis, the *glans,* is extremely sensitive. It contains numerous nerve endings that play a great part in the male orgasm.

In traveling to the outside, sperm must pass from each testis through the epididymis, vas deferens, ejaculatory duct, and urethra. During the male sexual climax, stored sperm in the seminal fluid of the seminal vesicles is forced through the ejaculatory ducts. Muscular contractions at the base of the penis force the seminal fluid past the prostate gland and bulbourethral glands, where it picks up more fluid, then through the urethral canal. This forceful ejection of fluid is called ejaculation. The material ejaculated consists of millions of sperm cells contained in a thick, alkaline fluid.

Although only one sperm actually fertilizes the ovum (egg), millions of sperm are necessary for fertilization of the egg to occur. It is not exactly known why so many sperm are necessary. About one-half teaspoonful (2.5 ml) of semen is usually ejaculated after three or four days of sexual abstinence. This volume of seminal fluid would normally contain 250 to 500 million sperm cells. A sperm count of less than 50 million sperm cells per ml of seminal fluid is considered by some to be inadequate for fertilization of an egg, although some studies indicate that conception has occurred when sperm counts are as low as 20 million per ml.

FERTILIZATION AND IMPLANTATION

Following ejaculation into the vagina, the sperm live approximately 48 to 60 hours if no spermicidal (sperm killing) chemical is present. After ovulation, the egg remains fertile (viable) for approximately six to 24 hours. Thus, for pregnancy to occur, intercourse should occur no more than 48 to 60 hours before ovulation or 24 hours after ovulation. (These are averages only; considerable variation exists in the survival time of both egg and sperm.)

At ovulation, the ovum is pushed out onto the surface of the ovary. Once the egg is in the fallopian tube, it moves rapidly for a few minutes due to smooth muscle contractions of the tube, which soon slow down. An egg usually takes a few days to reach the uterus. Fertilization, therefore, usually occurs in the fallopian tube.

Transport of sperm to the site of fertilization within the fallopian tube is extremely rapid; the first sperm usually arrive within 30 minutes of ejaculation. Movement of sperm is due, in part, to their "swimming ability." Movement of sperm is enhanced by the fluid pressure of ejaculation and the pumping action of intercourse. Contraction of the uterine muscles during and immediately after sexual stimulation also aids motility.

Several hundred million sperm may be deposited in the vagina, but few survive. Only a few thousand reach the fallopian tube. The initial contact between sperm and egg is probably due to random motion; no attracting chemicals seem to exist. When sperm and egg make contact, the sperm cell releases chemicals that allow it to enter the egg. The DNA-containing nuclei of the sperm and egg unite. The resulting cell contains 46 chromosomes (23 from the egg and 23 from the sperm), and fertilization is complete. If the egg is *not* fertilized, it slowly disintegrates.

The fertilized egg is now ready to begin its development as it continues its passage down the fallopian tube to the uterus. During its three- to four-day passage down the fallopian tube, the fertilized egg undergoes numerous cell divisions, while the uterine lining is being prepared to receive it. After the fertilized egg reaches the uterus, it floats in and is nourished by the intrauterine fluid for a few days. Approximately seven days after ovulation, implantation occurs. The developing embryo becomes completely embedded within the endometrium of the uterus. Ultimately, a combination of tissues (the placenta) develops and serves as the organ of nutrition and waste removal for the fetus. The fetus, attached to the placenta by the umbilical cord, floats in its completely fluid-filled cavity, and develops into a viable infant over a nine-month period. If fertilization of the egg does not occur, the inner lining of the uterus deteriorates and this debris, which sloughs off, is part of the waste of menstruation.

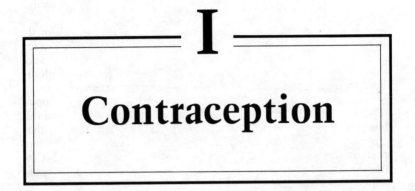

I

Contraception

1

Oral Contraceptives

INTRODUCTION

The development of the birth control pill began with clarification and understanding of the role of female hormones in ovulation and pregnancy in the early 1900s. Large scale clinical tests of "the pill" began in Puerto Rico in 1956. The first oral contraceptive contained relatively large amounts of synthetic estrogen and progestin and was determined to be effective in preventing pregnancy.

In June 1960, the U.S. Food and Drug Administration (FDA) formally approved use of the first combination (estrogen and progestin) birth control pill. Because of side effects associated with use of the early products, pharmaceutical manufacturers in the United States have substantially decreased the amounts of both hormones, thus minimizing side effects, while preserving effectiveness.

By the 1960s, the estrogenic component of the combination pill had been implicated in clotting disorders, and a "minipill," consisting of a progestin only, was evaluated as an oral contraceptive. Trials indicated that minipills produced fewer cardiovascular side effects than the combination pill, but the progestin-only pills are not without drawbacks, which will be outlined later in the chapter. Three progestin-only minipills are currently on the market (see Table 3).

The latest innovation in oral contraceptive therapy is the triphasic pill, which was introduced in 1984. The triphasic pill contains

15

TABLE 3
ORAL CONTRACEPTIVES AVAILABLE IN U.S.

Drug	Estrogen	Strength (mcg)*	Progestin	Strength (mg)**	Progestin Activity
Combination Pills (estrogen plus progestin):[1]					
Enovid-E	mestranol	100	norethynodrel	2.5	medium
Enovid-E 21[2]	mestranol	100	norethynodrel	2.5	medium
Norinyl 2 mg	mestranol	100	norethindrone	2.0	medium
Ortho-Novum 2 mg[2]	mestranol	100	norethindrone	2.0	medium
Ovulen	mestranol	100	ethynodiol diacetate	1.0	high
Ovulen 21[2]	mestranol	100	ethynodiol diacetate	1.0	high
Ovulen 28[3]	mestranol	100	ethynodiol diacetate	1.0	high
Norinyl 1 + 80[2,3]	mestranol	80	norethindrone	1.0	low
Ortho-Novum 1/80[2,3]	mestranol	80	norethindrone	1.0	low
Enovid 5 mg	mestranol	75	norethynodrel	5.0	medium
Demulin 1/50[2,3]	ethinyl estradiol	50	ethynodiol diacetate	1.0	high
Norinyl 1 + 50[2,3]	mestranol	50	norethindrone	1.0	low
Norlestrin 2.5/50[2,4]	ethinyl estradiol	50	norethindrone acetate	2.5	medium
Norlestrin 1/50[2,3,4]	ethinyl estradiol	50	norethindrone acetate	1.0	medium
Ortho-Novum 1/50[2,3]	mestranol	50	norethindrone	1.0	low
Ovcon-50[2]	ethinyl estradiol	50	norethindrone	1.0	low
Ovral[2,3]	ethinyl estradiol	50	norgestrel	0.5	high
Brevicon[2,3]	ethinyl estradiol	35	norethindrone	0.5	low
Demulin 1/35[2,3]	ethinyl estradiol	35	ethynodiol diacetate	1.0	high
Modicon[2,3]	ethinyl estradiol	35	norethindrone	0.5	low
Norinyl 1 + 35[2,3]	ethinyl estradiol	35	norethindrone	1.0	low
Ortho-Novum 1/35[2,3]	ethinyl estradiol	35	norethindrone	1.0	low

16

Ortho-Novum 10/11[5]	ethinyl estradiol	35	norethindrone	0.5	low
followed by	ethinyl estradiol	35	norethindrone	1.0	low
Ovcon-35[2]	ethinyl estradiol	35	norethindrone	0.4	low
Loestrin 1.5/30[2,4]	ethinyl estradiol	30	norethindrone acetate	1.5	medium
Lo/Ovral[2,3]	ethinyl estradiol	30	norgestrel	0.3	medium
Nordette[2,3]	ethinyl estradiol	30	levonorgestrel	0.15	medium
Loestrin 1/20[2,4]	ethinyl estradiol	20	norethindrone acetate	1.0	medium
Tri-Norinyl[6]	see footnote	------	------	------	------
Ortho Novum 7/7/7[7]	see footnote	------	------	------	------
Triphasil-21[8]	see footnote	------	------	------	------

Minipills (progestin only)

Micronor	------	------	norethindrone	0.35	low
Nor-QD	------	------	norethindrone	0.35	low
Ovrette	------	------	norgestrel	0.075	low

[1] Twenty-day regimen unless otherwise specified
[2] Available in 21 day regimen
[3] Available in 28 day regimen with 21 active and 7 placebo (inert) tablets.
[4] Also available with iron. Each of the 7 nonhormonal tablets contains 75 mg of iron as ferrous fumarate
[5] Ortho-Novum 10/11 is a biphasic oral contraceptive available in both 21 and 28 day regimen. In the 21 tablet cycle the first 10 tablets (35 mcg ethinyl estradiol and 0.5 mg norethindrone) are followed directly by the final 11 tablets (35 mcg ethinyl estradiol and 1.0 mg norethindrone). The 28 day regimen is exactly the same except that the active 10 and 11 day regimen is followed by 7 placebo (inert) tablets and the cycle begins anew.
[6] Tri-Norinyl is available in 21 and 28 day regimen. The first 7 tablets contain 35 mcg ethinyl estradiol and 0.5 mg norethindrone. This is followed by 9 tablets containing 35 mcg ethinyl estradiol and 1.0 mg norethindrone, then 5 tablets containing 35 mcg ethinyl estradiol and 0.5 mg norethindrone. Seven inert tablets are contained in the 28 day cycle.
[7] Ortho Novum 7/7/7 is available as a 21 and 28 day regimen. Each white and peach tablet contains 35 mcg of ethinyl estradiol. In both the 21 and 28 day regimen the white tablet contains 0.5 mg norethindrone, the light peach tablet contains 0.75 mg norethindrone and the peach tablet contains 1.0 mg norethindrone. The 28 day regimen contains seven green tablets which are inactive.
[8] Triphasil-21 is available as a 21 and 28 day regimen. The first 6 tablets (brown) contain 0.05 mg levonorgestrel and 30 mcg ethinyl estradiol, followed by 5 tablets (white) containing 0.075 mg levonorgestrel and 40 mcg ethinyl estradiol followed by 10 tablets containing 0.125 mg levonorgestrel and 30 mcg ethinyl estradiol. The 28 day regimen contains 7 green placebo tablets.
  * 1 mcg or microgram is one millionth of a gram.
  ** 1 mg or milligram is one thousandth of a gram.

both estrogen and progestin, but is designed with low doses of progestin in the pills taken at the beginning of a cycle. Larger doses of progestin are provided in the pills taken near the middle or end of the cycle. This approach to oral contraception more closely mimics the normal hormonal pattern.

Refinements in formulation and dosing of oral contraceptives over the past 25 years have resulted in reduced risk and excellent contraceptive effectiveness. The oral contraceptive remains an extremely useful and popular method of contraception.

EFFECTIVENESS OF THE PILL

The theoretical effectiveness of the combination pill (estrogen plus progestin) approaches 100%. In fact, it is slightly less than that due primarily to a tendency among some users to forget to take their pills or to take them on an erratic basis. In reality, the pregnancy rate among users of the combination pill is 0.1 to 0.34 pregnancy per 100 woman-years (1,200 menstrual cycles). No other contraceptive drug or device approaches the effectiveness of the combination pill.

The minipill (progestin only), if properly taken, is somewhat less effective than the combination pill, but as effective or slightly more effective than an intrauterine device (IUD). The pregnancy rate in minipill users is 0.5 to 1.5 pregnancies per 100 woman-years (1,200 menstrual cycles). In order to avoid some of the estrogen-induced side effects of the combination pill, particularly if you are a high-risk patient (smoker, obese, over age 35, have high blood pressure), you may wish to consider the minipill as an alternative to the combination pill. Sacrifice of a degree of effectiveness can increase safety.

USE OF THE PILL

Oral contraceptives are very popular. Over 150 million people worldwide have used oral contraceptives. In the United States, it is estimated that over 10 million women use oral contraceptives at a given time. This number represents about 20% of all married women in their reproductive years (between the ages of 15 and 44).

The oral contraceptive Ortho Novum® is the fourth most prescribed drug in America. Cost does not appear to be a barrier to its use. The average cost of a one-month cycle of oral contraceptive tablets is approximately $14.00.

American women clearly recognize oral contraceptives as an excellent approach to conception control. The reasons include effectiveness, ready availability, aesthetic acceptance to both sexual partners, convenient use, relatively low cost, and use that is independent of the act of intercourse.

HOW AN ORAL CONTRACEPTIVE WORKS

To understand how the pill works you must first understand the normal menstrual cycle. The "average" menstrual cycle lasts approximately 28 days and consists of four phases (see Figure 4). The first phase is the menstrual phase. This phase is followed by the proliferative phase, which is estrogen-dominated and produces a mature ovum (egg). The third phase of the menstrual cycle is ovulation, which usually occurs near the middle of a cycle (plus or minus several days in some individuals). The fourth phase, known as the luteal phase, is progesterone-dominated and ultimately results in the menstrual period if the egg is not fertilized.

The menstrual phase (phase I) usually lasts three to six days. Day one of the cycle begins with onset of the menstrual period. During this period the endometrial lining built up during the previous cycle is shed due to drops in estradiol (estrogen) and progesterone levels. If pregnancy had occurred, the endometrium would not have shed since hormone levels would be different; the developed endometrium would have been required to begin nourishing the developing fetus.

The proliferative phase (phase II) of the cycle (also known as the estrogenic or follicular phase) lasts until about the 14th day of the cycle. Release of follicle stimulating hormone (FSH) from the anterior pituitary gland in the brain results in the growth of ovarian graafian follicles (one of which will usually mature and release a viable ovum). The graafian follicle also secretes hormones (estrogens and small amounts of progesterone). Estradiol leads to regeneration

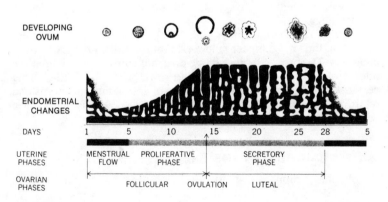

FIGURE 4

Phases of the menstrual cycle

of the previously shed endometrium of the uterus. High levels of estrogen at the end of the proliferative phase stimulate the release of luteinizing hormone (LH) from the pituitary gland, which causes the mature graafian follicle to rupture and release an ovum (phase III) for possible fertilization.

The ovum remains viable (fertilizable) for six to 24 hours. If fertilization does not occur, the cycle enters the luteal phase (phase IV); also known as the progestational or secretory phase. This phase lasts until the 27th or 28th day of the cycle. Pituitary LH transforms the ruptured graafian follicle into the corpus luteum, which secretes progesterone and some estradiol. Under the influence of progesterone, the endometrial glands of the uterus branch and their secretory function is initiated in anticipation of implanting a fertilized ovum. In the absence of pregnancy, the corpus luteum degenerates, and endometrial shedding (menstruation) begins a new cycle.

HOW THE PILL PREVENTS PREGNANCY

Oral contraceptives are available as either a *combination* product (those containing estrogen plus progestin) or a *progestin-only* product (minipill). The mechanism by which the two types of oral contraceptives prevent pregnancy are different. The *combination pill* (which includes the new triphasic pill) inhibits the release of pituitary follicle stimulating hormone (FSH) and luteinizing hormone (LH), thus preventing ovulation. Additionally, the combination pill thickens cervical mucus, inhibiting penetration of sperm into the uterus. The hormones in the pill retard implantation of a fertilized egg, in the unlikely event that ovulation and fertilization should occur, by interfering with the ability of the endometrium of the uterus to implant a fertilized egg.

The *progestin-only* pill (minipill) does not typically suppress ovulation, thus has a higher failure rate than estrogen-progestin combinations. The progestin dose alone does not substantially inhibit the release of FSH and LH; it appears to work primarily by thickening cervical mucus, thus retarding entrance of sperm into the uterus and retarding implantation of any egg that is fertilized by inducing a hostile endometrium.

CANDIDATES FOR USE OF THE MINIPILL

As the minipill is less effective than the combination pill, you may wonder why it is available. The minipill is most often used by women who cannot tolerate the estrogen in the combination pill, or who are at high risk for complications from estrogen use (for example, smokers, women over 35, women with high blood pressure, obese women, and women with a history of migraine).

Bothersome side effects of the minipill include a relatively high incidence of intermenstrual bleeding and spotting and occasional amenorrhea (absence of menstrual period). Because the minipill does not suppress ovulation, some physicians recommend a second method of contraception in midcycle, especially during the first three to six months of minipill use.

HOW ORAL CONTRACEPTIVES ARE ADMINISTERED

The effectiveness of all oral contraceptives depends on strict adherence to the dosage schedule. The possibility of pregnancy increases with each successive day that scheduled tablets are missed. Tablets may be taken with meals or on an empty stomach. Users are encouraged to take the tablet at intervals not exceeding 24 hours. Many women prefer to take the pill at bedtime so they do not have to carry the pills. Also, awareness of contraception may be higher on the part of the woman and the spouse at bedtime.

The combination birth control pill is taken once daily (preferably at the same time each day) for 20, 21, or 28 days (depending on the brand prescribed). The initial 20- or 21-day packet of the combination product is begun on the 5th day after the onset of menstrual flow. Menstrual flow will usually occur within two to three days after the last tablet is taken. The next pill packet is begun seven days after the last pill in the first pill packet was taken. This schedule should be followed even though spotting or breakthrough bleeding may occur during the cycle. If spotting or midcycle bleeding occurs for longer than two to three months, you should contact your physician. If menstrual flow does not occur when expected, pregnancy should be considered a possibility. The physician should also be contacted if a menstrual period is missed.

The 28-day packet of the combination pill is simpler to use because it eliminates the need to count the days between cycles. The 28-day pill packet usually consists of 21 tablets containing an estrogen and progestin and seven inactive tablets (placebos) or seven tablets containing an iron supplement. A pattern of daily, continuous pill-taking makes it easier for some women to remember to take their pills regularly.

The progestin-only minipill must be taken daily on a continuous basis. Use of the minipill would be started on the first day of a menstrual period. Once started, one tablet should be taken at the same time each day, every day of the year or until you decide that you no longer desire to use that method of contraception.

MISSED DOSES

If you miss one *combination tablet,* take it as soon as you remember, or take two tablets the next day, and resume the usual dosage pattern. If two consecutive tablets are missed, take two tablets daily for two days and resume the usual dosage pattern. If three consecutive tablets are missed, stop taking the drug and begin a new packet seven days after the last dose was taken. If two or three consecutive doses of the combination pill are missed, you should use an additional method of birth control for at least 14 days or until the start of the next menstrual period.

For the progestin-only *minipill,* the course of action is slightly different if doses are missed. If you miss one tablet, take it as soon as you remember, and then take the next tablet at the regularly scheduled time. If you miss two consecutive tablets, take one of the missed tablets, discard the other, and resume the usual dosage pattern. If you miss more than two consecutive tablets, discontinue the drug completely. Use an additional method of contraception any time two or more tablets are missed, until the menstrual period occurs, or until pregnancy is ruled out. If the menstrual period does not occur within 45 days, stop taking the drug regardless of circumstances and get a pregnancy test. Some women may wish to pursue a more conservative approach to missed doses since the minipill is less effective than the combination pill: this approach is to stop taking the minipill if even *one* tablet is missed and use an alternate method of contraception until the menstrual period occurs or pregnancy is ruled out.

If one or more doses of a *triphasic pill* (Tri-Norinyl, Ortho-Novum 7/7/7, or Triphasil-21) is missed, contact the prescribing physician for direction.

CHOOSING THE RIGHT PILL

As previously stated, the currently available oral contraceptives contain a synthetic estrogen plus a progestin (combination pill) or a progestin alone (minipill). Table 3 contains a list of oral contraceptives available in the United States, their content and strength.

Currently available combination oral contraceptives will contain one of two synthetic estrogens—mestranol or ethinyl estradiol. Mestranol is the less potent of the two, and is probably converted to ethinyl estradiol in the body. It takes 80 micrograms (mcg)* of mestranol to be equivalent to 50 micrograms (mcg) of ethinyl estradiol.

---

*1 microgram is one-millionth of a gram. 30 grams equals one ounce.

The content of estrogen in oral contraceptives varies widely. The combination products containing approximately 20 mcg of estrogen may be less effective than those containing higher amounts.

The progestin component of oral contraceptives, which may be used alone in a minipill or in combination with an estrogen, may consist of one of five different chemicals. Progesterone itself is relatively inactive when taken orally. The orally effective synthetic progestins used in oral contraceptives are norethindrone, norgestrel, ethynodiol diacetate, norethindrone acetate, and norethynodrel.

The progestin component has a considerable bearing on contraceptive effectiveness, and also assists in maintaining hormonal balance and normal menstrual flow. As Table 4 indicates, the progestins possess a great deal of chemical activity beyond the progestational activity. Given the potential of the various progestins to produce estrogenic (feminizing), antiestrogenic or androgenic (masculinizing) effects, the user may tolerate some progestins much better than others.

It is very important that a woman receive an oral contraceptive that is proper for her biochemical system. Often women experience drug-induced symptoms of estrogen excess or deficiency and/or progestin excess or deficiency. These symptoms can be extremely discomforting and are often avoidable if a more appropriate oral contraceptive is substituted.

Manifestations of oral contraceptive-induced estrogen excess or deficiency are included in Table 5. If any of these symptoms become troublesome or intolerable, they should be reported to your physician. Selection of another oral contraceptive with the appropriate amount of estrogen and/or progestin can usually minimize hormonal side effects without compromising contraceptive effectiveness. Appropriate integration of Tables 3, 4, and 5 of this chapter should guide you in selecting the oral contraceptive best for you.

WOMEN WHO SHOULD NOT USE ORAL CONTRACEPTIVES

Before prescribing any oral contraceptive, your physician must determine whether circumstances exist that would prevent use. These contraindications (conditions under which the drug should not be taken) may depend on whether the drug prescribed contains estrogen or not. Many adverse effects are dose-related; lower doses may minimize side effects. Smaller estrogen doses, for example, may decrease the incidence and/or severity of headaches, high blood pressure, depression, nausea, vomiting, and weight gain (see Table 5). Several studies suggest that combination pills with low to moderate

TABLE 4
PHARMACOLOGIC EFFECTS OF PROGESTINS USED IN ORAL CONTRACEPTIVES

Chemical	Activity			
	Progestin	Estrogenic	Antiestrogenic	Androgenic
Norgestrel/Levonorgestrel	+++	0	+++	+++
Ethynodiol Diacetate	++	+[1]	+[1]	++
Norethindrone Acetate	+	+	+++	++
Norethindrone	+	+[1]	+[1]	++
Norethynodrel	+	+++	0	0

The above effects can be minimized by adjusting the estrogen-progestin balance or dosage by selecting an appropriate product (see Table 3).

[1]Has estrogenic effect at low dose; may have antiestrogenic effect at higher doses.

Key: +++ Pronounced effect
     ++ Moderate effect
      + Slight effect
      0 No effect

Reprinted with permission of Facts and Comparisons Division of J. B. Lippincott, 1987.

24

TABLE 5
ACHIEVING THE PROPER HORMONAL BALANCE WITH ORAL CONTRACEPTIVE USE: SYMPTOMS OF EXCESS AND DEFICIENCY OF ESTROGEN AND PROGESTIN

Estrogen Excess	Estrogen Deficiency	Progestin Excess	Progestin Deficiency
—Hypermenorrhea (increased menstrual flow)	—Early cycle (days 1–14) spotting and bleeding	—Early cycle bleeding	—Late cycle (days 15–21) spotting and bleeding
—Dysmenorrhea (painful menstrual flow)	—Hypomenorrhea (decreased menstrual flow)	—Decreased length and volume of menstrual flow	—Dysmenorrhea (painful menstrual flow)
—Nausea and vomiting	—Amenorrhea (no menstrual flow)	—Increased appetite	—Amenorrhea (no menstrual flow)
—Cervical and vaginal mucorrhea (discharge)	—Hot flashes	—Weight gain	—Decreased breast size
—Hyperpigmentation	—Nervousness, jitters	—Lassitude, fatigue	
—Hypertension (high blood pressure)	—Susceptibility to vaginal fungal infections	—Oily scalp	
—Breast fullness and tenderness		—Acne	
—Fluid retention		—Hair loss	
—Headache		—Excess hair growth (total body)	
—Leg cramps		—Depression (mental)	
—Uterine fibroid growth		—Susceptibility to vaginal fungal infection	
		—Breast tenderness	
		—Delayed onset of period when pill discontinued	

25

estrogen content can decrease the risk of stroke, heart attack, clot formation, gallbladder disease, and other problems. Further research is needed to more fully determine the value of combination products with low to moderate estrogen content.

The progestins in combination pills have been implicated in a substantial increase in a type of cholesterol (low density lipoprotein) that has been linked to heart disease and stroke. For this reason, you (and your physician) should remember that there are combination oral contraceptives relatively low in progestin that are especially appropriate for women who already have an increased risk of cardiovascular disease (smokers, obese women, and women over 35 years of age, for example). Weight gain, depression, headache, and other minor, but troublesome, side effects associated with estrogens do not appear to occur when the progestin-only minipill is employed. The effect of the progestin-only minipill on increasing low density lipoprotein cholesterol has not been adequately evaluated.

Table 6 lists absolute and relative contraindications to combination oral contraceptives. A woman with an *absolute* contraindication is one in whom a condition exists that may be so severely complicated by use of oral contraceptives that they should not be used. A *relative* contraindication is one in which the woman and her physician consider all potential risks and benefits and decide whether potential benefits outweigh potential risks. The drug may or may not be utilized. Absolute and relative contraindications listed in Table 6 apply to the combination products containing estrogen.

HIGH-RISK WOMEN

Certain elements of health and life-style may increase risks for certain women taking oral contraceptives. Table 6 lists some of the specific risk factors associated with the use of oral contraceptives. Cardiovascular complications are of special concern. Most of the pill-related deaths occur in high-risk women. The amount of estrogen in the pill appears to be an important factor leading to cardiovascular complications. If you are a high-risk woman and insist on using the pill, you should consider a combination product containing a low dose of estrogen, or the progestin-only minipill. Progestin-only pills have not been thoroughly studied and cannot be presumed to be free of risk, however.

The mechanism by which the pill affects how blood clots is not known. In susceptible women, normal blood clotting may be adversely affected after one to three months of pill use. Possible health risks are superficial or deep clots in veins, clots in the lung (pulmonary emboli), strokes, high blood pressure, and heart attacks. If

TABLE 6
CONTRAINDICATIONS TO THE USE OF ORAL CONTRACEPTIVES

Absolute Contraindications[1]	Relative Contraindications[2]
Present or past thromboembolic (clotting) disease:	Smoking (more than 16 cigarettes per day)
Thrombophlebitis (inflammation of a vein due to a clot)	Obesity (greater than 30 pounds over ideal body weight)
Deep vein thrombosis (clot)	Age greater than 35 years
Stroke	Migraine headaches
Pulmonary embolism (clots in the lung)	High blood pressure (hypertension) more than 140/90 mm Hg
Myocardial infarction (heart attack)	Diabetes mellitus (both insulin-dependent and non-insulin-dependent)
Coronary artery disease (narrowing of arteries of the heart)	Gallbladder disease
Known or suspected cancer of uterus or breast or any estrogen-dependent cancer	Uterine fibroids
Known or suspected pregnancy	Seizure disorder (epilepsy, for example)
Past or present acute or chronic liver disease or tumors (benign or malignant)	Sickle cell disease
Any undiagnosed vaginal or uterine bleeding	Amenorrhea (no menstrual flow)
	History of jaundice during pregnancy
	Patients poorly motivated or unable to understand directions for use
	Young females in active growth phase
	History of mental depression
	Family history of early coronary artery disease
	High cholesterol and triglycerides (fatty substances) in the blood
	Presence of varicose veins

[1]Do not take the combination (estrogen-progestin) pill if any of these conditions exist!

[2]The pill may be taken under these conditions of increased risk, but you and your physician should determine whether potential benefits outweigh potential risks.

clotting defects or a tendency for these conditions does exist before initiating oral contraceptive therapy, the pill magnifies the risks.

Alterations in life-style (such as weight reduction, less smoking, and any change resulting in decrease in blood pressure or decrease in cholesterol levels in the blood) can minimize risks. Women over 35 to 40 years of age, especially where other risk factors are present (obesity, smoking, high blood pressure, for example) should probably not use the combination pill, as the risk of a heart attack or other serious cardiovascular problem is substantially increased. Oral contraceptive users who smoke are believed to be at least five times more likely to have a heart attack than nonsmoker users. Women who use the pill are strongly advised to avoid smoking.

If you are a diabetic, you may experience a poorer tolerance to glucose while taking the pill; doses of insulin or oral antidiabetic drugs may have to be adjusted accordingly. In addition, use of estrogen has been associated with elevated cholesterol and triglyceride levels. This drug-induced increase of lipids in the blood may increase the risk of heart attack or accelerate progression of coronary artery disease. It may also be difficult to regulate and control high blood pressure while on the pill.

The presence of varicose veins creates a substantially increased risk of superficial clots of the legs. The progestin component is generally implicated as the complicating factor in this case. Varicose veins do not seem to increase the risk of deep vein clots in users of the pill.

ADVERSE EFFECTS ASSOCIATED WITH USE OF ORAL CONTRACEPTIVES

Oral contraceptives are used by millions of women throughout the world and represent one of the most effective reversible methods of birth control. But the enthusiasm that accompanied their introduction has been dampened somewhat by continuing reports of serious and even life-threatening complications.

The pill has been one of the most studied drugs of all time. The Walnut Creek Drug Study took place over a 10-year period and involved over 16,000 women taking the pill. The study concluded that for young, adult, healthy, middle-class women the risks of pill use appear to be negligible. The presence of risk factors mentioned previously (Table 6) magnifies the possibility of adverse effects many times, however.

The overall incidence of adverse effects related to pill use is difficult to estimate because the complaints of many pill-users are vague. About seven percent of women stop taking the pill due to side effects. The most common adverse effect is nausea and/or vomiting, which occurs in about 10% of women during the first cycle. These symptoms usually disappear with time. Mild gastrointestinal side effects such as cramping and bloating are often reported. Blood pressure elevation occurs in five to six percent of women, and approximately six percent of women report some degree of depression. Less frequently reported adverse effects include breakthrough bleeding, spotting, absence of period, breast tenderness, rash, excess spotty pigmentation of the skin (melasma), migraine headache, intolerance to contact lenses, fluid retention, leg cramps, and increased appetite. You should report these and any other adverse effects to your physician. You and your physician should then jointly determine whether the pill should be continued.

Most pill-related deaths are due to cardiovascular complications—specifically heart attacks, strokes, and clots (especially clots in the lungs). The yearly death rate associated with pill use is approximately 3.7 per 100,000 users (1.8 per 100,000 nonsmokers and 6.5 per 100,000 smokers). This amounts to less than 400 pill-associated deaths per year in the United States. The negative aspects of pill use are frequently overplayed in the press. To put the mortality (death) figures in perspective, approximately 20.6 women per 100,000 die annually in childbirth. Pregnancy is, in fact, almost six times more likely to terminate in maternal death than pill use by nonpregnant women.

CARDIOVASCULAR COMPLICATIONS

Myocardial Infarction (Heart Attack)

An oral contraceptive user is two to three times more likely to experience a nonfatal heart attack than a woman who does not use the pill. Heart attacks are rare among 20- to 29-year-old women who do not take oral contraceptives (about 1 per 100,000 women per year). Use of the pill will increase this incidence to 3 to 4 per 100,000 women—still a low probability event. With advancing age, however, you should be more concerned about the association between heart attacks and pill use. It is estimated that in pill-users aged 40 to 44, 75 deaths annually per 100,000 women are due to heart attacks. Approximately 50 of these deaths are attributable to pill use.

One investigator examined the risk of heart attack relative to pill use and smoking. It was revealed that women who smoked more than 25 cigarettes per day, but did not take the pill, had a sevenfold increased risk for having a heart attack when compared with women who did not smoke. Women who took oral contraceptives but did not smoke were only at a fourfold higher risk. Smoking by itself is, therefore, almost twice as likely to produce a heart attack as pill use alone. Women who both smoke and take oral contraceptives are at a 39-fold higher risk to suffer a heart attack.

Other factors such as high blood pressure, high blood levels of cholesterol and triglyceride (fat), and diabetes also increase the risk of heart attacks in pill-users.

Pill-users who had high blood pressure and smoked were shown in one study to be 170 times more likely to be hospitalized for treatment of a heart problem than nonsmoking women who had normal blood pressure and did not take oral contraceptives. The presence of any three or more risk factors (see Table 6) appears to increase the risk of experiencing a heart attack approximately 128 times.

Thromboembolic Disorders (Clots)

During the early 1960s, a number of case reports suggested a relationship between oral contraceptive use and clot formation. In a controlled study of 46,000 British women, it was found that pill use increased the risk of clots in deep veins (deep vein thrombosis) at least fivefold and the risk of clots in superficial veins at least twofold because oral contraceptives elevate certain clotting factors in the blood. Estrogen seems to be the primary cause of increased clotting, although the role of the progestins in influencing clot formation has not been adequately studied.

Pill use is also associated with an increased risk of strokes due to clots and hemorrhage. Thrombotic strokes, believed to result from a clot blocking a blood vessel in the brain, occur at least four times more frequently in pill-users than nonusers. The risk of a stroke due to ruptured blood vessels in the brain (hemorrhagic stroke) is about two times higher in pill-users than nonusers. Although strokes may be very severe, only about 10 percent of strokes are fatal. The incidence of thrombotic strokes in pill-users is one in 10,000 yearly; the incidence of hemorrhagic stroke in pill-users is less than one in 20,000. Thus risks for strokes in pill-users are small if no other risk factors are present.

Risk of stroke can be magnified greatly by coexisting high blood pressure. Pill-users with blood pressure greater than 180/110 mm Hg are over 13 times more likely to experience a thrombotic stroke than those with normal blood pressure. The risk of hemorrhagic stroke increases more than 25-fold in severely hypertensive pill-users. If a woman has high blood pressure and desires to take oral contraceptives, it is critical that she control her blood pressure with diet, exercise, weight loss, and/or drug therapy, and have her blood pressure carefully monitored while on the pill.

Smoking does not appear to increase the risk of thrombotic strokes, but appears to increase the risk of hemorrhagic stroke seven-fold if the oral contraceptive user smokes more than one pack of cigarettes per day. Clots may migrate (travel) through the blood stream to parts of the body other than the brain or deep or superficial veins of the extremities (legs, arms). Clots that block blood vessels of the heart (coronary arteries) can produce serious heart attacks. Clots may also block tiny blood vessels in the lungs and create a severe threat to the respiratory system.

Hypertension (High Blood Pressure)

High blood pressure can increase risks for users of the pill. Oral contraceptives may cause high blood pressure. In a two-year study of 186 oral contraceptive users in Scotland, blood pressure increased in 88 percent of the women. Increased age, obesity, and a past history of hypertension make oral contraceptive-induced elevations in blood pressure more likely. When hypertension occurs, it becomes a risk factor that could precipitate a stroke or heart attack. Products containing lower doses of estrogens or progestin-only oral contraceptives should be considered in the presence of high blood pressure. If an appropriate lowering of blood pressure does not occur, an alternative form of contraception should be employed, or blood pressure lowering drugs taken. Blood pressure usually returns to what it was before taking the pill within one month to one year after stopping the pill.

LIVER TUMORS

Although rare, benign liver tumors have been associated with oral contraceptive use. Only about 200 cases had been reported up to 1981. Over half (54 percent) of women with liver tumors had used oral contraceptives for more than five years, but in 10 percent of the cases the pill had been used for only six to 12 months. Any abdominal mass or sudden onset of abdominal pain or tenderness in oral contraceptive users should be reported to the physician immediately.

GALLBLADDER DISEASE

In 1973 the Boston Collaborative Drug Surveillance Program reported a twofold increase in the incidence of gallbladder disease among pill-users under age 35. In another study, an increased risk of oral contraceptive-induced gallbladder disease appeared after two years of use, and doubled after four to five years of use. This rise in risk may be due to estrogen- or progestin-induced increases of certain forms of cholesterol in the bile. The cause and effect relationship between oral contraceptive use and gallbladder disease has been questioned, however, because the Walnut Creek Contraceptive Drug Study did not confirm the findings of the Boston Collaborative Study. If you are taking the pill and experience jaundice (yellowing of the skin and whites of the eyes) or if abdominal pain or gallstones develop, oral contraceptives should be suspected; you should contact your physician immediately and discontinuation of pill use should be considered.

NEUROLOGICAL DISORDERS

Headache is the most common neurological symptom associated with oral contraceptive use; approximately one in 10 pill-users report headaches. The headaches often resemble migraine headaches and may be associated with nausea, vomiting, and/or blurred vision. Women with a history of migraine may report more severe headaches while on the pill. Headaches associated with premenstrual syndrome, however, are often less severe.

Involuntary movement disorders are a rare side effect of pill use. Affected patients usually have a history of movement disturbances. Any woman with a history of movement disorder should report it to her physician. Symptoms usually disappear a few weeks after stopping the pill.

DERMATOLOGIC (SKIN) DISORDERS

Almost every drug is capable of producing a mild allergic reaction such as a rash. Oral contraceptives are no exception. Melasma, a patchy hyperpigmentation of the skin, occurs in about 70 out of 100,000 pill-users and is no cause for alarm. If a woman who develops melasma finds it cosmetically objectionable, she should try to avoid sunlight or consider discontinuing the pill. Acne may occur in women using oral contraceptives containing a progestin with high androgenic activity (see Table 4). An estrogen-dominant progestin should improve or eliminate acne. Hypersensitivity or allergy to sunlight may occur (although it is rare) in users of an oral contraceptive. Women should avoid or protect the skin from ultraviolet radiation (sunlight or tanning centers) if there is substantial intolerance to sunlight.

BEHAVIORAL CHANGES

Oral contraceptives have not been clearly and objectively implicated in causing mental depression. Symptoms of depression are frequently noted in users of oral contraceptives, however. Approximately six percent of users report symptoms indicating varying degrees of depression. Personality, situational factors, and a history of depression are often noted when pill-users report symptoms of depression. It is theoretically possible that estrogen-induced alterations in tryptophan metabolism may lead to decreased production of serotonin (a neurotransmitter) in the brain. A number of depressed users of oral contraceptives report relief of symptoms when they take 20 mg of oral pyridoxine (vitamin B_6) twice daily.

VISUAL DISTURBANCES

About one in five contact lens wearers who take oral contraceptives complain of tightness, burning, and itching. Decreased tear secretion and a change in the curvature of the cornea, similar to that occurring in pregnancy, is believed to be the cause of these side effects. There have been isolated reports of other visual disturbances that are believed to be induced by the pill. These include episodes of loss of vision, blurred vision, changes in color vision, light flashes, swelling of the retina, and clotting in the retina. Well controlled studies have failed to incriminate oral contraceptives; such adverse effects appear to be coincidental and unrelated to the drug.

WHAT TO DO IF YOU DEVELOP SYMPTOMS THAT MAY BE DUE TO ORAL CONTRACEPTIVE USE

This chapter provides detailed information on the positive and negative properties of oral contraceptives. A user of oral contraceptives should call her physician any time a discomforting symptom is thought to be due to the pill. No adverse effect induced by a drug is insignificant if it creates discomfort and disrupts the life-style of the user. Many of the minor side effects, such as excessive menstrual flow, painful menstruation, nausea, vaginal discharge, hyperpigmentation, breast tenderness, fluid retention, headache, nervousness, jitteriness, increased appetite, and fatigue are preventable (or can be made less severe) if the proper drug at the proper dosage is employed.

Symptoms that suggest a serious drug-induced adverse effect should be reported to your physician immediately. These include chest pain, lack of menstrual flow, painful menstrual flow, migraine headache, dizziness, fainting, blurred vision, double vision, pain in the extremities, difficult breathing, abdominal pain, mass in the breast or abdomen, jaundice, mental depression, acne, difficulty in controlling blood sugar if diabetic, and rash.

ORAL CONTRACEPTIVES AND CANCER

Beyond the rare association between oral contraceptive use and benign liver tumors, several studies have been conducted to determine whether the incidence of commonly occurring cancers in women are affected by oral contraceptives. Oral contraceptives have been in use long enough (over 20 years) to evaluate the relationship between use and frequency of cancer. Studies have focused on cancer of the breast, cervix, ovary, and endometrium (inner lining of the uterus).

The findings concerning pill use and cancer of the breast, ovary, and endometrium is reassuring. Based on several previous and ongoing studies, the FDA has concluded that there appears to be no increased risk of *breast cancer* with any oral contraceptive. Breast cancer will ultimately affect about one in 11 women and is the leading cause of death by cancer for women in the U.S. Even women who have taken the pill for up to 11 years do not appear to have an increased risk of breast cancer. Additionally, the pill does not appear to increase risk for breast cancer in women with benign breast disease or a family history of breast cancer. Patients with active breast cancer should not receive any estrogen-containing oral contraceptive, however.

Studies have demonstrated that oral contraceptives appear to have a protective effect against *endometrial cancer*. Endometrial cancer is the third most common cancer in U.S. women. Researchers have found that users of an estrogen-progestin combination pill for at least one year have half the risk for endometrial cancer than women who never took the pill. It is estimated that the combination oral contraceptive prevents about 2,000 cases of endometrial cancer per year. The protective effects of the combination pill appear to persist for at least 10 years after the pill is stopped.

The pill also appears to protect women from *ovarian cancer,* the fourth leading cause of cancer death in U.S. women. As with endometrial cancer, the pill seems to reduce the risk of ovarian cancer by approximately one-half. The pill, therefore, may prevent approximately 1,700 cases of ovarian cancer in the U.S. each year.

Oral contraceptive use does appear, however, to increase the risk of *cervical cancer.* In data from the Oxford Family Planning Association, of 6,838 women using oral contraceptives, 13 developed invasive cervical cancer. Nine of these had used the pill for more than six years. No cervical cancer, on the other hand, occurred in a control group of 3,154 women using an IUD. Additionally, cervical dysplasia (abnormal cell growth) occurred more frequently in the oral contraceptive group than the IUD group. The incidence of cervical cancer appears to be related to duration of oral contraceptive therapy; the incidence of cervical cancer was 0.9 per 1,000 woman-years in those using the pill up to two years, but 2.2 per 1,000 woman-years in those with more than eight years of pill use. Pill-users often have increased sexual activity, a known risk factor in cervical cancer. Whether this variable could have influenced findings is not known. Results are not conclusive, therefore, and further research is in progress.

It should be pointed out that the vast majority of cervical cancer can be effectively treated if diagnosed soon enough. All adult women should have regular (annual) cervical (Pap) smears, but this is particularly critical in patients using oral contraceptives.

Several studies have concluded that oral contraceptive users may have a slightly increased risk of developing *malignant melanoma*. It has been suggested that other factors, such as overexposure to sunlight, are actually responsible. The scarcity of data prevents any conclusive answer to this question.

Physicians have diagnosed greater numbers of benign *pituitary tumors* in young women over the past several years. The tumors are prolactinomas, that is, tumors that secrete greater than normal amounts of the hormone prolactin. As many of the patients were young women, a possible link between the pill and the tumor was evaluated. Researchers concluded that women using oral contraceptives were no more likely than any other women to develop prolactinomas, even when the pill had been used for up to five years.

ORAL CONTRACEPTIVES AND BIRTH DEFECTS

Any drug given to a pregnant woman during pregnancy has the potential to cause birth defects. Oral contraceptives are no exception. Use of oral contraceptives should be discontinued approximately three months before attempting to conceive, if possible. If that is not possible, it is recommended that the oral contraceptive be discontinued no later than the time of the first missed period. Use beyond two missed periods is unwise. Pregnancy is an absolute contraindication to the use of oral contraceptives.

One study of 11,468 babies, in which 432 (3.8%) were born to mothers who definitely or probably took estrogen or progestin during pregnancy, demonstrated that the risk of major malformation was 26% higher and risk of minor malformation 33% higher in the exposed group than in the nonexposed group. Estrogen-progestin combinations have been implicated as the cause of aborted fetuses with chromosome abnormalities, heart defects, limb defects, and neurological disorders. Oral contraceptive users who become pregnant while on the pill do not appear to be at increased risk of stillbirth, miscarriage, or ectopic pregnancy. The pill does not appear to influence sex ratio or birth weight.

Safe use of oral contraceptives in pregnancy has certainly not been established, nor is it likely to be, and what estrogens and progestins may do to a developing fetus has not been well defined. Most studies are based on viewing defects after birth and looking back for exposures that could cause the defect. Exposure to chemicals in the diet and environment, as well as to other drugs, could be responsible. The proper approach is to be as conservative as possible.

THE MENSTRUAL CYCLE AFTER PILL USE

After a woman stops taking oral contraceptives, there may be a delay before a normal menstrual period occurs. This is called post-pill amenorrhea (absence of period). Between one and 10 percent of oral contraceptive users will experience a delay in return of menstruation after stopping the pill. Women who experienced irregular menstrual cycles prior to the use of oral contraceptives are most likely to experience post-pill amenorrhea. In the majority of contraceptive users, menstruation occurs within 48 days to six months after discontinuing the drug. Ovulation resumes in many women during their first three post-treatment cycles.

As ovulation may occur before a menstrual period, and prediction of time of ovulation or menstrual flow is not possible, alternative methods of contraception must be employed immediately after discontinuing the pill if pregnancy is to be avoided. If post-pill amenorrhea continues beyond six months, it would be wise to contact your physician. Spontaneous return of menstruation may not occur for several months; drug therapy may be employed to induce ovulation and the menstrual cycle.

PREGNANCY AFTER PILL USE

Results of the Oxford Family Planning Study indicate that return of fertility after discontinuation of oral contraceptive therapy may be delayed a few months, especially in women who have not been pregnant before. Pill use does not appear to impair long-term potential for pregnancy, however.

ORAL CONTRACEPTIVES AND SEXUALLY TRANSMITTED DISEASES

Oral contraceptives do not appear to protect against any sexually transmitted disease except pelvic inflammatory disease (see Chapter 14). In fact, birth control pills may complicate the control of a number of sexually transmitted diseases. The pill changes the acidity of the vagina from acid to alkaline, which may increase the chance of infection with some bacteria or viruses.

ORAL CONTRACEPTIVES AND RHEUMATOID ARTHRITIS

A group of Dutch researchers have noted that the incidence of rheumatoid arthritis in women who use oral contraceptives appears to be approximately half that of nonusers. Further evaluation is

TABLE 7
MOST SIGNIFICANT DRUG INTERACTIONS WITH ORAL CON-TRACEPTIVES

Drug (use)	Possible Effect
Rifampin (antitubercular)	Decreased efficacy of contraceptive; increased incidence of breakthrough bleeding
Barbiturates (sleep aids)	Decreased efficacy of contraceptive
Phenytoin (seizure control)	Decreased efficacy of contraceptive; increased toxicity of phenytoin
Primidone (seizure control)	Decreased efficacy of contraceptive; increased toxicity of primidone
Isoniazid (antitubercular)	Decreased efficacy of contraceptive; increased incidence of breakthrough bleeding
Penicillin V (anti-infective)	Decreased efficacy of contraceptive; increased incidence of breakthrough bleeding
Tetracycline (anti-infective)	Decreased efficacy of contraceptive; increased incidence of breakthrough bleeding
Sulfonamides (anti-infective)	Decreased efficacy of contraceptive; increased incidence of breakthrough bleeding
Oral blood thinners	Decreased efficacy of blood thinners
Tricyclic antidepressants	Decreased efficacy of antidepressants
Blood pressure medicines	Decreased efficacy of blood pressure medicines
Tolbutamide (treats diabetes)	Decreased efficacy of antidiabetic drug
Ascorbic acid (vitamin C)	Increased effect of oral contraceptive

needed, however, before any protective effect of oral contraceptives against rheumatoid arthritis can be conclusively reported.

ORAL CONTRACEPTIVES AND OTHER DRUGS

Oral contraceptives can theoretically interact adversely with a number of other drugs. Table 7 lists only the more significant interactions between oral contraceptives and other drugs. These drugs *may* be given together, but appropriate adjustments of doses may be necessary to minimize any adverse effects from the combination.

CONCLUSION

Oral contraceptives are a very effective means of birth control if taken properly. Oral contraceptives have numerous side effects associated with their use, but the vast array of products available allows for selection of a product particularly suited to each individual woman. If a woman tolerates a particular oral contraceptive poorly, she should advise her physician. Adjustments in amounts of various ingredients may allow continued use with minimal or no discomfort.

Certain risk factors (age over 35 years, obesity, high blood pressure, diabetes) magnify the possibility that a serious adverse effect may be experienced by an oral contraceptive user. Taking these factors into account can minimize complications.

The decision of whether or not to use an oral contraceptive ultimately rests with you. The adverse consequences of oral contraceptive use have often been sensationalized. Elements of this chapter should assist you in deciding whether to use the pill, which pill to use, and how to monitor for pill-induced side effects.

2

The Intrauterine
Device (IUD)

INTRODUCTION

Much confusion has developed concerning the safety and effectiveness of the intrauterine device (IUD). The purpose of this chapter is to educate and inform you of the risks, benefits, values, and shortcomings of the IUD.

The first IUDs may have been small pebbles inserted into the uteri of camels by Arabs and Turks of ancient times who wanted to prevent pregnancies among their saddle animals during long desert journeys. The first true IUD was developed in 1909, was ring shaped, and was made of silkworm gut. The first widely used IUD was a ring of gut and silver wire used in Germany in the late 1920s.

Although the early crude IUDs lowered the incidence of pregnancy, their value was limited by an unacceptably high frequency and severity of complications, particularly infections. The medical attitude toward the IUD was extremely conservative until the late 1950s when technological advances prompted a reappraisal. The development of polyethylene, a biologically inactive plastic, and advances in antibiotic therapy, which dispelled fears of severe IUD-related infections, fostered much research into IUD use. During the 1970s, the medicated IUDs were developed. These devices contained either metallic copper or a progestational steroid.

The 1960s and 1970s witnessed rapid acceptance of the modern intrauterine device. Use of the IUD peaked around 1983, when approximately 1.5 million U.S. women utilized an IUD. That number has since fallen to below 1.0 million users. Although the IUD is second only to "the pill" in contraceptive effectiveness, serious questions about the safety of certain IUDs began to develop in the 1970s.

THE DALKON SHIELD

The Dalkon Shield® intrauterine device was introduced in 1970. The design of this IUD was apparently flawed, and the spiked, shield-like, nickel-sized, plastic IUD produced a very high incidence of complications that apparently contributed to at least 20 deaths and many serious illnesses. The Dalkon Shield® was withdrawn from the market in June 1974 because of a wave of lawsuits alleging damages such as perforation of the uterus, pelvic infection, pelvic inflammatory disease (PID), septic (infectious) abortion, infertility, and ectopic pregnancy.

The manufacturer of the Dalkon Shield®, the A.H. Robins Company, has since sought protection from its creditors under Chapter 11 of the federal bankruptcy law. At the time of filing for bankruptcy in 1985, the pharmaceutical company had settled 9,450 of 15,000 lawsuits brought by women claiming injury from the Dalkon Shield®. Claims cost A.H. Robins and its insurers over $500 million. The U.S. Bankruptcy Court then ordered A.H. Robins to conduct an international campaign to notify women who used the Dalkon Shield® that they had until April 30, 1986, to file a damage claim. Claims from over 300,000 women in the U.S. and 81 foreign countries amounting to hundreds of millions of dollars of alleged damages were filed.

If you are currently wearing an IUD inserted in the early to mid 1970s, you could be using a Dalkon Shield®. You should contact your physician for an examination if you think you are wearing a Dalkon Shield®. Prompt removal of the IUD should occur.

OTHER UNMEDICATED IUDs

Unmedicated IUDs, including the Lippes Loop®, Saf-T-Coil®, and Dalkon Shield®, were developed in the 1960s and early 1970s, and were made of chemically inactive polyethylene. The Lippes Loop® and Saf-T-Coil® (see Figure 5) could be molded and straightened for insertion. Due to the "memory" of the polyethylene, these IUDs returned to their original shape when released in the uterus. All unmedicated IUDs have now been withdrawn from the market, the most recent removal being the Lippes Loop® (September 1985).

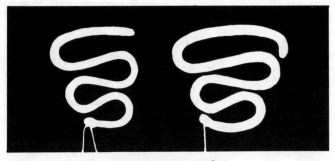

Lippes Loop®

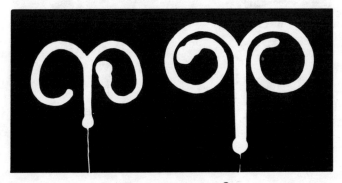

Saf - T - Coil®

FIGURE 5

Physical appearance of unmedicated intrauterine devices (actual size)

Removal of the Lippes Loop® and Saf-T-Coil® IUDs from the market was apparently not due to objective evidence of lack of safety or effectiveness, but rather to a preference in the marketplace for medicated IUDs, and difficulty experienced by manufacturers of IUDs in acquiring product liability insurance at an affordable premium due to the Dalkon Shield® situation.

MEDICATED IUDs

Medicated IUDs contain pharmacologically active substances, either metallic copper or a progestational steroid, that is slowly released into the uterine cavity. The only medicated IUD currently available in the U.S. is Progestasert®, which contains the hormone progesterone.

Unfortunately, the two copper-containing IUDs of high effectiveness and apparent safety have been voluntarily removed from the market by the manufacturer, G. D. Searle Company. The decision to

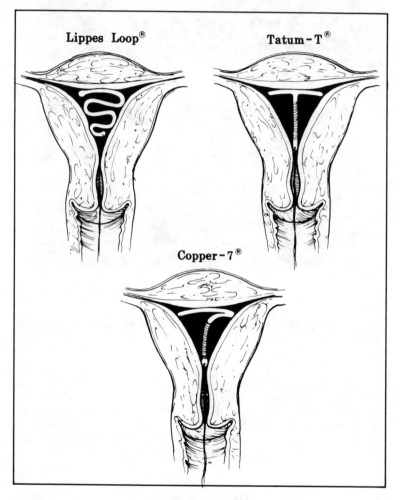

FIGURE 6

Appearance of selected intrauterine devices in utero

remove the copper-containing Copper-7® and Tatum-T® was not based on medical factors, but rather on business considerations. A litigious society, sensitized to real risks associated with use of the Dalkon Shield®, has contributed to the filing of approximately 775 suits over the last 12 years alleging damages from copper-containing IUDs.

Evidence that copper-containing IUDs pose medically unacceptable risks to potential users is lacking. Much of the litigation against the manufacturer of the copper-containing devices is unjustified, as is evidenced by the fact that 470 of 775 lawsuits alleging damages have already been settled. Only two judgments against the manufacturer have been rendered by the court. Searle asserts that it has full confidence in the safety and effectiveness of the Copper-7® and Tatum-T® when used according to FDA-approved prescribing information. No change in the status of the FDA's approval has occurred. Women currently using the copper-containing IUDs apparently need not have them removed prematurely.

PHYSICAL CHARACTERISTICS OF THE MODERN IUD

The appearance of selected intrauterine devices, as they appear in the uterus, are included in Figure 6. The shape of the IUD is very important. Modern IUDs (Figures 5 and 6) conform well to the normal anatomy of the uterus. They have significantly lower rates of expulsion, bleeding, perforation, pain, and infection associated with their use when compared to older IUDs.

The Progestasert® and Tatum-T® are T-shaped; the Copper-7® derives its name from its shape, which resembles the number seven. All modern IUDs have a string or tail of plastic thread. The thread should extend out of the cervix of the uterus into the vaginal canal so one can confirm the presence of the IUD by feeling for the string with a finger. Once the IUD is inserted, the physician will usually cut the thread, allowing approximately 2.0 inches (5.0 cm) of thread to protrude into the vaginal canal. This excess thread should not be pulled because this may dislodge a properly placed IUD.

If the thread cannot be felt, a physician should be contacted immediately. Most often, not enough thread was left by the physician who inserted the IUD, but the IUD is in its proper place. In some cases, the IUD may be tilted in the uterus and the thread drawn up into the uterine cavity. In this case, the IUD is still effective as a contraceptive, but the user has no way of being sure it is present. It is also possible that the IUD has been expelled without the user's knowledge. The consequence of expulsion is immediate loss of contraceptive protection and risk of pregnancy.

CHEMICAL CHARACTERISTICS

Unmedicated IUDs are made of inert polyethylene, do not release chemicals into the uterine cavity, and yet are approximately equal in contraceptive effectiveness to the medicated IUDs. The *copper-containing devices* include a plastic component which provides flexibility. The Copper-7® is made of pharmaceutical grade polypropylene with barium sulfate added so it may be seen by x-ray, if necessary. Coiled around the vertical stem is a pure copper wire providing approximately 200 square millimeters of exposed copper surface. The Tatum-T® is composed of polyethylene containing barium sulfate, with 120 milligrams (mg) of pure copper wire providing approximately 210 square millimeters of exposed copper wire wrapped around the vertical stem. The effective life of the copper containing IUDs is typically three years.

The Progestasert® is unique in that this T-shaped device (which is still on the market) consists of a polymer containing a reservoir of 38 mg of the hormone progesterone. Progesterone is continuously released into the uterine cavity at an average rate of 65 micrograms (mcg) per day for one year. Barium sulfate is dispersed throughout the plastic so the position of the IUD in the uterus can be determined by x-ray examination. The Progestasert® has an effective life of only 12 months and must be replaced annually.

HOW THE IUD WORKS

Although IUDs are used by millions of women throughout the world, the precise mechanism by which they prevent pregnancy is not absolutely defined. Research in animals has not been particularly useful, because the IUD appears to act somewhat differently from species to species.

In humans, the IUD produces numerous subtle cellular and biochemical changes in the endometrium, which lines the inner wall of the uterus. All unmedicated and copper devices produce a mild inflammatory or foreign body reaction in the uterus. This inflammatory reaction to a foreign body (the IUD) produces no discomfort or detectable symptoms in the user, but does cause changes in uterine fluid and the endometrium. After insertion of the IUD, numerous white blood cells appear in the uterine fluid and endometrium. These cells may literally consume or engulf sperm, the ovum, or a fertilized ovum not yet implanted. This proposed mechanism is very credible.

Another proposed mechanism, which may occur at the same time, delays or disrupts the normal hormonal cycle or directly affects the uterus, creating an endometrium that is not suited for implantation of a fertilized egg. If the fertilized egg is not implanted, it cannot be nourished and, therefore, dies.

The IUD produces a mild, but persistent, subclinical (no symptoms) endometritis (inflammation of the endometrium). There is presumably no bacterial or viral component to this inflammatory reaction. With shedding induced by the IUD, the epithelium of the endometrium never gets a chance to heal. Greater inflammatory changes with the copper devices, when compared to the unmedicated IUDs, have been noted, and this could account for the slightly greater contraceptive effectiveness of the copper-containing IUDs. Copper is also known to be toxic to sperm *in vitro* (in the test tube).

The Progestasert® IUD, due to its physical characteristics, also produces a foreign body reaction which promotes engulfment of sperm, egg, or fertilized egg. Like the copper-containing devices, its chemical reactivity also enhances its effectiveness. The small amount of progesterone released by Progestasert® each day (65 mcg) does not adversely affect the ovaries or retard ovulation. The progesterone level is not detectable in the blood and produces no side effects such as fluid retention, rash, acne, depression, or breast tenderness, which might occur if the drug were injected or taken orally. Progestasert® does, however, contain enough hormone to interfere with the hormone regulated cycle of the endometrium. The maintenance of higher than normal levels of progesterone in the uterus suppresses the proliferation of endometrial tissue. This artificially induced anti-estrogenic effect keeps the endometrium in a state in which implantation of a fertilized egg is unlikely.

EFFECTIVENESS

The IUD is one of the most effective modern methods of contraception (see Table 8). It is the most effective single contraceptive except for the oral contraceptive and, of course, sterilization or abstinence. All the values in Table 8 are theoretical effectiveness values; actual pregnancy rates may be higher if the contraceptive drug or device is not used strictly as directed.

COMPLICATIONS OF IUD USE

There are complications associated with use of the IUD, but the incidence of complications is not high. Complications of IUD use typically fall into one or more of the following categories:

1. Bleeding
2. Pain

3. Expulsion
4. Perforation or Embedment
5. Infection—Pelvic Inflammatory Disease
6. Ectopic Pregnancy
7. Vaginal Discharge
8. Spontaneous Abortion (Miscarriage) If a Uterine Pregnancy Occurs
9. Uterine Perforation If Inserted During Lactation
10. Impairment of Subsequent Fertility

BLEEDING

Increased uterine bleeding, often accompanied by lower back pain or abdominal pain, is the most frequent complication of IUD use. Bleeding of a minor nature is frequently associated with insertion of the IUD. If the IUD is inserted during the menstrual

TABLE 8
PREGNANCY RATE OF VARIOUS CONTRACEPTIVE METHODS*

Method	Number of Pregnancies per 100 Woman-Years**
Oral Contraceptive	
• combination estrogen-progestin ("the pill")	0.1–0.34
• progestin only ("minipill")	0.5–1.5
Intrauterine Device (IUD)	1.0–3.0
Condom	3.3–4.0
Condom with Spermicidal Agent	less than 1.0
Spermicidal Foam, Cream, or Jelly	3.0–4.0
Diaphragm with Spermicidal Agent	3.0–3.4
Coitus Interruptus (Withdrawal)	15.0–25.0
Rhythm	5.0–40.0
Douching	30.0–40.0

*Pregnancy rates are a composite derived from several studies by different investigators and are considered optimal. Actual pregnancy rates may be higher if the drug or device is not used strictly as directed.

**One woman-year is 12 menstrual cycles; therefore, 100 woman-years is 1,200 menstrual cycles. A pregnancy rate of 1.0 is one pregnancy per 1200 menstrual cycles.

NOTE: If no contraceptive method is employed, the pregnancy rate is 60–85 pregnancies per 100 woman-years.

period, the IUD-induced bleeding may not be noticed. If the IUD is inserted at another time within the cycle, you should expect some mild bleeding for one or two days after insertion, with intermittent spotting for several days within the first menstrual cycle. Such bleeding is considered normal; it is not a cause for concern unless severe pain is associated with the blood loss or unless the blood loss becomes chronic and is severe enough to produce anemia.

The copper-containing and unmedicated IUDs may produce small increases in blood loss at menstruation. The slight increase in menstrual blood loss, if it should occur, may produce some personal inconvenience, but rarely results in any clinical problem. The progestin-releasing device (Progestasert®) generally reduces menstrual blood loss by as much as 40 to 50 percent. This is approximately the same decrease in menstrual blood loss that is produced by "the pill." Women with a normally heavy menstrual flow or dysmenorrhea (painful menstruation) may tolerate the Progestasert® particularly well.

The menstrual period may be prolonged by three to four days if you use the Progestasert®. This prolonged bleeding may take the form of spotting. Breakthrough or midcycle bleeding (intermenstrual bleeding) is most likely if you use the Progestasert®. This bleeding is usually slight (one or two teaspoonsful; 5 to 10 ml) and tends to decrease with time elapsed after insertion.

Heavy and prolonged bleeding associated with pelvic pain may be associated with a serious pelvic infection or an ectopic pregnancy. If heavy and prolonged bleeding and/or pelvic pain persist, contact your physician immediately. Do not delay seeking appropriate medical attention.

PAIN

Mild pain is common in the few days after insertion of an IUD. The pain that occurs in the immediate post-insertion period is cramp-like, and may be felt in the lower abdomen or lower back. The pain is probably caused by contractions of the uterus as it tries to expel this foreign body. Contractions are strongest during the one to three days after insertion. The post-insertion pain is usually classified as mild to moderate and does not represent a cause for alarm. The pain is discomforting, however, and use of over-the-counter pain medication generally produces satisfactory relief of symptoms. It is appropriate to take aspirin or acetaminophen (Datril®, Tylenol®) to treat post-insertion pain. Doses of 650 mg (10 grains) of either aspirin or acetaminophen every four hours, as needed, are usually effective. Application of dry heat (heating pad) to the painful area of the back or abdomen may also be effective, and may be used alone or with aspirin or acetaminophen. Post-insertion pain should decrease over a three-day period. If pain lasts longer than three days or becomes severe and intolerable, contact your physician.

Chronic pain (lasting longer than three days) in the pelvic region should be considered a warning sign that some serious adverse event may have occurred, or is occurring, in the uterus. Chronic pelvic pain associated with abnormal bleeding is further evidence of an adverse condition that may be associated with the IUD. Chronic pelvic pain may be associated with an ectopic pregnancy, embedment of the IUD in the uterine wall, perforation of the uterine wall by the IUD, or an infectious and/or inflammatory condition. When pelvic pain lasts longer than three days, consult your physician.

EXPULSION

IUDs may be expelled spontaneously. Expulsion renders the woman immediately susceptible to pregnancy. The highest incidence of expulsion is within the first three months after insertion; approximately 50 percent of spontaneous expulsions occur during this time. Expulsions take place most frequently during menstruation, especially during the first menstrual period after insertion. When IUDs are reinserted, almost all will be retained with no further complication.

The single most important factor affecting expulsion rate may be the insertion technique and fit of the IUD in the uterus. Disorientation of the IUD in the uterus may provoke irritation and contractions which foster expulsion, especially during the first one to three months after insertion. The skill of the physician performing the insertion is a crucial factor. One group reported one-year expulsion rates of only one to two per 100 users compared to worldwide expulsion rates of five to 15 per 100 women per year.

Other factors which appear to influence expulsion rates are age of the user, parity (childbearing history) of the user, and, in some cases, time of insertion. Expulsion rates decline with the advancing age of the user. Among multiparous users (two or more normal births), expulsions are about twice as high under age 30 when compared to users 30 and over. Nulliparous women (women who have borne no offspring) have smaller uteri than parous women and have higher expulsion rates with all IUDs. An IUD should not be inserted immediately after delivery of a child, as expulsion rates are extremely high at this time. Insertion of the IUD between menstrual periods or during the menstrual period does not appear to have an adverse effect on expulsion rate.

Approximately 20 percent of IUD expulsions go unnoticed; therefore, users must monitor for the presence of the IUD. About one-third of pregnancies among IUD users occur after unnoticed expulsion. As a precaution, you should locate the tail (thread) of the IUD after each menstrual period, and check for the presence of the thread in the vaginal canal at least weekly for the first three to four months after insertion. You should also inspect sanitary napkins or tampons before discarding; the expelled IUD may adhere to these products.

The IUD may be completely or only partially expelled. With incomplete expulsion, the IUD may become lodged in the lower uterine cavity or the cervical canal. This greatly reduces contraceptive protection. In any situation where there is complete or partial expulsion, you should either refrain from intercourse or use another method of contraceptive protection until a new IUD is inserted.

PERFORATION AND EMBEDMENT

Although removal of an IUD that is embedded in the uterus or has perforated the uterus can be quite complex and invasive, it is important that this rarely occurring complication be placed in its proper context relative to incidence. It is reliably estimated that less than one-tenth of one percent (less than one in 1,000) of IUD users will experience embedment or perforation of the uterus. Most perforations begin or occur at the time of insertion, due to improper technique of insertion. The skill and experience of the physician is paramount to minimizing perforation. If the physician carefully measures the depth of the uterus and does not force the insertion, there is little chance of perforation.

INFECTION—PELVIC INFLAMMATORY DISEASE

Pelvic inflammatory disease (PID) is a general term for an ascending infection of the upper genital tract including the uterus, fallopian tubes, and ovaries. The term PID is used to refer to cases of acute infections ascending from the vagina or cervix. The organisms most frequently implicated are *Neisseria gonorrhoeae* and *Chlamydia trachomatis*. The gonorrhea-causing organism has been isolated from the endocervix of 45 to 70 percent of women in the United States with acute PID. *Chlamydia trachomatis* has been isolated from the cervix of 20 to 50 percent of U.S. women with acute PID. Often the episode of PID is due to a mixed infection of *N. gonorrhoeae, C. trachomatis,* and/or other abnormal bacterial or fungal components of the vaginal canal.

Studies in the U.S. and Sweden indicate that IUD users are about 1.5 to 4.0 times more likely to develop PID than sexually active women using no contraception. No significant differences in PID rates have been noted between the unmedicated and medicated IUDs.

The mechanism(s) by which IUDs increase the risk of developing PID is not known, but theories include the following:

1. The IUD produces a sterile inflammatory reaction in the endometrium and fallopian tubes that reduces resistance to the growth of disease-producing organisms.
2. The IUD alters normal menstrual bleeding, which may enhance bacterial growth.
3. Microorganisms may enter the cervix of the uterus by migrating up the thread (tail) of the IUD.
4. Microorganisms may be introduced into the uterus during insertion of the IUD.

Pelvic inflammatory disease (PID) can be an extremely serious medical disorder. Refer to Chapter 14 (Pelvic Inflammatory Disease) for detailed information on prevalence, causes, risk factors, signs and symptoms, complications, treatment, and prevention of PID.

ECTOPIC PREGNANCY

An ectopic pregnancy is any pregnancy arising from implantation of the fertilized ovum outside the cavity of the uterus. Sites of ectopic implantation include the fallopian tubes, ovary, and cervix, but about 98 percent of all ectopic pregnancies are tubal. Symptoms of a tubal pregnancy are amenorrhea (absence of a menstrual period), followed by dark and scanty vaginal bleeding or a disordered menstrual pattern, uterine bleeding, persistent and intense abdominal pain, and pelvic mass formation. Tubal pregnancies may be sudden in onset. Pain comes and goes, and backache may also be present. Abnormal uterine bleeding is present in 80 percent of cases, a pelvic mass can be felt in 70 percent, and approximately 10 percent of cases will lead to collapse and shock. In chronic tubal pregnancy, symptoms are less distinct. Blood leaks from the fallopian tube over several days, and a considerable amount of blood may pool in the peritoneal space in the abdominal cavity. Slight but persistent vaginal spotting may occur. Pain may occur, but is less intense than that associated with acute ectopic pregnancy.

There appears to be a very significant difference in ectopic pregnancy rates associated with the Progestasert® when compared to other IUDs. The pooled rate of ectopic pregnancy associated with all modern IUDs, except Progestasert®, is approximately one per 1,000 woman-years. The ectopic pregnancy rate in Progestasert® users is approximately five per 1,000 woman-years. Interestingly, the progestin-only oral contraceptive ("minipill") is associated with a higher ectopic pregnancy rate than the combination (estrogen-progestin) oral contraceptives ("the pill"). Progesterone appears to increase risk, but the mechanism is not known. Risk of developing an ectopic pregnancy also seems to increase as the period of IUD use increases. Although difficult to explain, increased risk of ectopic pregnancy seems to persist for up to one year after removal of the IUD.

Other factors which increase risk of developing an ectopic pregnancy are previous episodes of PID, history of ectopic pregnancy, or history of tubal surgery. IUDs should be avoided if one or more of these risk factors is present and another method of contraception is acceptable.

VAGINAL DISCHARGE

An inconvenience associated with IUD use in some women is a watery or mucus-like vaginal discharge. The vaginal discharge, if it should occur, is seldom serious enough to warrant removal of the IUD. The discharge is probably associated with mild inflammation of the endometrium. The copper-containing devices appear most likely to produce this side effect. Frequent bathing and drying of the vaginal area should minimize irritation and abnormal odor.

If vaginal discharge is associated with IUD use and is excessive to the point of soiling clothing, producing discomforting symptoms, or is very malodorous, this should be reported to your physician. These symptoms could be associated directly with use of the IUD, but may also be symptoms of pelvic inflammatory disease (PID) or an infection of the vaginal tract which may increase susceptibility to PID. Prompt treatment of the infection is necessary.

SPONTANEOUS ABORTION (MISCARRIAGE) IF A UTERINE PREGNANCY OCCURS

If a uterine pregnancy occurs with an IUD in place, the incidence of spontaneous abortion (miscarriage) is increased greatly. Approximately 50 percent of uterine pregnancies terminate in a spontaneous abortion if the IUD is not removed. This is three to five times the rate of spontaneous abortion in nonusers. Over one-half of spontaneous abortions appear to occur during the second trimester of pregnancy. Uncomplicated removal of the IUD early in pregnancy decreases the risk of spontaneous abortion by at least 50 percent. If the IUD is not easily removed, probing the uterus to remove the device may disrupt the pregnancy. In such cases, the IUD may be left in place if you want to continue the pregnancy. Close monitoring is essential, however, as such individuals are prone to pelvic infections and septic (infectious) abortion, and there is an increased risk of premature delivery, stillbirth, and low birth weight.

Serious physical and infectious complications of a first trimester spontaneous abortion are rare. Abnormal uterine bleeding is the most common adverse effect. Persistent and heavy bleeding requires prompt medical attention. All spontaneous abortions (miscarriages) should be reported to your physician.

The risk of experiencing a septic (infectious) second trimester spontaneous abortion in women with IUDs in place appears to be at least 25 times greater than in women without IUDs. Such a statistic makes a good case for prompt removal of an IUD as soon as a uterine pregnancy is confirmed.

UTERINE PERFORATION IF INSERTED DURING LACTATION

Embedment and perforation of the uterus by an IUD, regardless of type, appears to be more probable if the IUD is inserted during lactation. In one analysis, a 10-fold increased risk of uterine perforation was found among women who had been lactating at the time of IUD insertion when compared to women not lactating at the time of insertion.

Furthermore, a comparison was conducted evaluating the risk of difficult removal among women lactating and not lactating at the time of insertion. A difficult removal was found to be 2.3 times more likely in the group lactating at the time of insertion.

Lactation is evolving as a clear-cut risk factor for uterine perforation, and seems to contribute to a difficult removal if perforation occurs. Special caution should be exercised during insertion in lactating females.

IMPAIRMENT OF SUBSEQUENT FERTILITY

The effect of IUD use on subsequent fertility has not been extensively evaluated; most studies involve only IUD users who discontinued use to become pregnant. Among such women, the return to fertility is usually rapid, and approximately 70 percent conceive within 12 months. One study revealed that within two years after discontinuing IUD use, 92 percent of 258 women gave birth. Some women appear somewhat slow in recovering their fertility. Use of the IUD in healthy women does not appear to retard ultimate fertility, however. The same cannot be said for women who have experienced pelvic infection, spontaneous abortion, or ectopic pregnancy while using an IUD. Tubal scarring after such events can lead to reduced fertility or total infertility.

WOMEN WHO SHOULD NOT USE AN IUD

Numerous factors should be considered before one makes the decision to use or continue to use an IUD. The IUD is highly effective and does not require day-to-day action such as taking a pill or monitoring for signs of fertility. Effectiveness and convenience should not be the only criteria used in making a decision on IUD use, however.

A complete physical exam, including a pelvic exam, Pap smear, and other appropriate tests should assist in determining appropriateness of IUD use. Your physician should tell you, in understandable terms, how the IUD may affect your body, the effectiveness of the IUD, complications of IUD use, what to do if you cannot locate the thread or miss a menstrual period, signs of pelvic infection, and why the IUD may be an inappropriate contraceptive for you.

The IUD is contraindicated (not recommended) in the following situations:

1. Pregnancy or suspicion of pregnancy. Insertion of the IUD early in pregnancy will most likely cause the developing fetus to be aborted.
2. Acute pelvic inflammatory disease (PID) or a history of PID. Insertion of an IUD may worsen existing PID or promote the development or redevelopment of PID. Every episode of PID, no matter how quickly or successfully treated, increases the possibility of infertility due to tubal scarring and obstruction.
3. History of ectopic pregnancy. IUD use increases the probability that an ectopic pregnancy may occur.
4. Known or suspected malignancy of the genital tract. An IUD will only complicate diagnosis and/or management, possibly leading to bleeding that may progress to anemia, and/or increase the prospect of an infection of the genital tract.
5. Any gynecological bleeding disorder. If menstrual blood loss is excessive, the unmedicated and copper-containing IUDs may intensify blood loss, possibly to the point of inducing anemia. If blood loss is intermittent, this signals an abnormality of the reproductive tract that may be either malignant or nonmalignant.

Such an event should be reported to your physician immediately.

6. Any type of congenital (at birth) uterine abnormality or gynecological disorder which distorts the uterine cavity. Proper placement of the IUD may be difficult if the anatomy of the uterine cavity is not normal. Risks of IUD use under such circumstances are expulsion, embedment in the uterine wall, and/or perforation of the uterine wall.

7. Postpartum endometritis (inflammation of the endometrium), untreated acute cervicitis (inflammation of the cervix of the uterus), or infected abortion within the past three months. Insertion of any IUD into an environment that is inflamed, infected, or recently infected may lead to an infection or worsening of an existing infection.

8. Women whose immune system is suppressed due to drug therapy (such as chronic treatment of leukemia or numerous other forms of cancer or other diseases with corticosteroids). Such women may have substantially impaired ability to combat bacteria or viruses that may become infecting agents. IUD use further exposes such women to a potentially serious infection.

9. Blood coagulation defects. With the exception of Progestasert®, which decreases menstrual blood loss, IUDs may lead to increased menstrual blood loss. If a coagulation defect is superimposed on this situation, menstrual blood loss could be quite excessive. Additionally, women receiving prescription blood thinners, such as heparin or warfarin (Coumadin®), may experience a substantial increase in menstrual blood loss, or spontaneous blood loss if an IUD is employed.

10. Severe cervical stenosis (narrowing). If the canal or opening of the cervix of the uterus is abnormally narrow or partially obstructed and will not accommodate the IUD without severe trauma, the IUD should not be utilized.

While not contraindicated in women who have never borne a child, the IUD should be used cautiously in such women. There are definite risk factors which need to be assessed along with potential benefits. IUD use in women who have not delivered offspring has been associated with a higher incidence of pelvic inflammatory disease, higher rate of expelling the IUD, and a higher incidence of bleeding and pain when compared to women who have borne children.

INSERTION OF THE IUD

Once the decision has been made to utilize an IUD, the physician will measure the uterus, obtain a Pap smear, determine whether the patient is pregnant or not, determine the general health of the vagina and uterus, and inspect adjoining organs for inflammation and/or malignancy. There is no particular best time to insert an IUD; it can be inserted at the convenience of the user in most cases. Expulsion rates, perforation of the uterus, and infection rates may be higher if an IUD is inserted a few days after childbirth or immediately after a first trimester (first three months of pregnancy) spontaneous or induced abortion. This is typically a time of high user motivation, but it is best to delay insertion until the uterus has involuted (returned to normal size).

REMOVAL OF AN IUD

The frequency of IUD removal varies considerably from product to product. If you are wearing an unmedicated IUD, it may be worn for long periods of time (perhaps several years) if no complications develop. There is no particular limit to their duration of effectiveness. Annual checkups are strongly encouraged, however.

If you are wearing a copper-containing medicated IUD (Copper-7®, Tatum-T®), you must have it removed no later than 36 months after insertion. The copper-containing IUDs lose their copper, and some of their effectiveness, after three years. If you are diabetic and are wearing a copper-containing IUD, you should probably have it removed as soon as possible. Such IUDs in diabetics seem to corrode and experience accelerated encrustment; this may impair release of copper and the overall contraceptive effectiveness of the IUD. As the copper-containing IUDs are no longer available, when you have your Copper-7® or Tatum-T® removed, you will have to consider use of Progestasert® or another method of contraception.

The Progestasert® has the shortest duration of action of any IUD. The hormone progesterone is released consistently for at least 12 months. This device must be removed after 12 months of use. A new Progestasert® may be inserted, or an alternative method of contraception may be utilized.

Medical conditions that necessitate removal of the IUD include:

1. Pelvic pain or cramping. Such symptoms which occur in women previously tolerant to an IUD may indicate a serious complication such as uterine embedment or perforation, pelvic infection, or ectopic pregnancy.

2. Abnormal or excessive vaginal bleeding. Bleeding is frequently a symptom of a more serious complication, which may or may not be directly related to the IUD. Abnormal or excessive vaginal bleeding should be promptly reported to the physician.
3. Acute pelvic inflammatory disease that does not respond to antibiotics. The infection may be in the area immediately around the IUD, and treatment may be difficult unless the IUD is removed.
4. Displacement of the IUD from the uterus. If the IUD assumes an abnormal position in the uterus and produces pain, inflammation, and/or infection, it should be removed.
5. Pregnancy. Spontaneous abortion is likely (50 to 60 percent probability) in the first or second trimester in women who develop a uterine pregnancy while an IUD is in place. If the pregnancy is detected during the first 12 weeks of gestation, the IUD should be carefully removed if the thread is visible and the device moves easily.
6. Uterine or cervical malignancy. An IUD in a cancerous uterus can produce a host of complications (such as infection, embedment, perforation, bleeding, cramping, and pain) and should be removed as soon as possible after diagnosis.
7. Menopause. Women who pass through menopause while using an IUD should have the IUD removed; narrowing and shrinking of the uterus during menopause may make later removal of the IUD difficult.

MYTHS AND FALLACIES ASSOCIATED WITH USE OF AN IUD

The primary responsibility for educating you about the use of an IUD rests with your physician. Proper use and monitoring of IUD use is too important to leave to chance. Physicians report the following questions are among the most frequently asked when use of an IUD is being considered:

1. Can a copper-containing IUD protect me from acquiring gonorrhea or any other sexually transmitted disease if I have intercourse with an infected individual?

   The answer is an emphatic *no!* No protection against any sexually transmitted disease is conferred by any IUD.

2. If I wear an IUD, can I use vaginal tampons?

   Tampons may be used in women who wear an IUD. Tampons reside in the vaginal canal; the IUD is in the uterus.

3. Can an IUD interfere with sexual intercourse?

   The IUD does not interfere with sexual intercourse, although the male may be aware of the IUD thread in the vaginal canal during intercourse.

4. Do IUDs increase the incidence of cancer in the female reproductive tract?

   There is no evidence currently available which links use of an IUD with cancer of a woman's reproductive tract.

5. Will babies conceived during IUD use be deformed?

   There is no conclusive evidence that birth defect rates are higher in women who conceived while wearing an IUD vs. women who were not wearing an IUD when they conceived. The IUD does, however, greatly increase the risk of a spontaneous abortion (miscarriage) if it is not promptly removed. Premature delivery, stillbirth, and low birth weight are more common if the IUD is not removed during the pregnancy.

6. What should I do if I wear an IUD and miss a menstrual period?

   Return to your physician as soon as possible, since this suggests pregnancy and appropriate testing should be done. If pregnancy is confirmed, the IUD should be removed as soon as possible.

7. Can I douche if I wear an IUD?

   Yes. Douching should not dislodge or disrupt placement of an IUD.

8. How expensive are IUDs?

   IUDs are relatively inexpensive. The IUD and office visit should not cost more than $125.

9. Are IUDs the most effective contraceptive?

   IUDs are the most effective contraceptive *device*. The

oral contraceptive tablet is a *drug* and is the only contraceptive method (other than abstinence or sterilization) that is more effective than an IUD.

10. If I use an IUD, does my male sexual partner have to use a condom?

No. Use of a condom will, however, decrease the likelihood of pregnancy further, and will aid in preventing the spread of a sexually transmitted disease, if one should exist.

CONCLUSION

The IUD, while declining in availability and usage, is a very effective contraceptive device. Much of the current concern regarding use of modern IUDs is based on fear, misinformation, and sensationalism. When objectively reviewing effectiveness, risks, benefits, cost, convenience, simplicity, contraindications, reversibility, and aesthetics, it would not be surprising to see the IUD make a significant comeback in popularity and use.

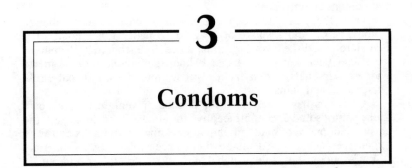

3

Condoms

INTRODUCTION

Historically associated with prostitution, illicit sex, and sexually transmitted disease, the condom has until recently been relegated to low status on the list of available contraceptive measures. Yet, it represents one of the most practical and effective methods of birth control available without a prescription.

Relatively simple to use, the mechanical principle of the condom is easily understood. A sheath of latex or animal skin membrane worn over the penis during coitus, the condom is the only widely available device that offers simultaneous contraceptive and disease protection for both men and women. Sales of condoms have increased dramatically because of the dual protection provided.

HISTORY OF THE CONDOM

The invention of the condom is considered by some as the beginning of modern contraception. The origin of the condom is unknown. The Egyptians wore a condom-like device almost 3500 years ago as a penis protector to ward off tropical disease and insect bites. Romans may have used a facsimile of a condom made from a goat's bladder, not so much for contraceptive purposes, but as protection against disease. Fallopius, in 1564, claimed that a linen sheath worn over the penis by 1,100 men protected them from syphilis with 100 percent effectiveness.

Over the years, the condom has assumed a large number of synonyms. Casanova spoke of it as "the English riding coat." The British returned the favor by calling it the "French letter." Condoms have also been known as bags, balloons, manhole covers, merry widows, personals, prophylactics, pros, protectives, raincoats, rubbers, safes, and skins.

Condoms have been used for disease prevention for well over four centuries and as a contraceptive for almost three centuries. The early condoms were made of animal intestinal membranes and were expensive. The expense made them accessible only to the rich. "Skin" condoms are still available in today's marketplace and remain relatively expensive when compared with modern latex condoms. However, they are preferred by some who claim skin condoms transmit sensation better than rubber condoms.

The first rubber condoms were marketed approximately 100 years ago. Although the flexibility and impermeability of rubber made it an excellent material for use as a barrier contraceptive, approximately 75 percent of those produced in the late 19th and early 20th century were defective. The Federal Food, Drug and Cosmetic Act of 1938 authorized the Food and Drug Administration (FDA) to regulate and inspect condom production standards. Since that time, condom quality has undergone a profound improvement.

At about the time the FDA assumed responsibility for condom production standards, the latex manufacturing process was developed. Latex is much easier to work with than dissolved rubber. Condoms made from latex are thinner, stronger, and last longer than natural rubber.

Merle Youngs, a drugstore products salesman during the 1920s, began a condom manufacturing company that adhered to strict quality and production standards. Youngs convinced pharmacists to stock his product by supplying a high quality condom. He also helped remove many U.S. laws designed to restrict condom use through a series of court suits.

TYPES OF CONDOMS AVAILABLE

Two basic materials are used to produce condoms available in today's marketplace—the cecum (intestinal pouch) of an animal and latex. The vast majority of users prefer condoms made of latex. Only one percent of all condoms produced worldwide are made from animal intestinal tissue. Condoms from animal sources are more popular in the U.S., accounting for approximately five percent of U.S.

condom sales. "Skins" differ from latex condoms in a number of ways (see Table 9).

Many users of skin condoms maintain that skins provide greater sensitivity. Skins derived from intestinal tissue of the lamb are not elastic and may not always fit securely on the penis. Because of this feature, skin condoms may be more easily lost upon withdrawal from

TABLE 9
SELECTED CHARACTERISTICS OF LATEX VS. SKIN CONDOMS

Characteristic	Latex	Skin*
Colors	Transparent Black Blue Green Purple Red Turquoise Yellow	Opaque
Lubricated Unlubricated	Yes Yes	Yes No
Plain-end Reservoir-end	Yes Yes	Yes No
Porosity	Air- & water-tight	Unknown
Shank	Straight-sided Contoured Rippled	Straight-sided
Sizes	Small** Medium*** Large	————
Texture	Plain Ribbed Rough Surface	Plain
Thickness	.06 mm	.04–.07 mm

*Skin condoms are derived from intestinal tissue of animals.

**Recently introduced in China.

***Not generally available in U.S., except through mail-order houses, and promoted as "fitting snugger for extra sensitivity."

the vagina. If kept in a lubricated container, skins seldom shrink, whereas latex condoms can shrink significantly if exposed to heat and/or prolonged storage. Skins are 2 or 3 times more expensive and more difficult to test for strength.

Modern latex condoms are thin, flexible, and well lubricated. Latex condoms are also available without lubrication, as well as in a variety of colors, shapes, and textures (see Table 9). Those who have a negative opinion of condoms based on hearsay may find modern latex condoms to their liking.

Lubricated condoms are used and preferred by the vast majority of condom users in the U.S. Condoms may come lubricated from end to end, or only at the tip and partially down the shank. They are recommended for use if vaginal penetration is difficult or painful due to lack of natural moisture in the vaginal canal. Some experts maintain that lubrication may reduce friction stress on the condom during coitus (intercourse). Table 10 lists the features of most available condom brands.

Condoms are available with a "dry" or a "wet" lubricant. Dry lubricants are less messy, odorless, and used often with transparent and colored condoms. Wet lubricants evaporate quickly, have a slight odor, and are used with opaque and skin condoms.

Unlubricated condoms, with or without a reservoir-end, are probably least preferred by users. Some who use unlubricated condoms prefer to rely on natural vaginal lubrication. Some men and women maintain that lubricated models provide too much lubrication. Others prefer to apply a lubricant that fits their individual needs. It should be pointed out, however, that insufficient lubrication is the biggest reason for condom tearing and subsequent leakage. Only nonallergenic lubricants, such as K-Y Jelly®, should be used with condoms. Petroleum-based lubricants, such as Vaseline®, mineral oil, and cold cream, should not be used because they may weaken the rubber, causing decreased elasticity, leakage, and decreased contraceptive effectiveness.

"Reservoir-end condoms" have a nipple-like tip at the closed end to hold ejaculated semen. Condoms with a reservoir-end are available with or without a lubricant. Most users prefer a condom with a reservoir-end.

Contoured condoms come in two varieties, flared or narrowed down (see Figure 7). The flared version has a wider end which allows more freedom of movement inside the condom. Narrowed-down condoms are constricted just behind the glans of the penis for a more snug fit. Contouring appeals to as many as one in five condom users.

Condom size is becoming more important to users, and represents a significant advantage of latex condoms over "skins." Different sizes of condoms are available to accommodate differences in penis size between American and Asian men. The average penis length and

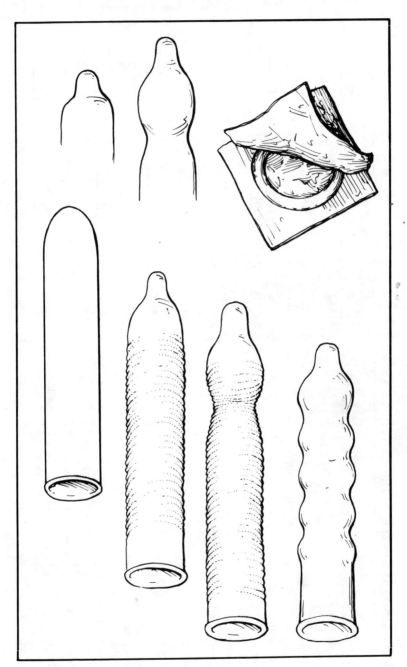

FIGURE 7
Various shapes and textures of condoms

63

TABLE 10
CONDOM BRANDS AVAILABLE IN THE UNITED STATES*

Brand Name	Supplier	Type	Reservoir-End	Special Shape	Textured
Conceptrol Shields	Akwell	Latex	Yes	Narrowed	——
Conceptrol Shields Unlubricated	"	"	Yes	Narrowed	——
Conture	Warner-Lambert	"	——		Ribbed
Excita Sensitol	Schmid	Latex	Yes	Flared	
Fetherlite	Schmid	Latex	——		
Fetherlite w/Natursol	"	"			
Fiesta Sensi-Color	Schmid	Latex	Yes		
Fourex	Schmid	Skin	——		
Guardian	Youngs	Latex	Yes		
Horizon Conture	Akwell	Latex	Yes	Narrowed	
Horizon Nuda	"	"	Yes		
Horizon Prime	"	"	Yes		
Horizon Prime Unlubricated	"	"	Yes		
Horizon Stimula	"	"	Yes		Ribbed
Hugger	Ansell	"	Yes		
Lifestyle**	——		——		——
Naturalamb	Youngs	Skin	——		——
Nuda	Warner-Lambert	Latex	——		——
Nuform Sensi-Shape	Schmid	Latex	Yes	Flared	——

64

Nuform Sensi-Shape Unlubricated	"	"		Flared	
Prime	Ansell	"	Yes		
Ramses	Schmid	Latex	Yes		
Ramses Extra**	"	"	Yes		
Ramses Unlubricated	"	"			
Ramses Sensitol	"	"	Yes		
Rough Rider	Ansell	"			Studded
Sheik Plain End #22	Schmid	Latex			
Sheik Reservoir-End Lubricated #54	"	"	Yes		
Sheik Reservoir-End Unlubricated #28	"	"			
Stimula	Warner-Lambert	"	Yes		Ribbed
Tahiti	Akwell	Latex	Yes		
Trojan-Enz	Youngs	Latex	Yes		
Trojan-Enz Unlubricated	"	"			
Trojans	"	"	Yes		
Trojans Unlubricated	"	"			
Trojan Guardian	"	"	Yes		
Trojan Plus	"	"	Yes	Narrowed	
Trojan Plus 2**	"	"	Yes		
Trojan Ribbed	"	"	Yes		Ribbed

*Except where indicated, all brands shown above come with a lubricant.

**Lubricant also contains a spermicidal chemical. The contraceptive value of the spermicide in the lubricant has not been clearly established. Such products should not be used in place of a vaginal spermicide plus condom.

width in American men is roughly 10 to 15 percent greater than for Asian men. As a result, some condoms are now produced in sizes. Each size is slightly longer than the average penis length in the countries where it is most likely to be used. The width is somewhat narrower than the average penis width. U.S. manufacturers promote the smaller condom (generally available only through mail-order houses) as a "snugger fit" condom.

Colored condoms are a relatively new addition to the condom market and have boosted sales significantly. Textured condoms are another variation. The surface around the circumference of a textured condom may have dots, ribs, or other projections.

More recent developments include condoms bathed in a "desensitizer," such as benzocaine (Ramses®, NuForm®) that supposedly helps "aid in temporarily prolonging time for ejaculation." If you are allergic to topical anesthetics, sunscreen products, sulfa drugs, or hair dyes, you should avoid use of this type of condom. Condoms bathed in a spermicidal lubricant (Ramses Extra®, Trojan Plus 2®, Lifestyle®) may appeal to couples desiring extra lubrication and added contraceptive protection.

Condoms are most economical when purchased in quantity. Purchasing condoms by the dozen, three dozen, or by the gross (144 condoms) can save up to 20, 30, and 50 percent respectively over the price per condom in the three pack. Condoms cost from 30 cents to over $2.00 each, depending on the brand, type, and quantity purchased.

ADVANTAGES OF CONDOM USE

THE CONDOM AS A CONTRACEPTIVE

The condom is a very effective and practical method of contraception. It is the oldest form of male contraception and remains the only *device* available to be used by men for this purpose. Vasectomy is the only other measure of contraception currently available exclusively to males. A safe, reversible method of contraception, the condom requires no medical supervision and produces virtually no adverse effects. Only oral contraceptives and the IUD are considered more effective than condoms as a single contraceptive method.

Over the years, condom contraceptive effectiveness has been somewhat misrepresented due to poor results shown in several crudely conducted studies from the 1930s through the 1950s. Even with some lingering doubt and confusion, the condom is very popular in the U.S. Over 4.5 million men and women rely on condoms for contraceptive protection. This is fewer than the number using oral contraceptives, but more than any other single form of birth control except for voluntary sterilization.

Failure of most barrier methods of contraception is a result of:

1. Product Failure—pregnancy occurred even though the product was used correctly and consistently.
2. User Failure—pregnancy occurred as a result of incorrect or inconsistent use of the product despite adequate instructions.
3. Provider Failure—pregnancy occurred because the provider did not supply adequate instructions for use.

Product failure of condoms represents the theoretical or expected effectiveness of condom use. This is a measure of the likelihood that a condom may break or leak, resulting in conception.

User failure does occur with condom use. Erroneous application of the condom is rarely the cause of contraceptive failure, however. Conception most often occurs from inconsistent use. Factors affecting consistency of condom use, and therefore condom effectiveness, are age, whether they are used to delay or prevent birth, age at marriage, religion, family income, level of education, length of marriage, and length of use. Age and length of time the method was used were the factors that influenced condom effectiveness most. Young couples are more likely to use condoms inconsistently and are less likely to use them for extended periods (more than six months).

Provider failure may occur when inadequate directions for use are provided with the condom package. Although condoms are relatively simple to use, the instructions for use are important (see Table 11). To the credit of major manufacturers in this country, at least a limited set of directions for use accompany each condom package.

EFFECTIVENESS OF THE CONDOM

Effectiveness of the condom as a contraceptive can be as high as 97 percent when condoms are used properly. Overall, the theoretical rate of effectiveness, when condoms are used correctly, ranges from 0.5 to 3.0 pregnancies per 100 woman-years. Modern studies have placed the effectiveness of condoms during actual use between 3.0 and 4.0 pregnancies per 100 woman-years. This figure is the number of times pregnancy occurred due to product failure and/or user failure.

OTHER IMPORTANT POINTS TO REMEMBER

- Condoms should *not* be tested by inflating or stretching them before use. The chances of weakening or damaging the wall of the condom are much greater than finding a defect.

• As an added precaution to reduce the risk of sexually transmitted disease, wash the penis and surrounding area immediately after withdrawal.

Men vary in their ability to anticipate or control ejaculation. This may be the reason most pamphlets describing how to use condoms advise the user to place the condom over the penis before any genital contact. Some experts state that motile sperm do not exist in the clear fluid involuntarily released from the penis during sexual arousal. This has not been proven, however. Insertion and withdrawal prior to ejaculation, and without benefit of the condom, may result in pregnancy. If the condom is being used for contraceptive purposes only, you may believe you can anticipate or control ejaculation and you may choose to wait until just prior to male orgasm before placing the condom on the penis. If uncertainty exists about general self-control and control of ejaculation, it is wise to use the condom before any genital contact.

On the other hand, if a condom is used for prevention of a sexually transmitted disease (STD), it *must* be worn before any genital contact occurs. Even brief contact with syphilis or herpes lesions or with discharge containing the organism producing gonor-

---

TABLE 11
HOW TO USE CONDOMS

---

1. Keep an adequate supply of condoms on hand. Store in a cool, dry place. Use one at every intercourse. Do not reuse.
2. For maximum protection against sexually transmitted disease, place the condom on the penis *before* any genital contact or penetration. Handle gently. Keep the condom away from sharp fingernails.
3. Condoms unroll in one direction. Place the condom over the head of the penis with the rolled portion out.
4. As it is unrolled, hold about 1/2 inch of space at the end for ejaculated semen if the condom does not have a reservoir-end.
5. Slowly unroll the condom over the entire length of the erect penis.
6. If additional lubrication is desired, lubricate the outside of the condom with a water-soluble lubricant such as K-Y Jelly®, or contraceptive jelly. *Do not use Vaseline, cold cream, mineral oil,* or any other type of petroleum-based product.
7. After ejaculation, withdraw the penis while it is still erect. Grasp the rim of the condom firmly at the base of the penis during withdrawal to avoid slippage and spilling of sperm in the vaginal canal.
8. Examine the condom for tears. If a tear has occurred, insert a spermicidal foam, cream, or jelly into the vaginal canal immediately.

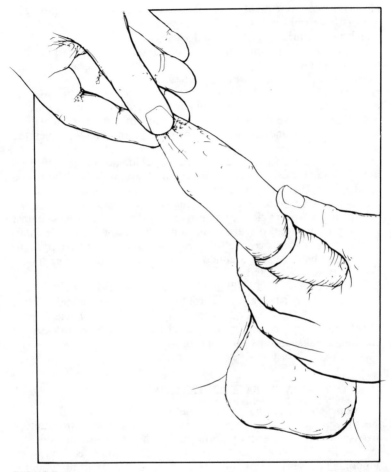

FIGURE 8

Placement of condom demonstrating the space at the closed end that will collect the ejaculate

rhea from the vagina or the male or female urethra may be sufficient for transfer of STD.

It is also generally recommended that air be expelled from the ½ inch space left at the end of the condom (see Figure 8). When the space is filled with air, some maintain the ejaculate may produce excess stress at the condom tip, or semen may be forced down the side of the penis. This recommendation may be a holdover from the days when condom quality was dubious. It is unlikely that the force of ejaculation would break or tear today's high quality latex condoms, which are surprisingly strong and elastic.

Since a certain amount of manual dexterity is needed to fit a condom, persons with coordination disabilities or paralysis of the upper extremities may find them difficult, if not impossible, to use. It is possible to overcome this problem if both partners are involved in use of the contraceptive. The problem of placement can not only be overcome, but also can be a part of the lovemaking if the female is more dexterous and assists in placement of the condom over the penis.

If you desire to reduce the risk of accidental pregnancy even further, you may use a spermicidal cream, foam, or jelly along with a condom. In theory, with combined use it is possible to increase effectiveness up to 99 percent. Along with increased contraceptive effectiveness, spermicides may provide additional protection against sexually transmitted disease. Insertion of a spermicide before intercourse may also prove useful if you choose to wait just prior to ejaculation before using a condom—especially if ejaculation should occur before anticipated.

Some experts find it difficult to justify combining the two contraceptives if insistence on the routine use of a spermicide deters couples from using the condom correctly. Even if a spermicidal agent is not used with a condom, one should be kept on hand in case the condom breaks or slips off while in use.

THE CONDOM IN DISEASE PREVENTION

Repeated studies have shown that condoms are very effective in the prevention of gonorrhea and most other sexually transmitted diseases (STDs). One study performed with 246 Australian soldiers serving in Vietnam revealed quite convincingly the effectiveness of condoms in disease prevention. Out of this group, 55 used condoms consistently. Not one soldier contracted an STD. On the other hand, of the 191 soldiers who did not always use condoms, 35 percent became infected with an STD.

Pelvic inflammatory disease (PID), an infection of the uterus, fallopian tubes, and adjacent structures, is often caused by STDs. The end result of PID is often infertility or ectopic pregnancy. Sperm may provide transportation through the cervix for some or all of the organisms that cause PID. Sperm and the infecting organisms are prevented from entering the cervix when the male uses a condom. Women whose partners use condoms are 70 percent less likely to develop PID than women who use the IUD or birth control pill for contraception.

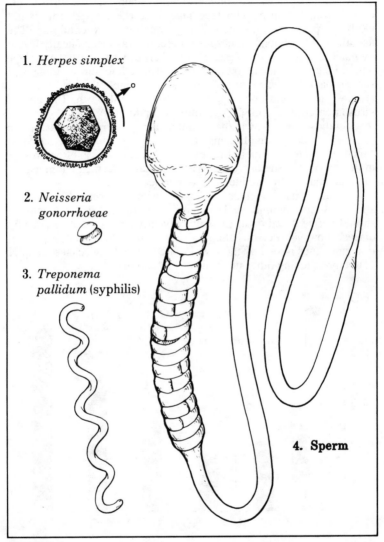

1. *Herpes simplex*

2. *Neisseria gonorrhoeae*

3. *Treponema pallidum* (syphilis)

4. Sperm

FIGURE 9

Relative size of the sperm cell in relation to some common sexually transmitted disease organisms

Condoms may afford some protection against herpes virus transmitted from sexual contact (see Figure 9). The herpes virus is not likely to pass through today's high quality latex condoms. The usefulness of condoms in herpes protection was mechanically tested by placing condoms impregnated with herpes virus around a syringe with plunger. A nutrient broth was pushed into the condom and sucked back by the plunger 50 times to resemble the act of coitus. Herpes virus could not be found in the nutrient broth. The herpes virus apparently cannot pass through a condom.

Studies have shown that women using barrier contraceptive methods, such as diaphragms, are less likely to develop cervical cancer than other women. Interestingly, herpes virus is often present in the cervical tissue of women with cervical cancer. Condom use by the male may further reduce risk of cervical cancer.

Condom use by male homosexuals has increased protection against Acquired Immune Deficiency Syndrome (AIDS). Condoms should not be relied on as the sole preventive measure of this deadly disease, however. Persons at high risk for AIDS should follow prevention guidelines issued by the U.S. Public Health Service (see Chapter 11) before seeking other methods of protection.

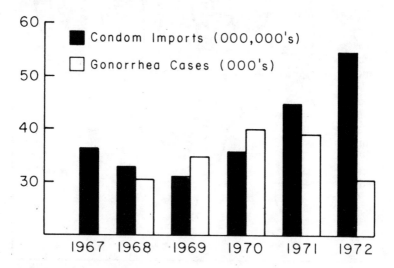

FIGURE 10

As the number of condoms available in Sweden began to drop (1967 to 1969), the number of reported cases of gonorrhea began to rise (1968 to 1970). From 1970 to 1972, as the number of condoms available grew, the number of reported cases of gonorrhea diminished.

Vaginal infections, such as trichomonas infections, are common among women between the ages of 15 and 44, and are treated effectively with prescription drugs such as metronidazole (Flagyl®). In many cases, successful treatment is dependent upon having both the female and the male partner treated simultaneously. If simultaneous treatment does not take place, the infection is passed back and forth between sexual partners. Condoms may be useful during treatment of vaginitis as an added safeguard against this "Ping-Pong" effect.

In 1972, the Swedish Association for Sex Education sponsored a national program to encourage the use of condoms. Repeal of laws restricting the advertising of contraceptives paved the way for open promotion. As a result, the number of reported cases of STD dropped markedly as condom imports were increased between 1969 and 1972 (see Figure 10).

Women must bear the entire risk and burden of experiencing an adverse drug reaction when using contraceptive measures such as "the pill" and the IUD; some women find the freedom from side effects when the male uses condoms quite desirable. Women often suffer physically from a sexually transmitted disease (STD) more than do men.

Those who have many different sex partners may find the disease protection aspect of condoms particularly appealing. Teenagers between the ages of 15 and 19 account for 25 percent of all reported cases of gonorrhea, almost 18 percent of all births, and over 30 percent of all abortions. Use of planned methods of contraception which require prescriptions, such as birth control pills, diaphragm, or an IUD, are sometimes avoided by teenagers, whose attitudes about sexual intercourse are often casual, irresponsible, and unsophisticated. Some teenagers avoid or delay planned contraceptive methods because they do not fully appreciate the risks of unprotected intercourse. The condom is simple to use, inexpensive, readily available, and should be considered by teenagers, if they engage in intercourse. Condoms can be purchased in a pharmacy without a prescription or a medical examination and can be kept in a pocket or purse for quick use. Carrying and using a condom may be less traumatic for teenagers and parents alike when the trauma resulting from a sexually transmitted disease, unwanted birth, or abortion is considered.

OTHER ADVANTAGES OF CONDOM USE

In addition to contraception and disease protection, condoms possess a number of other advantages. For a small percentage of users, the condom actually increases coital sensitivity. For most couples, however, condoms reduce sensation. Decreased sensation is an advantage for men who experience premature ejaculation. Condoms have also been reported to help overcome aesthetic objections to intercourse during menstruation. Other couples find condoms convenient for short-term use, such as between marriage and a planned pregnancy or between pregnancies. Condoms are often used prior to switching to a more permanent method. For example, after the birth of a child a couple may have to wait until vaginal muscles have recovered from delivery and the uterus has returned to normal size before a diaphragm or IUD is used. Condoms can provide a viable temporary contraceptive alternative in situations such as this.

Condoms have proved useful in treating infertility in some women who are infertile due to an allergy to sperm. Between 10 to 30 percent of unexplained infertility may be due to antibodies produced by the woman which inactivate sperm. Researchers believe that sperm antibodies may be produced when sperm comes into contact with cervical tissue. In one study, five women had their partners use condoms for two to six months. Unprotected intercourse was then timed to coincide with ovulation. All showed a significant reduction in sperm antibody count during condom use. Three of these women became pregnant. A number of questions remain unanswered about the use of condoms with infertility therapy. Nevertheless, it is estimated that women with a high sperm antibody count can increase the chance of conception by 20 to 30 percent if condoms are used by the partner for at least three months or until the antibody count drops. The probability of pregnancy is still small. But considering how inexpensive condom therapy is, and its freedom from side effects, the condom may be helpful to some infertile couples.

As previously stated, barrier methods of contraception, particularly diaphragms and condoms, may protect against cervical cancer. Cervical cancer appears to be initiated or promoted by a sexually transmitted agent, possibly herpes. Barrier methods limit transmission of this agent.

LIMITATIONS TO CONDOM USE

Although the advantages of using condoms are numerous, less than 10 percent of sexually active men and women use them in the United States. Decreased sensitivity during coitus, interrupted love-making, and messiness were the reasons most often given by both users and nonusers for not using condoms.

Years ago U.S. condoms were among the thickest in the world. This perpetuated the complaint that condoms dulled sensitivity and mutual sensation. Decreased sensitivity is becoming less of a problem as the thickness of modern latex condoms is reduced. The success of the ultrathin condom in Japan calls for close examination of current U.S. standards for condom thickness.

Although occasional complaints associated with condom use cannot be completely eliminated, some of them can be minimized. For example, if condoms interrupt lovemaking, the problem can be at least partially overcome by involving the female partner in the process of placing the condom over the penis. The new "dry" silicone-based lubricants are making condoms less messy than wet lubrication.

Unpleasant odor has been reported by some users. Skin condoms are cited most often for objectionable odor. Lubricant from latex condoms may possess a pungent odor. For couples finding condom odor a deterrent to their use, scented condoms are now available from mail-order houses in the U.S.

Condom packages have improved a great deal over the years, but a few problems remain. Condoms usually come in packages of three, with perforations between each envelope to facilitate separating them. The perforations between packets in some brands have been found to be inadequate, as two packets would open instead of one. If two packets become unsealed, do not save the second condom for future use.

Storage next to a hot radiator or hot air duct may cause accelerated deterioration. Deterioration of condoms can be accelerated by prolonged exposure to oxygen, ozone, and ultraviolet light. U.S. manufacturers point out that foil packages protect condoms from these hazards. There is little doubt that foil packages protect condoms from oxygen and ozone. The same may not be true in the case of ultraviolet light. Although most packages are sufficiently opaque to resist sources of ultraviolet light, such as sunlight or fluorescent light, some brands have a window on one side of the packet. Condoms with this type of packaging should not be left near sunlight or fluorescent light.

PREVALENCE OF CONDOM USE

It is estimated that worldwide over 40 million couples rely on condoms, making them the most widely used *mechanical* contraceptive in the world. However, they continue to be underutilized in those areas that could benefit most from condom use. In developing countries where fertility rates are high, and in developed countries among young couples at great risk of STD, condom use is low. Additionally, condoms are used more in urban than in rural areas— perhaps due to a higher concentration of retail outlets in urban areas. The bulk of condom use is concentrated in a few areas. Nearly two-thirds of all condoms are used in industrialized nations (see Figure 11).

Condom use is highest in Japan, where 70 to 75 percent of all

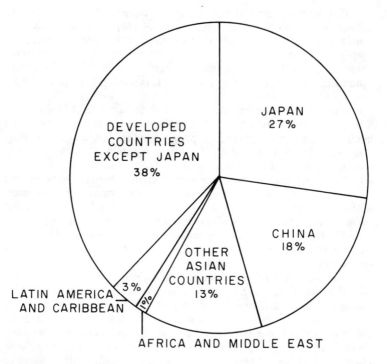

FIGURE 11

Percentage of condom users in areas of the world in 1981

couples using contraception rely on condoms. The introduction of an ultrathin condom in Japan in 1970 increased sales over 43 percent in one year.

The most interesting aspect of Japan's approach to marketing condoms is the "condom lady," who goes from door to door selling condoms to Japanese housewives. This approach has segmented the market, with men buying condoms in pharmacies and women purchasing them in their homes from "condom ladies." The result of this novel approach is that housewives now account for almost 20 percent of all condom sales in Japan. The high rate of condom use in Japan may also stem from psychological conditioning. Many Japanese women do not like to touch their genitals. Therefore, spermicides and diaphragms are not widely used. Additionally, the use of estrogen as an oral contraceptive is illegal in Japan.

Condom use is most often started in this country upon the initiative of a couple interested in conception control. In the past, condoms were not routinely recommended by the family doctor or by family planning clinics. A majority of health professionals don't consider condoms a medical device. However, that attitude is changing gradually as advantages of condoms become more widely known.

Condom sales in the U.S. increased dramatically in the mid-1980s. The condom remains the most easily obtainable contraceptive for teenagers. Young women may find modern methods, such as the birth control pill, more acceptable. Some may find condoms disagreeable because, unlike most other forms of contraception, the condom must be disposed of—sometimes serving as an unpleasant reminder of an indulgence.

The inability of the condom to become substantially more popular in the U.S. may be a result of legal and cultural restraints. Between 1868 and 1873, a series of state and federal laws, including the Comstock Act, declared condoms and information about their use obscene and illegal. The long-term association of condoms with prostitution and STD has persisted in the minds of many middle-aged and older couples. The widespread distribution of condoms to servicemen during World War II for disease prevention only helped to strengthen the negative connection.

A Supreme Court decision in 1977 declaring any ban on advertising or sale of condoms unconstitutional made outdated state laws and local ordinances restricting condom sales or dissemination of information regarding condom use obsolete. Prior to 1977, requesting condoms from a "secret" place behind the pharmacy counter was a ritual most males purchasing condoms experienced. This was quite embarrassing for some men. The move to openly display condoms in pharmacies has done much to make the condom more acceptable and accessible.

Open display of condoms is accepted by women as well as men. For many women, condoms are nothing more than another item on the shopping list. Approximately 40 percent of all condoms sold in U.S. pharmacies are now purchased by women.

It is likely that condom promotion will increase in media such as daily newspapers and even appear on television. The open promotion of feminine hygiene products, contraceptive vaginal suppositories, and spermicidal agents in the mass media is making advertising of other contraceptives more acceptable.

MANUFACTURING AND TESTING OF CONDOMS

Most condoms are manufactured under carefully controlled, highly automated conditions that result in a high degree of quality. As a result of federal regulations, a batch of condoms (not to exceed 150,000 condoms) may include no more than 0.25 percent substandard units—a drastic improvement from pre–World War II days when 75 percent of all condoms produced were defective. U.S. manufacturers supply over five billion condoms annually. The average couple who are regular users of condoms use about 2 condoms per week, or about 100 condoms a year.

CONCLUSION

The condom offers a completely reversible, widely available, relatively inexpensive, and easy-to-use means of birth control. The proven safety and effectiveness of the condom as a contraceptive, and as a disease preventative, distinguish it from some other methods of birth control. Despite legal and moral constraints imposed on condoms during the late 19th and early 20th century, use of condoms is increasing.

4

Barrier Methods:
Diaphragm and
Contraceptive Sponge

INTRODUCTION

New attention is being focused on one of the oldest and simplest forms of contraception—a barrier in the vagina. This chapter addresses use of the diaphragm and contraceptive sponge. While risks associated with the oral contraceptive and IUD are minimal for most women, adverse publicity has convinced some women that trading high contraceptive effectiveness afforded by the pill and IUD for the safety of less effective barrier methods is the proper action. Barrier methods are a useful alternative to the pill and IUD.

The vaginal barrier methods of contraception offer both advantages and disadvantages. Advantages of the diaphragm and contraceptive sponge include the following:

1. Effective when properly used
2. Reversible
3. Safe, with no serious physical adverse effects with long-term use
4. Controlled by user and used only when needed

5. Usable during menstruation (although not recommended with the contraceptive sponge)
6. Protective to some extent against sexually transmitted diseases (STDs) and pelvic inflammatory disease (PID)
7. Usable in nursing mothers since lactation is unimpaired

Disadvantages of the diaphragm and contraceptive sponge include the following:

1. Relatively high accidental pregnancy rate. A high degree of user motivation to use the product consistently and carefully is required with each act of intercourse.
2. Anticipation of the sexual act or interruption of sexual activity to use. Impairs spontaneity.
3. Manipulation of genitalia, for which some women have an aversion, is necessary.
4. Relatively expensive if used frequently.
5. If spermicide is also used (as with a diaphragm), some women complain of the messiness.
6. Need to leave in place several hours after intercourse (six hours).
7. Insertion and removal may prove troublesome for some women.

HISTORY OF BARRIER METHODS OF CONTRACEPTION

ANCIENT HISTORY

For centuries women have used vaginal methods of contraception. Vaginal plugs consisting of gums, leaves, fruits, seed pods, chopped grass, rags, oiled bamboo pulp, pulp of figs and pomegranates, beeswax, paper, solid waste of animals, and sponges have been inserted into the vagina to block access to the ovum by sperm. These devices blocked the opening of the cervix to varying degrees. The highly acid nature of certain plant constituents produced a serendipitous spermicidal action. History does not record the complications from use of such contraceptive devices, but it is certain they were associated with numerous adverse effects of an infectious and/or inflammatory nature.

RECENT HISTORY

The first modern female barrier contraceptive devices were the diaphragm and cervical cap. The first cervical cap was developed in

1838 by a German physician. Another German physician developed the diaphragm in 1880. Most U.S. physicians did not endorse these methods because they felt the methods were too complicated and involved excessive genital manipulation. It was not until the 1920s that diaphragms became readily available and were utilized extensively in the U.S.

PEAK USE

During the first half of the 20th century, diaphragms and condoms were the most commonly used contraceptives in the U.S. In 1955, 25 percent of white, married couples using contraception in the U.S. relied on the diaphragm for birth control; 27 percent relied on the condom. Growing use of these two barrier methods was due primarily to increased availability and a general acceptance of birth control by society. Use of vaginal barrier methods peaked in the 1950s.

CURRENT ACCEPTANCE

As oral contraceptives and intrauterine devices became widely available in the 1960s, use of barrier methods rapidly decreased. By 1965 only 10 percent of white, married couples using contraception relied on the diaphragm; by 1976 this number had declined to three percent. During the late 1970s, however, publicity about the potential side effects of oral contraceptives and the IUD stimulated renewed interest in vaginal contraceptive methods. The popularity of the diaphragm has increased substantially, and public acceptance of the relatively new contraceptive sponge is good. Among more than a million mostly young, first time contraceptive users in the U.S., 12.9 percent chose the diaphragm in 1980 compared with 5.7 percent in 1975. Among California women receiving family planning services in state funded clinics, diaphragm use increased from 7.1 percent in 1976 to 12.8 percent in 1979. Use was greatest in young women (age 25 to 29), increasing from 10.1 percent in 1976 to 15.8 percent in 1979.

DIAPHRAGM

PHYSICAL CHARACTERISTICS OF THE DIAPHRAGM

Diaphragms are shallow, rubber domes with a firm but flexible outer rim. When fitted properly, the diaphragm fits snugly between the recess behind the pubic bone and the posterior vaginal wall and covers the opening of the cervix completely (see Figure 12). Diaphragms are produced in sizes ranging from 50 to 105 mm in diameter. The most commonly used sizes are between 65 and 80 mm.

There are three major types of diaphragm. These are the flat-spring, coil-spring, and arcing diaphragm. The flat-spring diaphragm is the original diaphragm and has a flat metal band in the rim. The coil-spring diaphragm has a wire spiral within the rim. Both are well suited for women with good vaginal muscle tone and an adequate vaginal recess behind the pubic arch. The flat-spring diaphragm exerts slightly more pressure against the vaginal wall than the coil-spring diaphragm and is better suited for use in women who have a shallow recess behind the pubic bone. Both the flat-spring and coil-spring diaphragms fold flat for insertion. The arcing diaphragm has a sturdy, firm rim that folds into an arc, which some women find easier to insert. The arcing diaphragm may be especially useful in women with poor vaginal muscle tone, bulging of the bladder into the vagina (cystocele), bulging of the rectum into the vagina (rectocele), a long uterine cervix, and/or a tilted uterus.

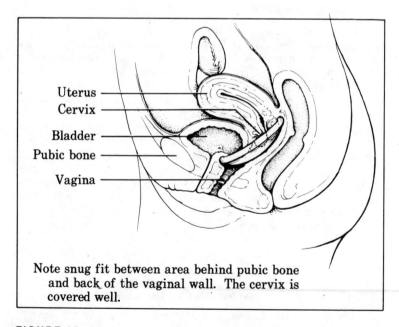

Uterus
Cervix
Bladder
Pubic bone
Vagina

Note snug fit between area behind pubic bone and back of the vaginal wall. The cervix is covered well.

FIGURE 12

Demonstration of a properly fitted diaphragm

PREVENTION OF PREGNANCY BY A DIAPHRAGM

When properly fitted, the diaphragm covers the opening of the cervix and helps prevent entry of sperm into the uterus. The fact of the matter is, however, a diaphragm used alone will not fit snugly at all times during intercourse. Coital movement and/or coital position may allow openings through which sperm can gain entry into the uterus. It is, therefore, critical that in order for a diaphragm to be effective *it must be used with a spermicide*.

A diaphragm may be inserted up to six hours before intercourse, but before it is inserted, one to three teaspoonfuls of spermicidal cream or gel *must* be placed in the dome and spread around the rim (see Figure 21, Chapter 5). The diaphragm may then be inserted. If the diaphragm is in place more than two hours before intercourse, application of additional spermicide in the vaginal canal near the cervix is recommended for optimal protection. Once inserted, the diaphragm must be left in place for at least six hours after intercourse, but no longer than 24 hours after intercourse. If intercourse is to take place again within 24 hours, and the diaphragm is still in place, an additional applicator full of spermicide must be inserted into the vagina prior to intercourse.

EFFECTIVENESS OF THE DIAPHRAGM

When properly fitted and inserted, a diaphragm can be highly effective. First year failure rates in the range of only two to three pregnancies per 100 woman-years have been reported. Range of failure varies from two to 20 per 100 woman-years. The typical failure rate for the population at large is probably in the range of 4.2 to 4.8 pregnancies per 100 woman-years. Lowest failure rates occur in women highly motivated to prevent pregnancy, older users, and women who have had very good instruction and/or experience with vaginal methods of contraception. High failure rates occur if the diaphragm is misused or not used, and most failures occur during the first six months of use.

FITTING A WOMAN FOR A DIAPHRAGM

To be effective, a diaphragm must be properly fitted to the individual user. The person doing the fitting may be a physician or another trained person. Paramedical workers are most likely to have the time to educate and train women in proper diaphragm use. If a nurse or other health worker needs assistance in fitting a diaphragm, a physician may be called.

DETERMINING THE CORRECT SIZE AND TYPE OF DIAPHRAGM

To determine the correct size and type of diaphragm you need, a pelvic examination is required. A review of anatomical features and determination of vaginal muscle tone will aid your physician in selecting the flat-spring, coil-spring, or arcing diaphragm. To determine correct size, a measurement is made of the diagonal length of the vaginal canal from the area behind the pubic bone to the rear of the vaginal canal. This is accomplished in three steps (see Figure 13).

Diaphragms must be fitted carefully. One that is too small may slip out of place. One that is too large may buckle, producing discomfort for you and/or your male sexual partner. The largest size diaphragm that will fit evenly in the vaginal canal, without your being aware of its presence, is the one usually chosen.

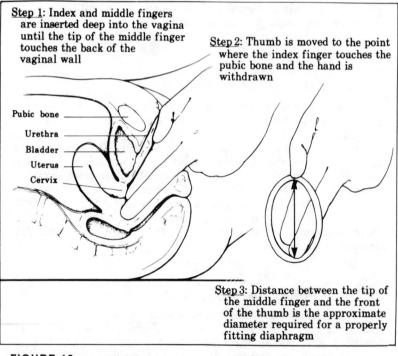

FIGURE 13

Steps for fitting a diaphragm

Vaginal muscle tone is affected by many factors including number of births, body weight, pelvic surgery, abortion, and psychological state during fitting. If you have given birth, you are likely to require a larger diaphragm than a woman who has not given birth. Childbirth stretches the vaginal canal. If you used a diaphragm prior to pregnancy and delivery of offspring, you should be refitted after each birth if you intend to continue using a diaphragm. This measurement should not take place until about six weeks after delivery. A gain or loss of 15 or more pounds also requires a refitting. If you undergo pelvic or abdominal surgery, you should be refitted, as organs and tissues may redistribute. If a second trimester abortion occurs, a refitting should occur about four weeks later. Tension during the initial fitting may cause vaginal muscles to tighten. This may lead to fitting of a smaller diaphragm than is actually required.

You should have a follow-up exam one to two weeks after the initial fitting. You may be asked to come for this exam with the diaphragm in place so the fit can be checked. It is wise to use a supplemental contraceptive, such as a condom, along with the diaphragm plus spermicide until the follow-up visit. Once a proper fit is confirmed, diaphragm plus spermicide should confer adequate contraceptive protection if properly used.

WHEN THE DIAPHRAGM CANNOT BE USED

There are some medical conditions which may prohibit use of a diaphragm. Many of these conditions involve abnormal anatomy of the vagina, cervix, or uterus. Diaphragms cannot be used if there is very poor vaginal muscle tone, severe bulging of the bladder into the vagina (cystocele), severe bulging of the rectum into the vagina (rectocele), or collapse of the uterus into the vagina. If you have just given birth, you should not rely on a diaphragm as a contraceptive for at least six weeks and until you are refitted. Women with chronic, recurrent urinary tract infections may have their condition aggravated by a diaphragm. Rare allergy to the rubber of the diaphragm, or to the spermicide, is a contraindication to use. If you have a psychological aversion to manipulating your genitalia, you should not use this device.

INSERTION AND REMOVAL OF A DIAPHRAGM

Insertion

Although the diaphragm may be inserted with the dome up, most women insert it with the dome down to keep the spermicide from

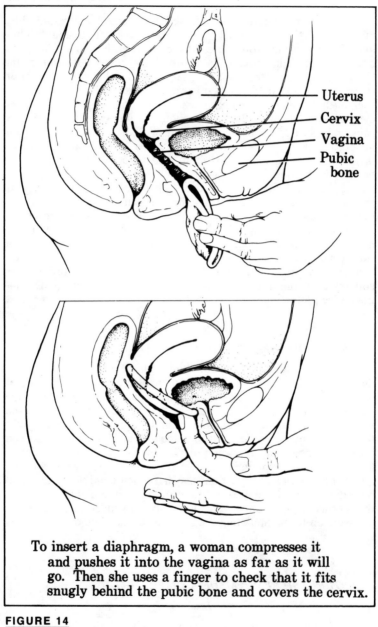

Uterus
Cervix
Vagina
Pubic bone

To insert a diaphragm, a woman compresses it and pushes it into the vagina as far as it will go. Then she uses a finger to check that it fits snugly behind the pubic bone and covers the cervix.

FIGURE 14

Insertion of a diaphragm

86

falling out of the dome. One to three teaspoonfuls (a three- to five-inch ribbon) of spermicidal cream or jelly is placed inside the dome. A thin layer should be spread around the rim. *Spermicide must be used!* The best fitting diaphragm does not press against the vaginal wall tightly enough to completely prevent passage of sperm. It may be inserted up to six hours before intercourse.

To insert the diaphragm, you may assume one of four positions—sitting on the edge of a chair, lying flat on the back with knees bent, squatting, or propping one leg up on a toilet seat or seat of a chair. Holding the spermicide-containing diaphragm in one hand, the rim should be pinched together using the index and middle fingers and the thumb. With the labia spread by your other hand, the diaphragm is then inserted into the vagina as far as it will go (see Figure 14). The forward rim is then pressed behind the ridge created by the pubic bone. If you are standing, the diaphragm is inserted almost horizontally; if you are lying down, its insertion is almost vertical.

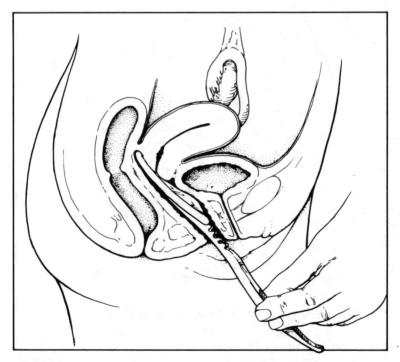

FIGURE 15

Insertion of diaphragm with plastic introducer

If you want to avoid touching a "messy" diaphragm or the genitalia, a specially designed plastic inserter (introducer) is available (see Figure 15). The introducer has calibrated notches that correspond to diaphragm size. The rim of the diaphragm is hooked onto the introducer and inserted into the vagina. By giving the introducer a quarter turn, the diaphragm is disengaged and the introducer removed. You must then use your finger to push the forward rim of the diaphragm behind the pubic bone and determine whether the cervix is covered.

Once inserted, you must check to see if the diaphragm is in the proper place. The cervix can be felt by the index finger, through the dome of the diaphragm (see Figure 16). The cervix feels like the tip of the nose with a dimple in the center. Avoid perforating the diaphragm with a fingernail.

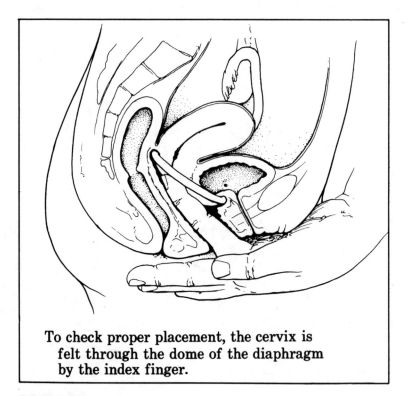

To check proper placement, the cervix is felt through the dome of the diaphragm by the index finger.

FIGURE 16

Demonstration of technique for determining proper placement

Removal

The diaphragm should be left in place for at least six hours, but no longer than 24 hours, after intercourse. Removal six hours after intercourse virtually assures that no live sperm have survived exposure to the spermicide; if left in place more than 24 hours, the probability of infection is increased. An additional application of spermicide should precede each additional act of intercourse. Douching should not occur while the diaphragm is in place; the liquid may dilute and remove the spermicide, and the force of the liquid may propel viable sperm under the diaphragm and into the uterus. The diaphragm is usually removed by hooking an index finger behind the forward rim and then pulling down gently (see Figure 17).

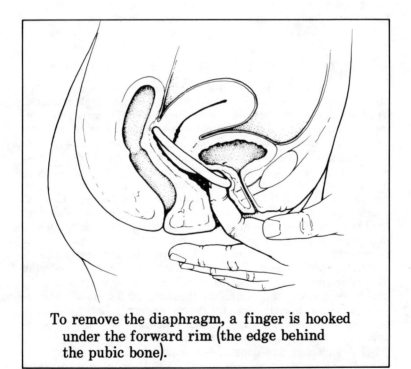

To remove the diaphragm, a finger is hooked
under the forward rim (the edge behind
the pubic bone).

FIGURE 17
Removal of the diaphragm

CARE OF THE DIAPHRAGM AFTER REMOVAL

If properly cared for, diaphragms may last two years or more. It is usually recommended, however, that a new diaphragm be obtained every year or whenever defects are recognized or suspected. Upon removal, you should gently wash the diaphragm with mild soap and warm water. The diaphragm should be patted dry very gently and dusted with cornstarch or unscented talcum powder. This will protect the rubber from deterioration. Exposure of a diaphragm to scented products, hot water, heat, bright light, oils (such as Vaseline® or mineral oil), metals (such as copper, zinc, or silver), and printing inks (such as on newspaper) may erode the latex. You should store the diaphragm in a protective container.

Before the diaphragm is reused, it should be checked for holes, tears, fissures, and cracks. Such defects normally appear near the rim. Inspection by holding the diaphragm up against light, or placing water inside the dome, should indicate any defects. If the rubber is puckered or uneven, a new diaphragm should be obtained.

SIDE EFFECTS ASSOCIATED WITH USE OF THE DIAPHRAGM

The diaphragm plus spermicide seldom produces serious side effects. Side effects may include irritation by latex rubber, vaginal irritation due to the spermicidal agent, mild allergic reaction, or increased frequency of urinary tract irritation and/or infection.

Urinary tract infections in sexually active women usually manifest themselves as urethritis (inflammation of the urethra secondary to infection) and cystitis (inflammation of the bladder secondary to infection) and have been linked to intercourse during menstruation, past history of infection, higher than average frequency of intercourse, and diaphragm use. The reasons for a higher rate of urinary tract infection in diaphragm users may be due to (1) irritation, which may promote an infection, from the rim of the diaphragm pressing against the urethra, (2) introduction of bacteria into the vagina or urethra due to handling of genitalia during insertion and removal of the diaphragm, and (3) blockage of the passage of urine out of the bladder by pressure on the urethra, thus creating a stagnant environment promoting bacterial growth. There is an increased risk of vaginal infection and erosion of the vaginal mucosa if you leave the diaphragm in place longer than 24 hours.

It is logical to consider whether diaphragm use may increase the risk of toxic shock syndrome (TSS). Data to date only suggest a possible link between diaphragm use and TSS. Two of the 1,000 cases reported between January 1980 and June 1981 occurred in diaphragm users. Four U.S. cases of TSS occurred in diaphragm users in 1981 and 1982. Three cases occurred in young women who had their diaphragm in place from 24 hours to three days. Some investigators have reported that the spermicide (chemical which inactivates sperm) nonoxynol-9 may inhibit growth of *Staphylococcus aureus,* the organism believed to cause most cases of TSS. Use of a diaphragm with spermicide may, therefore, actually decrease the risk of developing TSS. More research is needed before the role of the diaphragm in producing or preventing TSS can be defined, however.

DIAPHRAGM-INDUCED PROTECTION OF WOMEN AGAINST SEXUALLY TRANSMITTED DISEASE (STD) AND PELVIC INFLAMMATORY DISEASE (PID)

It appears that both spermicides and diaphragms may protect women against many STDs and against PID. Nonoxynol-9 is toxic to the organism that causes gonorrhea and may inhibit other bacteria. A two-year study of 241 women found that spermicide users had a gonorrhea rate about one-fourth that of oral contraceptive users. The protective action of spermicides appears to be enhanced by diaphragms, which prevent organisms from reaching the upper vagina and cervix. Because they protect against STDs, spermicides and diaphragms probably protect against PID. A study of 306 PID patients, and over 1,175 controls, revealed that spermicide users faced 60 percent of the risk of PID compared to those who did not use spermicide; diaphragm users faced 40 percent of the risk. The combination of diaphragm plus spermicide may confer additional protection.

ROLE OF DIAPHRAGMS IN PROTECTING WOMEN AGAINST CERVICAL CANCER

Diaphragms appear to have substantial ability to protect against cervical cancer. Cervical cancer may be initiated or promoted by a sexually transmitted agent, possibly a herpes or papilloma virus. By limiting transmission of these organisms, the incidence of cervical cancer has been shown to be substantially decreased. The incidence of cervical cancer or cervical dysplasia (abnormal cells) in women at large is 0.73 cases per 1,000 woman-years; the incidence in women who used a diaphragm for at least five years was 0.17 cases per 1,000 woman-years, a greater than fourfold decrease.

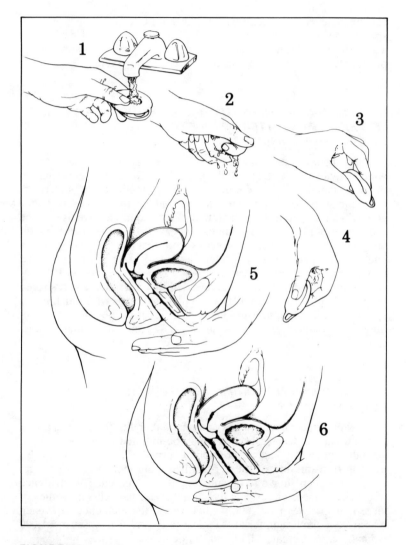

FIGURE 18
Steps for inserting the Today® vaginal contraceptive sponge

1. The sponge may be inserted any time up to 24 hours before intercourse. When ready to insert, remove the sponge from the airtight inner pack and hold in one hand with the "dimple" side up. The loop should dangle under the sponge. The sponge should feel slightly moist. Wet it more with a small amount (about two tablespoons) of clean tap water.
2. Squeeze the sponge gently to remove excess water. It should feel moist and soapy, but not dripping wet.
3. Fold the sides of the sponge upward with a finger along each side to support it. The sponge should look long and narrow. Be sure the string loop dangles underneath the sponge from one end of the fold to the other as shown.
4. Bend wrist and point the end of the folded sponge toward the vagina. Be sure you can see the fold when you look down at it and the string dangles below.
5. From a standing position, squat down slightly and spread legs apart. Use free hand to spread apart the labia. You may also stand with one foot on a stool or chair, sit cross-legged, or lie down. The semisquatting position seems to work best for most women. Slide the sponge into the opening of the vagina as far as the fingers will go. Let the sponge slide through the fingers, deeper into the vagina.
6. Use one or two fingers to push the sponge gently up into the vagina as far as it will go. Be careful not to push a fingernail through the sponge. Check the position of the sponge by sliding your finger around the edge of the sponge to make sure the cervix is not exposed. You should be able to feel the string loop.

CONTRACEPTIVE SPONGE

PHYSICAL CHARACTERISTICS OF THE CONTRACEPTIVE SPONGE AND HOW IT WORKS

The Today® vaginal contraceptive sponge was approved by the FDA in 1983. The sponge is a soft, white, resilient, water-absorbing polyurethane foam. It is biologically compatible with the vaginal environment and formulated to feel like normal vaginal tissue. It is slightly concave and round. The sponge is smaller and thicker than a diaphragm and comes in only one size designed to fit comfortably and snugly in the upper vagina with the concave side covering the cervix. Approximately one gram (1,000 mg) of the commonly used spermicide, nonoxynol-9, is incorporated throughout the sponge. The sponge has a ribbon loop for ease of removal.

The Today® sponge is sold over-the-counter, requires no medical supervision for use, and is disposable. The sponge has three different types of contraceptive action. The spermicidal activity is due to the nonoxynol-9 impregnated in the sponge. The spermicide is activated by moistening the sponge with about two tablespoonfuls (one ounce) of tap water. The sponge should be squeezed gently to remove excess water and then inserted. Absorption of vaginal secretions and compression during intercourse will cause release of the spermicide into the upper vagina. About 200 mg of spermicide is released over 24 hours.

The sponge has an absorption action also. The sponge-like polyurethane is open celled and allows absorption of sperm. The number of sperm available for fertilization is thus reduced.

The sponge also has a blocking action as it covers the entrance to the uterus from the vagina. Its shape allows it to function much like a diaphragm. The fit will not generally be as good as a diaphragm, however, as the sponge is available in only one size and is not rigidly held against the vaginal wall and over the cervix.

INSERTION AND REMOVAL OF THE CONTRACEPTIVE SPONGE

The manufacturer recommends folding the sponge in half and pushing it high into the vagina (see Figure 18). The softness of the sponge may make it more difficult to insert than a diaphragm. It is also difficult to check for correctness of positioning. If the strap attached for ease of removal is turned the wrong way, it may be difficult to remove the sponge.

The sponge may be inserted up to 24 hours before intercourse. Once inserted, the sponge is immediately protective and may be used for 24 hours, regardless of the frequency of intercourse. It must be left in place for at least six hours after intercourse, even if it has been in place for 24 hours, so that viable sperm will be inactivated or destroyed before it is removed. At that time, the sponge should be removed and discarded. It should not be reused.

Proper removal involves following the steps shown in Figure 19. The Today® contraceptive sponge is both soft and strong, but pulling too hard or too quickly on the removal loop may cause it to tear. If this occurs, rather than pull on the loop, grasp the sponge between two fingers and remove slowly and gently. The sponge should be disposed of in a waste container; do not flush it down a toilet.

It is unlikely that the sponge will fall out of the vagina. It may be pushed down to the vaginal opening during a bowel movement or other internal straining. If this occurs, simply push the sponge back into the vagina as far as it will go with a finger. Discard the sponge if it falls completely out.

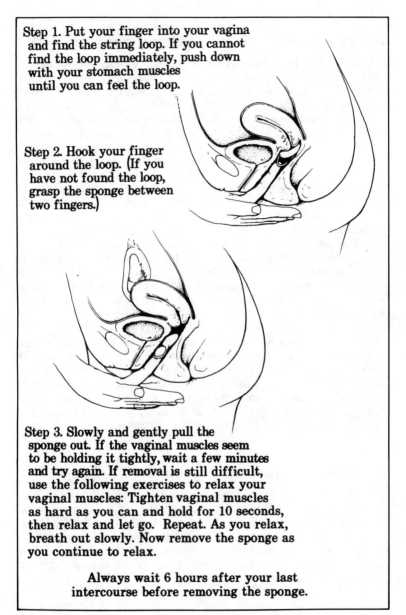

Step 1. Put your finger into your vagina and find the string loop. If you cannot find the loop immediately, push down with your stomach muscles until you can feel the loop.

Step 2. Hook your finger around the loop. (If you have not found the loop, grasp the sponge between two fingers.)

Step 3. Slowly and gently pull the sponge out. If the vaginal muscles seem to be holding it tightly, wait a few minutes and try again. If removal is still difficult, use the following exercises to relax your vaginal muscles: Tighten vaginal muscles as hard as you can and hold for 10 seconds, then relax and let go. Repeat. As you relax, breath out slowly. Now remove the sponge as you continue to relax.

Always wait 6 hours after your last intercourse before removing the sponge.

FIGURE 19

Steps for removing the Today® vaginal contraceptive sponge

EFFECTIVENESS OF THE CONTRACEPTIVE SPONGE

Two recently completed trials of the contraceptive sponge reported pregnancy rates of 9 to 27 per 100 woman-years. (As defined earlier, 1 woman-year is 12 menstrual cycles. 100 woman-years is 1,200 menstrual cycles). These trials allowed use for 48 hours, rather than the recommended 24 hours, and may be higher than what might be seen with the currently marketed product with use restricted to a 24-hour period. Canadian and British studies indicated a pregnancy rate of 27.3 per 100 woman-years for the sponge compared to 10.2 for diaphragm users. In U.S. trials, the sponge has been compared to diaphragm plus spermicidal jelly or cream. The pregnancy rate for sponge users was 16.8 per 100 woman-years, and 12.5 per 100 woman-years for diaphragm users. Under certain conditions, the sponge approaches the diaphragm plus spermicide in effectiveness.

The pregnancy rate from the sponge in a subgroup of women who had borne children was 21.1 per 100 woman-years compared to 12.5 in a group of women who had not borne children. Other studies support this finding. The sponge, therefore, appears most effective in women who are nulliparous (have not borne children). Women who have given birth may require a larger diameter barrier device (e.g. diaphragm) to assure a relatively snug fit in the upper vagina. You should consult your physician before using the contraceptive sponge, or any method of birth control, after childbirth or abortion. All vaginal contraceptive methods are highly dependent on user motivation, consistency, and careful use if optimal effectiveness is to be achieved. Current data suggest that the contraceptive sponge is not as effective as a diaphragm plus spermicide. Further data will lead to definitive conclusions regarding relative effectiveness.

SAFETY OF THE CONTRACEPTIVE SPONGE

The contraceptive sponge appears to be as safe as any other spermicide-containing barrier contraceptive. No serious adverse effects have been reported in patients using nonoxynol-9. The most commonly documented side effects of the contraceptive sponge are allergic-type reactions, vaginal irritation, and vaginal itching. One U.S. study found that four of 100 sponge users discontinued use because of allergic-type reactions, compared with 0.7 per 100 diaphragm users. In addition, about eight per 100 sponge users, compared with about three per 100 diaphragm users, discontinued use because of vaginal discomfort such as soreness, itching, dryness, and stinging. In another study, involving 719 women in the U.S., only 12 (1.7%) discontinued use of the sponge because of itching, irritation, or rash, and only 14 (1.9%) discontinued use because of allergic-type reactions. Leaving the sponge in place for long periods can cause irritation, discharge, disagreeable odor, and possible infection. If vaginal burning or itching persists, you should consult your physician.

A consumer group has expressed concern that the contraceptive sponge was not adequately tested for possible cancer causing effects. Nonoxynol-9 has been used in vaginal spermicides by millions of women for over 20 years and has been declared safe by the FDA. However, 2,4 toluenediamine (2,4-TDA) can occur as a contaminant during the polymerization of polyurethane. Precautions have been taken by the manufacturer to prevent formation of this known carcinogen. Sensitive analyses have failed to detect any carcinogen in the sponge. If carcinogens were present, the amounts would be so small it would be extremely unlikely that cancer would occur as a complication.

If you notice a foul odor when the sponge is removed, do not be concerned unless the odor persists. It is not uncommon for material placed in the vagina to produce an odor when exposed to normal vaginal fluid and/or semen. If the odor persists, however, it may indicate an infection, and a physician should be consulted.

No toxic shock syndrome (TSS) was reported among several thousand users of the sponge in multicenter trials before marketing, but 13 cases of TSS in contraceptive sponge users were reported from 1983 through 1984, and additional cases have been reported since. A cause and effect relationship between sponge use and TSS has not been proven, however. In four of the cases, the women left the sponge in place more than 30 hours. The spermicidal ingredient in the sponge is believed to be hostile to the growth of *Staphylococcus aureus,* the organism thought to be responsible for causing TSS. If, however, you use the contraceptive sponge, you should report any two or more of the warning signs of TSS (such as sudden onset of high fever, vomiting, diarrhea, body rash similar to sunburn, muscle aches, dizziness, or low blood pressure) to your physician immediately. If you experience difficulty in removing the sponge or sponge fragments, you should consult a physician or call the toll free VLI Hotline at 800-223-2329, a service of VLI Corporation, manufacturers and distributors of the sponge. (Call 800-222-2329 in California.) The absolute risk of TSS in women who use the contraceptive sponge remains to be determined, but use of the sponge during the menstrual period or immediately after childbirth is not recommended.

ACCEPTANCE BY THE PUBLIC

The sponge has been well accepted by the public. Over 17 million contraceptive sponges were sold in the U.S. in less than one year. Eighty-six percent of women surveyed at the end of clinical trials said the Today® contraceptive sponge would be their contraceptive method of choice in the future. Although it appears somewhat inferior to diaphragm plus spermicide in contraceptive effectiveness, the following factors account for its popularity:

1. A greater degree of spontaneity than is possible with some other vaginal contraceptives or the condom. The contraceptive sponge may be inserted up to 24 hours in advance of intercourse. It provides continuous protection, regardless of frequency of intercourse, during the 24-hour period. Intercourse can take place immediately after insertion.
2. In contrast to foams, creams, jellies, and vaginal suppositories, the contraceptive sponge is not messy to use.
3. The contraceptive sponge may be purchased without a prescription and does not require fitting or insertion by a physician. It can be inserted quickly and easily by the user.
4. Neither partner can detect the presence of the sponge during use.
5. The sponge contains no hormones. The active ingredient, nonoxynol-9, has been in widespread use for over 20 years.
6. A woman can swim or bathe while wearing the contraceptive sponge.
7. Clinical trials indicate the contraceptive sponge may approach the effectiveness of the diaphragm plus spermicide when used properly.
8. Clinical trials have established the safety of the sponge when used as directed.

CONCLUSION

Vaginal barrier methods of contraception offer alternatives to other methods of contraception. They are neither the most nor least effective contraceptive method. They are of low risk potential relative to oral contraceptives and the IUD. Risk and benefit considerations, relative to other contraceptive methods, should guide you in selecting vaginal barrier methods.

5

Spermicidal Gels, Creams, and Aerosol Foams

INTRODUCTION

Spermicidal foams, creams, and gels represent an often overlooked, yet viable alternative method of contraception. Classified as barrier contraceptives, spermicides are used both alone and in combination with other methods of contraception. Spermicides differ from most other devices in their class (condoms, diaphragms, and cervical sponges and caps), because they provide both a physical and a chemical barrier against conception. Although oral contraceptives and the IUD have eclipsed spermicides in popularity, spermicides remain an important part of conception control and family planning.

HISTORY OF SPERMICIDAL DOSAGE FORMS

Spermicidal (sperm killing) agents are certainly not a new idea. Vaginal contraceptive preparations have been used for almost 4,000 years. As early as 1850 B.C. the Egyptians employed pessaries (vaginal tampons) made of crocodile or elephant dung, lactic and boric acid, various oils, honey, and natron (native sodium carbonate) as vaginal contraceptives.

At the turn of the 20th century, most vaginal spermicides in use were not very effective. Although many of these preparations were highly acidic, and did inhibit sperm, a strong dose often caused severe irritation to the woman. Homemade spermicidal preparations included vinegar and water mixtures, butter and margarine, and soaps and detergents. None of the home remedies possessed the combined safety and effectiveness of today's spermicidal agents.

In the 1920s, a significant advance in vaginal contraception occurred. The German pharmaceutical industry introduced an effervescent tablet that would foam after contacting vaginal moisture. However, a relatively effective spermicidal agent was not available until the introduction of phenylmercuric acetate (PMA) in 1937. The mercury-containing spermicides were later removed from the market due to potential adverse effects.

The 1950s marked the advent of surface-active agents (surfactants) for use in spermicides. For the first time, spermicidal products became an alternative method of birth control that offered both safety and effectiveness. Since the introduction of surfactants as spermicides, no significant advances in development of more effective spermicidal agents have taken place.

CHARACTERISTICS OF SPERMICIDES

Vaginal contraceptives are substances placed in the vagina prior to intercourse to prevent sperm from fertilizing the ovum. They prevent pregnancy by acting as a physical barrier keeping sperm from entering the cervical opening and/or by providing a direct spermicidal chemical action.

Spermicidal preparations now come in a variety of forms (see Table 12). To understand how they work, it is necessary to know the two basic components of spermicides, an inert base (inactive ingredient) and a spermicidal agent (active ingredient). The inert base comes in the following three forms: aerosol foams, creams or gels (jelly), and suppositories (vaginal).

THE DOSAGE FORM

Aerosol foams are the most popular form of vaginal spermicide. They are available either in pressurized cans with an applicator or in pre-loaded ready-to-use applicators for easier handling and application. Like creams, but unlike suppositories and gels, aerosol foams do not require a waiting period after vaginal insertion prior to intercourse.

Creams and gels are recommended for use only with a diaphragm. After the initial act of coitus, subsequent acts require another application of the spermicide, with the diaphragm left in place. Spermicidal creams and gels come with an applicator, which facilitates placement high into the vagina near the cervical opening.

Suppositories are not recommended for use alone as a contraceptive spermicide. The manufacturer of the first foaming suppository available in the U.S. was reprimanded by the FDA after making claims that the product was effective after vaginal insertion for up to *two* hours. Package claims now inform the user to insert another suppository if intercourse has not taken place within one hour. Encare Oval®, S'Positive®, Intercept®, and Semicid® are the suppository products available (see Tables 12 and 13). Both melt when exposed to body heat and moisture. Their effectiveness has not been well documented.

Drawbacks of vaginal contraceptive suppositories outweigh any possible advantages, such as being easier to carry and less messy. The user is required to wait at least 10 minutes, or longer, before intercourse to allow suppositories to foam. Suppositories require moisture to foam, thus their effectiveness is dependent upon the amount of vaginal moisture present. Finally, suppository dispersion is more dependent upon coital movement than other spermicidal dosage forms.

THE SPERMICIDAL AGENT

The active ingredient, or spermicidal agent, immobilizes sperm cells. Today's spermicidal ingredients are surface-active agents or surfactants. Surfactants immobilize sperm cells by rupturing or removing the outer membrane of the sperm cell, similar to the manner in which dishwashing liquid removes an oily film from a plate. Although containing surfactants, household and personal hygiene products are *definitely not* recommended for use as vaginal contraceptives. Presently there are two active spermicidal chemicals marketed in the U.S. that possess proven safety and contraceptive effectiveness, nonoxynol-9 (most commonly utilized) and octoxynol-9.

SAFETY OF SPERMICIDES

An attractive quality of spermicides is their relative safety. Anxiety over side effects from oral contraceptives and the IUD has caused some women to turn to vaginal spermicides for contraceptive protection.

TABLE 12
SPERMICIDAL PREPARATIONS AVAILABLE IN THE U.S.

Product	Manufacturer	Base	Active Ingredient		Comments
Because®	Schering	foam	Nonoxynol-9	8 %	
Conceptrol®	Ortho	gel	"	4 %	b
Conceptrol®	"	cream	"	5 %	b
Dalkon	Robins	foam	"	8 %	
Delfen®	Ortho	foam	"	12.5%	
Emko®	Schering	foam	"	8 %	a
Encare®	Thompson Medical	suppository	"	2.27%	
Gynol	Ortho	jelly	Octoxynol	1 %	b
Gynol II®	Ortho	jelly	Nonoxynol-9	2 %	b
Intercept®	Ortho	suppository	"	100 mg	
Koromex®	Holland-Rantos	cream	Octoxynol-9	3 %	b
Koromex®	" "	foam	Nonoxynol-9	12.5%	
Koromex®	" "	jelly	"	3 %	b
Koromex Crystal Clear Gel®	" "	gel	"	3 %	b
Koromex II®	" "	jelly	Octoxynol-9	1 %	b
Koromex II®	" "	cream	"	3 %	b
Koromex II-A®	" "	jelly	Nonoxynol-9	2 %	b
Ortho-Creme®	Ortho	cream	"	2 %	b

Ortho-Gynol®	"	jelly	Octoxynol-9	1 %	b
Ortho-Gynol II®	"	jelly	"	2 %	b
Ramses® 10 hour	Schmid	jelly	Nonoxynol-9	5 %	b
Ramses Extra®	Schmid	condom	"	5 %	c
Semicid®	Whitehall	suppository	"	100 mg	
S'Positive®	Jordan-Simmer	suppository	"	5.67%	
Today Sponge®	VLI Corp.	sponge	"	1 gram	d

a—Available in a box of 6 pre-loaded applicators
b—For use with a diaphragm
c—Latex condom that uses spermicide as lubricant
d—Vaginal sponge impregnated with nonoxynol-9

TABLE 13
SELECTED CHARACTERISTICS OF VAGINAL SPERMICIDES

Characteristic	Dosage Form			
	Aerosol Foams	Jellies	Creams	Vaginal Suppositories
Dispersion	Most rapid & thorough	Rapid and thorough when in contact with vaginal secretions	Poor, tend to remain where discharged	Poorest and slowest
Interval between application and intercourse	No waiting necessary	2–3 min. to liquefy	2–3 min. to liquefy	15 min. to dissolve and disperse
Physical Characteristics	Vanishing quality; not lubricating	Liquefy at body temperature; very water soluble	Firmer consistency than jellies; lubricating	Melt at body temperature
Administration Requirements	Insertion with applicator high into vagina	Insertion with applicator high into vagina	Requires careful placement with applicator high into vagina	Requires careful placement with fingers high into vagina
Shelf Life	Longest due to protection from environment	—	—	Requires protection from heat and humidity

104

Allergic reactions to spermicides are rare. Spermicides are not strongly acidic and, therefore, rarely cause irritation to the vagina or penis. Should irritation occur in either partner, use of the spermicide should be discontinued, and a physician should be consulted. Foaming suppositories generate heat when dissolving, which some couples find annoying.

Several years ago, it was suggested by some researchers that spermicides may be the cause of birth defects. Spermicides normally rupture the sperm cell. Some scientists believe that the outer membrane of some sperm cells may only be weakened and their genetic message (DNA) altered by chemical contraceptives. Should such a weakened sperm cell fertilize the ovum, it is theoretically possible that its altered genetic structure could cause a defective conception. There is also concern that if some of the spermicidal agent was absorbed into the bloodstream, it could reach the ovum or developing embryo and damage it.

After reviewing available data, the National Institutes of Health (NIH) and the National Institute of Child Health and Human Development (NICHD) concluded there was no significant difference in birth defect rates between infants whose mothers used spermicides and infants whose mothers used some other form of contraception. Based on the same data, the FDA denied a request to require a printed warning on spermicidal products warning about possible birth defects from spermicide use. At present there is no proof that spermicides cause birth defects.

EFFECTIVENESS OF SPERMICIDES

Effectiveness is often the greatest single consideration for choosing a method of contraception. However, if you are worried about the possible side effects that may occur from more popular methods, such as oral contraceptives, spermicides offer a viable alternative relative to safety. As with most other methods of contraception, the incidence of pregnancy is based on product, user, and provider failure.

The pregnancy rate reported for spermicides has been as low as 0.3 and as high as 40 per 100 woman-years. More realistically, when spermicidal foams are consistently used correctly, the incidence of pregnancy ranges from 4.2 to 4.8 per 100 woman-years (see Table 14). Pregnancy rates with other spermicides used alone, and in combination with other contraceptives, are also included in Table 14.

Effectiveness of any spermicidal product is dependent upon how well it disperses in the vagina and over the cervical opening. The inert base (cream, gel, or aerosol foam) is designed to hold the active ingredient in the vagina next to the cervix. Additionally, it forms a physical barrier over the cervix which functions to prevent sperm from entering the cervical opening. Of all the various spermicidal products available, aerosol foams and creams disperse best.

Vaginal suppositories dissolve unpredictably, probably because they require moisture to foam or body heat to melt. Successful distribution also depends on coital movements. One study revealed little or no foam generated by the Encare Oval® contraceptive suppository in 9 out of 20 women 15 minutes after vaginal insertion, and the suppository was removed almost fully intact.

Vaginal fluids are normally acidic and may themselves inhibit sperm. During sexual arousal, increased cervical and vaginal secretions create a less acidic, almost neutral environment in the vagina which promotes sperm motility and viability. Suppositories dissolve better under acidic conditions. The less acidic environment of the vagina that occurs during sexual arousal may not allow for maximum contraceptive protection from vaginal contraceptive suppositories.

The amount of spermicide required to stop sperm in 20 seconds is more than what several of the products that have been tested contained in a single dose. The product showing the lowest relative potency, indicating that it was *not* superior to other products tested, was a suppository containing only 2.27 percent nonoxynol-9. The product with the highest relative potency was Delfen Contraceptive®, an aerosol foam containing 12.5 percent nonoxynol-9. If a vaginal spermicide is to be used alone as a contraceptive, you should consider products that contain at least 8 percent of an active spermicide (nonoxynol-9 or octoxynol-9).

Since dispersion of the base and the amount of spermicide contained in the product are so essential for successful contraception, aerosol foams are considered the more effective dosage form. It is for these reasons that instructions for use in this chapter (see Table 15) outline only how to use aerosol foams when spermicides are the sole contraceptive method employed.

Although no method of contraception can guarantee 100 percent protection, to gain maximum effectiveness it is essential that spermicidal foams be used strictly according to directions (see Table 15). Several human factors can affect how well directions are followed and, thus, the level of contraceptive protection that can be expected. These factors include:

1. Motivation of the user
2. User's social and educational background

TABLE 14
USUAL CONTRACEPTIVE EFFECTIVENESS OF SPERMICIDES WHEN USED ALONE AND WHEN USED WITH OTHER CONTRACEPTIVE METHODS

Method Used	Pregnancies per 100 Woman-Years*
**Spermicidal Foams (alone)	4.2– 4.8
***Spermicidal Creams & Gels (alone)	4 –40
Condom with Foams, Creams, and Gels	1 – 4
Diaphragm with Creams and Gels	2 – 8

*1,200 menstrual cycles

**containing 8 percent or more of spermicidal chemical

***use of spermicidal creams and gels as a sole means of contraception is not recommended due to chemical nature of the inert base and relatively low concentration of spermicidal chemical.

NOTE: Rates of pregnancy were derived from separate studies conducted by different investigators in several groups. Comparisons cannot be made with absolute precision.

3. Willingness of sexual partners to share contraceptive responsibility
4. Experience in using the contraceptive method

The theoretical effectiveness rates of spermicidal foams vary from the actual effectiveness rate for several reasons. Some of the mistakes made when using aerosol foams include:

1. Not using the foam before every act of sexual intercourse (even during supposedly infertile days of the month)
2. Not interrupting lovemaking to use the foam
3. Not reapplying the foam for subsequent acts of coitus, or not reapplying the spermicide during prolonged sessions of intercourse (more than one hour)
4. Not inserting the spermicide far enough into the vagina
5. Using too little foam
6. Not shaking the can enough to disperse the spermicidal agent evenly
7. Failing to notice that the container is empty
8. Failing to have the spermicide on hand when needed

9. Allowing coitus to take place in a position which allows the spermicide to drain out from the vagina
10. Douching too soon after intercourse (wait at least 8 hours)
11. Inserting the spermicide into the rectum instead of the vagina

When used correctly, vaginal spermicides have a high rate of effectiveness. If appropriate instructions for use are provided by a health professional (the most logical choice being a pharmacist), contraceptive effectiveness can be as high as 95 percent. With the introduction of oral contraceptives and the IUD, health care providers deemphasized spermicides as a contraceptive alternative. Since spermicides do not require a prescription or medical supervision, they are often overlooked by family planning personnel. Some physicians assume that when you request a form of contraception,

---

TABLE 15
DIRECTIONS FOR USING AEROSOL FOAM SPERMICIDES

1. Shake the can 20 times before using to ensure that bubbles form and the spermicidal chemical is mixed well with the foam. Several brands of aerosol foam come in pre-loaded applicators which are ready to use (see Table 12).
2. If the foam comes in a separate container, the applicator is filled to a designated mark by applying pressure directly onto the top of the container or by tilting the applicator.
3. It is essential that spermicides be inserted *before* coitus. Spread the labia apart. Insert the applicator into the vagina about 3 or 4 inches (about 2/3 the length of the applicator), or until it will not go any further. Withdraw the applicator about half an inch, press the plunger, and deposit the foam completely. (See Figure 20.) Then withdraw the applicator from the vagina completely, without pulling out the plunger so as not to suck foam back into the applicator.
4. Regardless of the time of the month, spermicides should be used each and every time intercourse takes place. *Each application* of aerosol foam provides enough *protection for only one act of intercourse.* Another applicatorful must be reinserted high into the vagina for subsequent or prolonged (more than one hour) acts of intercourse.
5. Clean the applicator with soap and warm (not boiling) water. Shake applicator to remove excess water.
6. Keep a spare container on hand. With some brands it is difficult to tell if the container is empty or about to run out.
7. Insert a tampon to keep the foam from dripping out should intercourse

occur immediately prior to going to work, shopping, walking, or exercising.

8. Do not douche* for at least eight hours after the last act of intercourse so as not to remove the spermicide and allow viable sperm cells that may be located in the vaginal canal to enter the cervix.

9. Keep this and all medications out of the reach of children.

---

*NOTE: Douching is not recommended as a means of contraception. It is possible for sperm to reach the cervix within 90 seconds after ejaculation. Therefore, it is unlikely that a douche can be performed in time to remove all sperm from the vagina. The possibility exists that douching can push sperm *into* the cervix. Douche liquid will also *dilute* the concentration of spermicide.

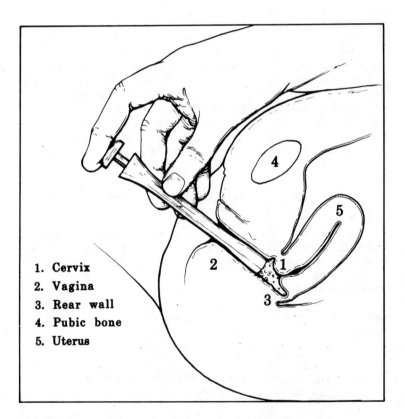

1. Cervix
2. Vagina
3. Rear wall
4. Pubic bone
5. Uterus

FIGURE 20

Anatomical presentation of spermicidal aerosol foam application

you have already considered nonprescription alternatives. Many physicians find it easier, and no doubt faster, to prescribe an oral contraceptive. You should encourage discussion with your physician and not simply accept a quick prescription for an oral contraceptive until all available contraceptive methods have been reviewed.

The pharmacist is an often overlooked source of family planning information. Pharmacists receive more formal education about prescription and nonprescription drugs and health care devices than any other health professional. If you wish to use a nonprescription contraceptive method, but are undecided about which method to use, or if you are confused about the proper use of a chosen method, a pharmacist may be of assistance.

Instructions for spermicide use vary slightly from product to product. You should read package instructions carefully before use. If instructions for use are not clear, consult a pharmacist or physician.

With some spermicidal products it is unclear if the manufacturer is recommending the product for use with a diaphragm or alone. Recommendations for use without a diaphragm are usually printed plainly on the package label. Advocating use of creams, gels, and vaginal suppositories with low concentrations of spermicidal chemicals as sole contraceptive agents is somewhat similar to recommending a condom with only one tiny hole in it. To the credit of most manufacturers, the package inserts for their creams and gels clearly state they should only be used with a diaphragm (see Table 12).

EFFECTIVENESS OF SPERMICIDES IN COMBINATION WITH CONDOMS

If both methods are used correctly, simultaneous use of condoms and spermicides can yield a pregnancy rate as low as 1 per 100 woman-years. However, in actual use the enhanced contraceptive protection can be negated if the additional expense of using two methods becomes a burden causing inconsistent use of the more effective condom, or if using both methods becomes so complicated and troublesome that the more effective condom is not used correctly.

EFFECTIVENESS OF SPERMICIDES WHEN USED WITH DIAPHRAGMS OR CERVICAL CAPS

Spermicides are used to aid insertion and proper placement of the diaphragm. Table 16 outlines the steps for proper use of spermicides with a diaphragm. As with condoms, simultaneous use of the diaphragm with a spermicidal cream or gel should increase the degree

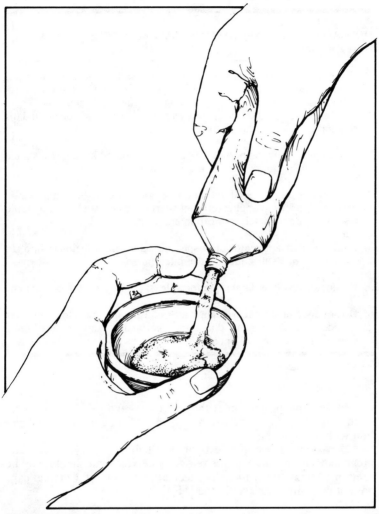

FIGURE 21
Placement of spermicidal cream in diaphragm

TABLE 16
HOW TO USE SPERMICIDAL CREAMS AND GELS WITH A DIAPHRAGM

---

1. Place at least one teaspoonful or tablespoonful (the amount varies from product to product—READ DIRECTIONS CAREFULLY) of spermicidal cream or gel into the dome of the diaphragm (see Figure 21) that will cover the cervix, and spread a little spermicide around the rim and the outer surface of the diaphragm.

2. The diaphragm with spermicide placed as outlined in step one should be inserted six hours or more prior to intercourse.

3. If intercourse is planned within 6 to 8 hours, leave the diaphragm in place and insert an applicatorful of spermicidal cream or gel high into the vagina immediately prior to intercourse.

4. Insert another applicatorful of spermicidal cream or gel high into the vagina for *each* subsequent act of intercourse.

5. Do not remove the diaphragm for at least six hours after intercourse.

6. Do not douche for at least eight hours after intercourse. Douching may dislodge the diaphragm, dilute the spermicide, and possibly force sperm into the cervical opening.

---

of contraceptive protection. Although creams and gels are used most often with diaphragms, aerosol foams may also be used in combination with a diaphragm.

Occasionally sperm find their way behind a cervical cap and pregnancy can occur. For this reason, a cervical cap should only be used in combination with a spermicidal cream or gel. Cervical caps are not presently available in the U.S.

SOME OF THE NONCONTRACEPTIVE BENEFITS OF SPERMICIDES

Growing concern over increased risks associated with the more effective methods of contraception, such as oral contraceptives and the IUD, has caused an increase in sales of vaginal spermicides. Spermicides are preferred by many users because they do not reduce coital sensation as condoms may. Spermicides are easy to use, easy to understand, widely available, and do not require a prescription, medical examination, supervision, or medical follow-up. Most vaginal spermicides are purchased in pharmacies, with about 20 percent being bought in nonpharmacy outlets. Spermicides cost about 30 to 60 cents per dose.

Vaginal spermicides apparently offer some measure of protection against gonorrhea, genital herpes, and possibly other sexually transmitted diseases. One study suggests that women using spermicides consistently are 75 percent less likely to develop gonorrhea. Recent reports have suggested that spermicides may prevent common vaginal infections, such as trichomoniasis.

The combined use of spermicides and condoms could provide a greater degree of protection against sexually transmitted disease (STD) than either method used alone. If you must choose between the two methods, the condom is the more effective method in preventing the spread of STD.

Situations in which vaginal spermicides may prove useful include:

1. Use as a contraceptive prior to and during the first month of oral contraceptive therapy.
2. Use as a vaginal lubricant by couples who may require additional lubrication.
3. Use as a convenience by women who have intercourse infrequently.
4. Use by a diaphragm user who has intercourse a second time before the diaphragm is removed.
5. Use as a backup method to have at home if you stop or run out of oral contraceptives, or should your IUD be spontaneously expelled.
6. Use for the first several months after IUD insertion, when expulsion of the IUD is most likely to occur.
7. Use as a supplemental contraceptive during the period of the month ovulation is most likely to occur. For example, a condom and spermicide may be used simultaneously during the most fertile days.
8. Use immediately, should a condom tear, leak, or slip off during intercourse.
9. Use for protection against certain sexually transmitted diseases. Combined use with a condom is recommended for maximum protection.
10. Use as a contraceptive when the condom is not desired by the male and/or the female.
11. Not having to fit anything before or remove anything after intercourse when using spermicides is an attractive feature to some couples.

LIMITATIONS TO USING SPERMICIDES

Drawbacks reported with spermicide use include:

1. Spermicides are a nuisance for women and men who do not want to interrupt lovemaking or apply the spermicide prior to coitus.
2. Spermicides are not appealing to women who do not like sex or have an aversion to touching their genitals.
3. The waiting period required for suppositories to dissolve is not liked by some couples.
4. The heat generated by suppositories is not liked by some men and women.
5. Couples who engage in oral sex may find the taste of spermicides unpleasant.

CONCLUSION

Vaginal spermicides represent one of the safest methods of conception control. Growing concern over the potential adverse effects from other contraceptive methods has generated renewed interest in spermicides. Additionally, when used alone or in combination with other barrier contraceptives, vaginal spermicides can be highly effective if used properly and consistently. They continue to offer a useful method of birth control for a variety of life-styles when used alone or in combination with other barrier methods (such as the condom and diaphragm).

6

Other Contraceptive Methods

INTRODUCTION

Numerous contraceptive methods, other than those previously presented, may be employed. These include rhythm (periodic abstinence), withdrawal, douching, and postcoital contraception (utilizing diethylstilbestrol or an IUD). Rhythm, withdrawal, and douching are considered "high-risk" methods of contraception. Postcoital contraception is employed under special circumstances, rather than routinely. Each of these approaches to contraception is presented in this chapter.

RHYTHM (PERIODIC ABSTINENCE)

The rhythm or periodic abstinence method of birth control involves abstinence from sexual relations during the fertile period of the female menstrual cycle. The effectiveness of this method of birth control depends largely upon a couple's motivation to avoid pregnancy and on the woman's ability to recognize and interpret signs and symptoms of the fertile period. Once the fertile period is identified, women may either abstain from intercourse during this time, or the male or female may employ another method of contraception.

Other names for the rhythm or periodic abstinence method of birth control include natural family planning and organic, cooperative, calendar, temperature, and cervical mucus birth control.

Abstinence during the fertile period is the only method of family planning approved by the Roman Catholic Church. The papal encyclical *Casti Connubii* (1930) and particularly the encyclical *Humanae Vitae* (1968) have promoted periodic abstinence by Catholic couples while condemning "artificial means" of birth control.

THE BIOLOGICAL BASIS FOR THE RHYTHM METHOD OF CONTRACEPTION

The rhythm method is based on certain biological facts. Awareness of these facts is essential to properly understanding and acceptably utilizing periodic abstinence (rhythm) as a birth control method. Among these facts are the following:

1. A woman normally produces one fertilizable egg during each menstrual cycle.
2. Ovulation typically occurs about 14 days before the next menstrual period begins, regardless of the length of the cycle. A two day variance either way may occur, so one may conclude with some degree of assurance, but not with certainty, that ovulation occurs 12 to 16 days before the onset of the menstrual period (blood flow).
3. The egg has an active life of six to 24 hours. Some experts believe the egg may remain viable for up to 36 hours. It is during this period of time that an egg may be fertilized by sperm.
4. Sperm are capable of surviving in the female reproductive tract for at least 48 to 72 hours. Some experts believe deposited sperm may survive for up to five days. During this period sperm may fertilize the egg.
5. The time of ovulation may be predicted with some degree of accuracy because once ovulation occurs, the hormone progesterone is produced in increasing amounts and causes a slight rise in body temperature. This temperature elevation is not immediately useful, but if menstrual cycles are regular and of fairly constant length, several months of carefully recording body temperature cycles may assist in pinpointing and predicting the time of ovulation in subsequent cycles.
6. The character of cervical mucus undergoes changes throughout the menstrual cycle. By being aware of changes that occur at or near the time of ovulation, a

woman may avoid intercourse or unprotected intercourse during this fertile time.

7. Levels of luteinizing hormone (LH) surge just prior to ovulation. This surge is detectable in the urine using monoclonal antibody testing.

The conclusion which may be drawn from these facts is that there is only a period of about six days each month when intercourse may lead to pregnancy. This includes the five days when sperm may be present in the female reproductive tract, and the 24 to 36 hours after ovulation when the egg is fertilizable.

Predicting when ovulation will occur will allow you to avoid intercourse or use alternate contraceptive methods during the "unsafe period." Recognizing when ovulation has occurred will serve as a guide in determining when unprotected intercourse may be resumed.

TECHNIQUES INVOLVED IN UTILIZING THE RHYTHM METHOD EFFECTIVELY

There are five basic techniques for predicting when ovulation will occur or when ovulation has occurred. These techniques include the calendar method, the temperature or thermal method, the cervical mucus method, the sympto-thermal method, and the in-home ovulation test. All of these techniques assist in identifying the fertile period, but none are absolutely precise. Furthermore, it may be necessary for some couples to abstain or use alternate contraception for one-fourth to one-half of a menstrual cycle and sometimes longer, depending on the rhythm technique employed.

CALENDAR METHOD

The calendar method is the oldest rhythm technique, and involves attempts to calculate safe days and fertile days based on the length of previous menstrual cycles. If women had regular menstrual cycles, the calendar method would be somewhat more reliable. Women could then readily predict the safe days well before ovulation, the fertile days surrounding ovulation, and the safe days after ovulation and could restrict intercourse accordingly. This could be done because we know that ovulation generally (not absolutely) occurs 12 to 16 days before the onset of the next menstrual period, the period of viability of released sperm is from 48 hours to five days, and a released egg is fertilizable (viable) for 24 to 36 hours.

The value of the calendar method is questionable in reality, however, because few women have menstrual cycles of consistent length. In a study of an average of 13 cycles in 30,000 women, it was found that approximately two-thirds (20,000) of these women had irregular menstrual cycles, varying in length from 23 to 31 days. Other studies indicate that cycles vary by an average of seven to 13 days for the peak reproductive years. Even greater variations occur in teenagers and women approaching menopause. The wider the variation in length of menstrual cycle, the more prolonged the period of abstinence must be.

CALCULATING SAFE DAYS USING THE CALENDAR METHOD

The calendar method is not a dependable method of birth control unless the length of menstrual cycles have been recorded for the previous nine to 12 months and unless the strictest methods for calculating safe days are employed. The calendar method involves calculating the earliest safe days of the menstrual cycle and the latest safe days of the menstrual cycle.

To calculate the early safe days one should subtract 14 from the length of the shortest menstrual cycle noted over the past nine to 12 months since ovulation usually occurs approximately 14 days prior to the first day of the menstrual period (blood flow). Now subtract at least three more days to allow for the period of viability of sperm. One may wish to subtract five days instead of three as an added precaution since there is some documentation that deposited sperm have remained active for up to five days in the female reproductive tract.

If, for example, the shortest menstrual cycle over the past nine to 12 months was 26 days, the most conservative calculation to determine the early safe days would involve subtracting 16 and five from the length of the cycle (26 days). This allows for ovulation 16 days prior to the onset of the period and a five day life span for sperm. Such a woman could, with a significant degree of contraceptive assurance, engage in unprotected intercourse from day one (the first day of her menstrual flow) to day five of the cycle. This could involve engaging in intercourse during menstrual flow, but such a practice is objectionable to many men and women.

To calculate the late safe days of the cycle, one should subtract 14 days from the length of the longest menstrual cycle noted over the past nine to 12 months. Two days should then be added to the number obtained in the event that ovulation occurred 12 (rather than 14) days prior to the first day of the following cycle. Then add one day to allow for a 24-hour period of viability of the egg (add two days to cover a 36-hour period of viability).

If the longest menstrual cycle over the past 9 to 12 months was 32 days, the most conservative calculation to arrive at the late safe days would involve subtracting 14 from the length of the longest cycle (32 days). The number derived is 18. To this number we should add four days (two days to compensate for a "late" ovulation, and two days to allow for a 36-hour life span for the released egg). The final number is then 22, which represents the last probable day of fertility. Unprotected intercourse could be resumed, in this case, on day 23 of the menstrual cycle.

Using this method for a hypothetical woman whose shortest menstrual cycle over the past nine to 12 months was 26 days and whose longest cycle was 32 days, the conservatively calculated unsafe or fertile period would be from day 6 through day 22 of subsequent menstrual cycles. This prolonged period (17 days—about three times the length of the actual fertile period), which requires either abstinence or alternate methods of contraception, is considered undesirable by most individuals.

TEMPERATURE (THERMAL) METHOD

Unlike the calendar method, which depends primarily on the regularity of the menstrual cycle, the temperature or thermal method depends upon identifying a single event—the rise in basal body temperature (BBT) that signals that ovulation has occurred.

When ovulation occurs, a woman's basal body temperature may drop slightly. This is followed by a rise in body temperature of 0.5 to 1.0 degree Fahrenheit over the next two to three days (see Figure 22). The rise in temperature, which begins one to two days after ovulation, is in response to rising levels of the hormone progesterone. Unprotected intercourse should not take place at any time between the onset of the menstrual period and ovulation, as the temperature method does not predict when ovulation will occur; it only indicates that ovulation has occurred. This method cannot assist in determining early safe days, but it is helpful in predicting late safe days. A three day wait after the temperature begins to rise is intended to assure that the egg is no longer fertilizable. For the highest degree of contraceptive effectiveness, unprotected intercourse should not occur from the onset of the menstrual period until three days after temperature elevations have been recorded. The safe days are considered the post-ovulatory phase, usually 10 to 12 days before onset of the next period. Thus, the temperature method requires abstinence, or alternative contraception, for more than half of the menstrual cycle.

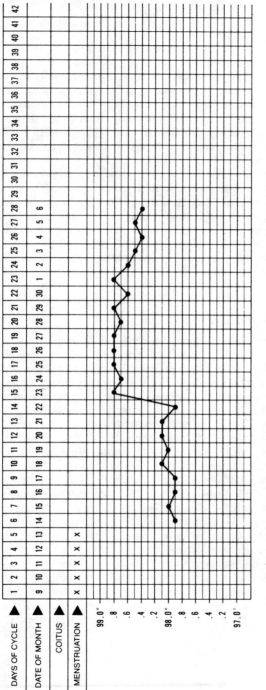

- A persistent temperature rise for three days is considered to be adequate evidence that ovulation has occurred if other temperature elevating factors are absent.

- Safe days of the above cycle would be days 17 - 28.

FIGURE 22

Basal body temperature record

RECORDING OF TEMPERATURE

The effectiveness of the temperature method depends on how carefully daily temperatures are taken and recorded, how well one recognizes temperature increases, and how well the temperature rise correlates with ovulation.

Great care is required in obtaining basal body temperature. Although a fever thermometer may be used to acquire body temperatures, a basal thermometer is easier to read than a fever thermometer. A fever thermometer has a temperature scale from 94 to 106 degrees Fahrenheit, and is graduated in two-tenths degree increments. The scale on a basal thermometer is 96 to 100 degrees Fahrenheit, and graduations are in one-tenth degree increments. Basal thermometers, also known as rhythm, sex, and pregnancy thermometers, are available in most pharmacies without a prescription.

A woman must be extremely meticulous and consistent in acquiring basal temperature readings. The following steps are recommended:

1. Shake the thermometer down the night before or immediately after use.
2. Record temperature the first thing upon awakening in the morning after at least five hours of uninterrupted sleep and before getting out of bed. Basal body temperature is the body temperature at complete rest. Slight activity may cause a rise in body temperature. Do not eat or drink anything before taking the basal body temperature.
3. Acquire the temperature daily and at the same time each day. It is not necessary to obtain temperatures during the menstrual period. Begin recording when menstrual flow stops.
4. Temperature readings may be taken orally or rectally, but the same method must always be used. Rectal readings are usually more reliable.
5. Leave the thermometer in place for five minutes.
6. Record the temperature on the temperature chart immediately by placing a dot where the horizontal date column joins the vertical temperature column (see Figure 22). Connect dots with a straight line.
7. If you miss a day, or have to arise from bed before the temperature is acquired, make a note on the temperature chart.

Numerous factors other than ovulation may alter body temperature. Illness may confuse temperature readings substantially. Bacterial infections (such as a respiratory infection, urinary tract infection, or sore throat) and viral infections (such as colds or influenza) may produce low to moderate increases in body temperature. Emotional tension and lack of sleep may also lead to slight elevations. It is wise to avoid unprotected intercourse for at least three days after you are sure an illness has passed, and basal temperatures are again reflective of hormonal changes and ovulation. If the illness was severe, ovulation may be early or late in the subsequent cycle, and appropriate precautions should be observed.

CIRCUMSTANCES UNDER WHICH THE TEMPERATURE METHOD IS UNRELIABLE

Irregular menstrual patterns and situations where ovulation is delayed or erratic render the temperature method unreliable and/or ineffective. Such situations commonly exist in adolescent women, women approaching menopause, immediately after giving birth, immediately after abortion, during lactation, after prolonged periods of using oral contraceptives, and in women experiencing anorexia nervosa. Furthermore, the temperature method will not prove reliable unless you are highly motivated to acquire basal temperatures in a proper and consistent fashion, accurately record the temperatures, and interpret the data accurately. Unprotected intercourse during the pre-ovulatory period is unwise if the temperature method is used because this method does not assist in predicting when ovulation may occur; its value is in indicating when ovulation has occurred.

CERVICAL MUCUS METHOD

Advocates of this technique claim convenience and simplicity as its advantages. This technique involves recognizing and correctly interpreting the significance of changes in the nature and quantity of cervical mucus during various phases of the menstrual cycle. This method can be used to predict when ovulation most probably occurs or will occur. To practice this method, women must learn to differentiate between sensations of "dryness," "moistness," and "wetness" during the phases of the menstrual cycle.

STAGES OF THE MUCUS CYCLE THROUGHOUT THE MENSTRUAL CYCLE

In the early days of the cycle, when estrogen levels are low (the five or six days after menstrual flow), mucus secretions are scant, and the vagina is relatively dry. As ovulation approaches and estrogen levels increase, the volume of cervical secretions increase, and the vagina feels moist. The character of cervical secretions also change from a thick, pasty, sticky fluid to a slippery, clear, thin, stretchy type of mucus near the time of ovulation. The early secretions that are creamy, thick, and pasty are somewhat acid and of a molecular structure that may retard sperm passage into the uterus. The more abundant, clear, thin, stretchy secretions that exist immediately prior to ovulation are alkaline, and represent a more favorable environment

TABLE 17
CHARACTER OF CERVICAL MUCUS DURING VARIOUS PHASES OF A TYPICAL 30-DAY MENSTRUAL CYCLE

Phase	Approximate Days of Cycle	Character of Mucus
Menstrual	1–5	Mucus may or may not be present, but presence is obscured by menstrual flow.
Postmenstrual	6–10	Little if any mucus present. These days are often called "dry days." If present in small amounts, it is quite sticky and thick. Women may report sensation of vaginal moistness, but not wetness.
Early pre-ovulatory days	11–13	Volume of mucus present is greater. Mucus is cloudy, yellowish or white, thick, and very sticky. Women may report vaginal moistness, but not wetness.
Immediately before, during, and immediately after ovulation	14–17	Volume of mucus is high. Mucus appears clear. It is slippery, wet, elastic, and stretchy with the consistency of raw egg white. This mucus is very lubricative, alkaline, and a favorable environment for sperm. Women may report a sensation of vaginal wetness.
Post-ovulatory days	18–30	Volume of cloudy, sticky mucus is small. Toward the end of this phase women may report little or no vaginal moistness. Days 21 to 30 are often classified as "dry days."

for sperm. This type of mucus is very characteristic. It is akin to raw egg white in consistency, and can be stretched between the thumb and forefinger into a clear, shiny strand before breaking. No other mucus produced during the cycle has this stretchy character. After ovulation, mucus again becomes cloudy, thick, sticky, and creamy. The volume of cervical mucus secretion tends to diminish after ovulation. Table 17 characterizes cervical mucus during various phases of the menstrual cycle.

DETERMINATION OF THE FERTILE OR UNSAFE PERIOD USING THE CERVICAL MUCUS METHOD

Figure 23 provides a rough indication of the fertile and infertile periods of a menstrual cycle as determined by the cervical mucus method. Note that specific days are not assigned to the various segments of the graph in Figure 23 because lengths of menstrual cycles are so variable.

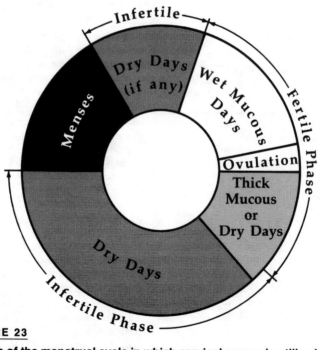

FIGURE 23

Phases of the menstrual cycle in which cervical mucus is utilized to predict fertile and infertile periods

"Dry days" may immediately follow menstruation, usually last for four to five days, and are considered infertile days. Unprotected intercourse may occur on these days, but intercourse on consecutive days is not advised as expelled semen may interfere with the character of mucus for up to one day. When the mucus is present in detectable amounts and is sticky, cloudy, thick, and yellowish to white in coloration, you should abstain from unprotected intercourse. This type of mucus indicates that ovulation is imminent. Avoidance of unprotected intercourse is vitally necessary when the cervical mucus becomes clear, slippery, wet, stretchy, of raw egg white consistency, and the woman experiences the highest degree of vaginal moistness or wetness. These symptoms are associated with the immediate pre- and post-ovulatory days and the day of ovulation. The several days following ovulation may be associated with mucus that is cloudy, thick, and sticky. These days should be considered to be in the fertile phase, but as these secretions diminish and the woman notes less vaginal moistness and a return of "dry days," a couple may resume unprotected intercourse.

PRECAUTIONS TO OBSERVE WHEN USING THE CERVICAL MUCUS METHOD

There are numerous precautions which should be observed if the cervical mucus method is to be optimally effective:

1. Even though "dry days" are discussed within the context of the cervical mucus method of contraception, the vagina is never entirely dry. Dryness, moistness, and wetness are relative terms. You will have to learn the relative character of your cervical mucus during the menstrual cycle to determine the difference between "fertile mucus" and "infertile mucus."
2. Before relying on the cervical mucus method, you should learn your pattern of mucus secretion over a period of at least six months.
3. It is highly advisable to keep a daily written record of the character of cervical mucus utilizing a chart similar to that used to record basal body temperatures (see Figure 22). Use of terms such as dry, wet, cloudy-sticky, wet-clear, wet-white, milky, profuse, scant, slippery, watery, or stretchy are most useful in describing the mucus and predicting events occurring in the reproductive system.
4. Coordinating the character of cervical mucus with basal

body temperature charts can increase the probability of predicting times of fertility and infertility during a cycle.

5. If you have short menstrual cycles, you may not experience any "dry days" after menstrual flow ceases. If mucus is present immediately upon cessation of the menstrual period, the entire period from the start of menstruation through the several moist days after ovulation should be considered fertile days.

6. Self-examination requires touching cervical mucus. Merely noting a feeling of vaginal wetness, or observing discharge on underclothing, is not enough. You should wipe the vulva with a tissue before urinating, remove mucus from the vulva with a finger, or insert a finger into the vagina to obtain a sample of mucus from the cervix. Cervical mucus should be placed between the thumb and forefinger and evaluated for color, thickness, stickiness, and stretchiness.

7. Cervical mucus should not be checked when one is sexually aroused because thin vaginal lubrication could be mistaken for "fertile mucus."

8. Sperm and seminal fluid will obscure the true character of cervical mucus; it may be necessary to wait up to 24 hours after intercourse to determine the true nature of the mucus.

9. Do not engage in unprotected intercourse during the pre-ovulatory period unless mucus is absent. If mucus is present immediately after menstruation, it may indicate an early ovulation.

10. After ovulation, the mucus should return to the dry or sticky type. Four days after wet, stretchy cervical mucus dries up is generally considered the beginning of the infertile phase of the cycle. This should correspond to the third day of elevation of basal body temperature. If a woman uses both methods, and one method suggests safety while the other suggests fertility, consider the day an unsafe one.

11. Women with active vaginal infections, one or more sexually transmitted diseases, or cervical erosion may have abnormal vaginal discharge and cervical mucus patterns. The cervical mucus method of contraception will prove unreliable and should not be utilized until the pathology is effectively diagnosed and treated.

SYMPTO-THERMAL METHOD (STM)

The sympto-thermal method (STM) of contraception combines various techniques for identifying the fertile period, especially cervical mucus or calendar methods to predict the beginning of the fertile period, and cervical mucus or basal body temperature methods to predict the end of the fertile period. If the sign or signs of one method are difficult to interpret, they may be checked against another method. The use of reliable multiple indices of symptoms and basal body temperature can improve the reliability of the rhythm approach to contraception while minimizing the impact of variables which could destroy the validity of a single method. Any combination of cervical mucus, calendar, and basal body temperature methods should prove more effective than any single rhythm method.

Symptoms other than cervical mucus and basal body temperature may be helpful, but they are not consistent. These include abdominal pain (associated with ovulation); intermenstrual bleeding; self-observed changes in the position, texture, moistness, and dilation of the cervix; breast tenderness; edema; mood changes; and several other symptoms. These symptoms are not precise predictors of ovulation and should not be relied upon.

IN-HOME OVULATION TEST

The in-home ovulation test has joined the growing list of self-diagnostic devices sold over-the-counter in pharmacies to predict time of ovulation. Such tests are highly accurate, sensitive, fast, convenient, and relatively economical. In-home ovulation testing may replace the more traditional approaches to pinpointing ovulation (such as calendar method, thermal method, cervical mucus method, and sympto-thermal method).

Three home ovulation tests are the Ovu Stick®, Ovutime®, and First Response®. The tests use monoclonal antibodies which detect the increase in levels of luteinizing hormone (LH) just prior to ovulation. It is this rise in levels of LH that causes ovulation, which usually occurs 24 to 36 hours following the initial increase in LH.

The tests use special test sticks which measure levels of LH in the urine. Urine collection cups are included in the kit. The urine is checked daily for several days within each cycle. The color change on the test stick indicates the level of LH present in the urine. The first significant change in color indicates the LH surge, which is predictive of ovulation within 24 to 36 hours. Color charts are included in the kit.

Excellent instructions for proper use are contained in the package. If, however, assistance in interpreting instructions is needed, you are encouraged to seek the advice and counsel of your pharmacist or physician.

EFFECTIVENESS OF THE RHYTHM (PERIODIC ABSTINENCE) METHOD OF CONTRACEPTION

Pregnancy rates are high when the rhythm (periodic abstinence) method is utilized as the sole method of preventing pregnancy. This method is considered "high risk." Pregnancy rates generally range from 5 to 40 per 100 woman-years. Whether the high pregnancy rate is due primarily to method failure or user failure has not been determined, although failure to utilize the various techniques properly is the most probable cause of failure.

ADVANTAGES OF THE RHYTHM (PERIODIC ABSTINENCE) METHOD

There are advantages to the rhythm (periodic abstinence) approach to contraception, but they tend to be overshadowed by disadvantages. Advantages include:

1. No physical side effects are associated with this approach to contraception.
2. It is relatively inexpensive.
3. It has no adverse effect on long-term fertility.
4. It is acceptable to the Roman Catholic Church and, therefore, morally acceptable to couples who wish to adhere to the teachings of the Catholic Church.
5. It may be a more esthetically acceptable approach to contraception than intercourse-related methods such as condoms, diaphragms, spermicidal chemicals, and the vaginal contraceptive sponge.
6. Users may be trained in proper use by qualified health care workers who are nonphysicians. No prescription is required.
7. Training in the rhythm methods increases awareness and knowledge of reproductive processes and can assist couples in achieving pregnancy and spacing births as well as preventing pregnancy.
8. Responsibility for effective use of rhythm methods may be shared by both sexual partners, thus fostering cooperation and communication.

DISADVANTAGES OF THE RHYTHM (PERIODIC ABSTINENCE) METHOD

Each technique involved in the rhythm methods of contraception has distinct disadvantages. Among these are the following:

1. All rhythm techniques are considered "high risk" and are associated with high pregnancy rates.
2. Certain methods require daily monitoring of bodily functions and charting of symptoms. This meticulous daily attention to monitoring body function and predicting fertile (unsafe) and safe times may prove too bothersome and disruptive of a life-style.
3. Many months of records and charts must be kept before using some rhythm methods of birth control.
4. Women with irregular menstrual cycles have difficulty using some rhythm methods.
5. Rhythm methods will not be successful unless both sexual partners cooperate.
6. Prolonged periods of sexual abstinence required by this approach to contraception may add stress to a marital relationship.
7. Douching, vaginal and uterine infection, semen, and use of vaginal spermicides (foams, creams, jellies) may make interpretation of cervical mucus patterns difficult.
8. Disease-induced fever may impair interpretation of a basal body temperature chart.

WITHDRAWAL (COITUS INTERRUPTUS)

Withdrawal involves removal of an erect and stimulated penis from the vagina and the area of the external female genitalia prior to ejaculation. Emission of large amounts of sperm does not take place in the vagina. Withdrawal (coitus interruptus) is probably one of the most common forms of "contraception" employed worldwide and among U.S. teenagers. Withdrawal, also known as the "pulling out" and "French" method, is mentioned in this book only to point out what a high-risk and poor contraceptive method it is.

UNRELIABILITY OF THE WITHDRAWAL METHOD

Withdrawal leads to a pregnancy rate of between 15 and 25 pregnancies per 100 woman-years. It is extremely unreliable and cannot be recommended as a means of contraception.

WHY THE WITHDRAWAL METHOD IS SO UNRELIABLE AND UNSATISFACTORY

There are many reasons why withdrawal is so unreliable. Among these reasons are those included below:

1. The stimulated male penis will discharge, without the male's conscious control, secretions through the urethra that are rich in sperm. These involuntary urethral secretions released prior to ejaculation, but while the erect penis is in the vaginal canal, may lead to sperm migration to and through the cervical opening, and to ultimate fertilization of an egg. The probability of pregnancy is greatest when ejaculate is released into the vagina at the time of orgasm, *but* only one sperm cell is required to actually fertilize an egg. Advocates of the withdrawal method seldom appreciate the fact that involuntary urethral secretions of the male, which are released during sexual excitation, may contain adequate sperm to produce pregnancy. Furthermore, sperm in urethral secretions may enter the cervix of the uterus when deposited on the woman's external genitals, as well as when released in the vagina.
2. In spite of good intentions, few males possess the self-control and split second timing required to remove the stimulated penis from the vagina immediately prior to ejaculation. When this method fails and the female becomes pregnant, most men offer up an excuse such as "I didn't know orgasm was going to occur when it did."
3. The withdrawal method grants the woman little control of either intercourse or contraception. She cannot assist the male significantly in anticipating the appropriate time to withdraw. Her role is a passive one, yet she must experience much of the psychological and all of the physical stress of an unwanted pregnancy.
4. Sexual gratification is seldom achieved by either sexual partner when the withdrawal method is employed. The male may experience an orgasm and ejaculate outside the vagina. The female would seldom achieve a simultaneous orgasm, yet is exposed to the risk of an unwanted pregnancy. It is seldom possible for one or both sexual partners to achieve a satisfactory sexual response when both must worry whether the male will "make it out in time."

DOUCHE

EFFECTIVENESS OF DOUCHING AFTER INTERCOURSE AS A CONTRACEPTIVE

Mechanical flooding and flushing of the vagina immediately after intercourse to remove ejaculated semen is extremely unreliable as a means of conception control. Douches should be viewed as liquids to be used as feminine hygiene aids, not contraceptives.

A survey of women who relied on douching for contraception revealed a pregnancy rate of 36 per 100 woman-years. A 1939 survey found that 39 percent of U.S. women using douching for contraception experienced an unwanted pregnancy within a year. Current studies place the pregnancy rate in the range of 30 to 40 per 100 woman-years when douching is the sole contraceptive method employed. Failure to use any contraceptive method generally yields a pregnancy rate of 60 to 85 pregnancies per 100 woman-years. Clearly, douching is little better than using nothing to prevent pregnancy.

The theory of douching immediately after intercourse is based on the concept that a quick and thorough vaginal irrigation will wash semen from the vagina before sperm can enter the uterus, thus preventing fertilization of an egg. Douching alone cannot be effective, however, because if there are no other barriers to passage of sperm into the cervix (such as a diaphragm, condom, vaginal contraceptive sponge, or spermicidal foam, cream, or jelly), sperm may reach the cervix within 90 seconds of ejaculation. Active sperm may be well into the cervix of the uterus within 1.5 to 3 minutes after intercourse. Sperm has been found in the fallopian tubes 30 minutes after insemination. It is, therefore, highly improbable that douching can be initiated quickly or thoroughly enough to remove all traces of sperm from the vagina before some sperm enter the cervix of the uterus. Some investigators believe that the mechanical force of instilling douche fluid into the vagina may actually propel sperm toward the cervix, thus speeding the rate by which sperm gain entry into the cervix. Furthermore, if a spermicidal foam, cream, or jelly is used prior to intercourse, the douche liquid may dilute or remove the active spermicide, thus decreasing its contraceptive effectiveness.

SAFETY OF DOUCHING

Douching, as an approach to feminine hygiene, can be safe if irritating chemicals are not employed and if the frequency of douching is not excessive. Douching too frequently may remove protective bacteria from the vaginal tract and lead to infections. Douches used as contraceptives have historically been irritating and/or corrosive. It had been thought that use of douching agents containing soap suds, household disinfectants and cleansers, alum, mercury bichloride, and other caustic chemicals might be spermicidal. Apparently they were not. Carbonated soft drinks, notably Coca Cola®, have been popular contraceptive douches in developing countries although they are neither effective nor safe. Douches should not be viewed as contraceptives.

POSTCOITAL CONTRACEPTION—THE MORNING-AFTER PILL

Postcoital contraception means applying a contraceptive measure after intercourse. The objective is to prevent a potential pregnancy from progressing.

Most attention has focused on estrogens, progestogens, and the IUD. Neither progestogens nor the IUD have been approved by the FDA for use as a postcoital contraceptive. Postcoital administration of the estrogen diethylstilbestrol (DES) has been tested and approved by the FDA as a postcoital contraceptive (morning-after pill).

PREVENTION OF PREGNANCY BY DIETHYLSTILBESTROL (THE MORNING-AFTER PILL)

Diethylstilbestrol (DES) apparently prevents pregnancy by interfering with implantation of the fertilized egg in the endometrium (inner uterine lining). Exactly how DES retards implantation is not well understood. The orally administered DES may interfere with the normal estrogen-progesterone balance in the body, thus producing biochemical and cellular changes in the inner lining of the uterus and thereby preventing a fertilized egg from being implanted. Another theory is that DES administered after intercourse may slow or speed transport of the ovum through the fallopian tube to the uterus. Premature or late arrival may interfere with implantation, should the egg be fertilized. If implantation does not occur, the fertilized egg is either resorbed or eliminated as cervical debris.

TAKING THE MORNING-AFTER PILL

DES has been approved by the FDA for use in emergency cases, such as rape and incest, but the medical community may, and often does, interpret "emergency" fairly liberally. Very young women, women who were intoxicated when intercourse occurred, imminent risk to fetus if pregnancy occurs, fitness of female to be a mother, and a host of other situations and factors may be viewed by the physician as legitimate emergency conditions which warrant use of the morning-after pill.

DES should be administered as soon as possible after intercourse, preferably within 24 hours and definitely within 72 hours. Use more than 72 hours after intercourse will probably not prevent implantation of a fertilized egg. Twenty-five milligrams (mg) of DES must be taken *twice* daily for five consecutive days. If vomiting occurs within four hours, another dose of DES must be taken because the previous dose may not have been completely absorbed. If nausea and vomiting is a problem, this should be reported to the physician. An antinausea medication may be taken one hour before DES to help prevent nausea and vomiting. The full five day course of therapy (50 mg per day) must be completed to avoid pregnancy!

EFFECTIVENESS OF THE MORNING-AFTER PILL IN PREVENTING PREGNANCY

If taken strictly as prescribed, DES is an effective postcoital contraceptive. In a study of 1,217 cases in which DES was properly taken, and there were no other episodes of unprotected intercourse in the cycle, no pregnancies occurred. In a summary of 10,500 cases, the failure rate was 0.4% (42 pregnancies). Only four pregnancies appeared to be due to failure of the method. Thirty-eight of the 42 pregnancies were apparently due to other episodes of unprotected intercourse in the cycle, full doses of DES were not taken, or DES therapy was started too late.

ADVERSE EFFECTS COMMONLY ASSOCIATED WITH THE MORNING-AFTER PILL

The side effects of postcoital DES are similar to those associated with estrogens in "the pill" (see Chapter 1). Because the daily dose of DES required for contraception is large (approximately 50 times the amount of estrogen the body normally produces in a day), the frequency of side effects is high. Sixteen to 24 percent of women will experience nausea and/or vomiting. Seven out of 10 women will experience one or more of the following side effects: nausea, vomiting, headache, breast tenderness, and menstrual irregularities. About one-third of women who take DES as a postcoital contraceptive will not experience side effects.

ECTOPIC PREGNANCY RATE WITH THE MORNING-AFTER PILL

When postcoital DES fails, the ectopic pregnancy rate is approximately one in 10, versus one in 200 under normal circumstances. This higher than normal incidence of ectopic pregnancy may be due to a DES-induced slowing of the passage of the egg through the fallopian tube. Implantation thus takes place at a site other than the uterus.

DES AND VAGINAL CANCER IN THE FEMALE OFFSPRING OF THE MOTHER WHO USED THE MORNING-AFTER PILL UNSUCCESSFULLY

It is highly unlikely that DES, when administered postcoitally (after intercourse) at a dose of 25 mg twice daily for five consecutive days, will cause genital cancer in female offspring resulting from a treatment failure. If, however, a developing female embryo is exposed to DES during the sixth week of gestation or later, she may face a higher than usual risk of developing a rare form of genital cancer later in life.

Time of exposure is crucial to possible association between DES and cancer in offspring. The critical time is the sixth week of pregnancy or later because it is at or near the sixth week that the genital tract of the embryo begins to form.

POSTCOITAL CONTRACEPTION—THE IUD

PREVENTION OF PREGNANCY WITH AN IUD IF INSERTED AFTER UNPROTECTED INTERCOURSE

Although not yet approved by the FDA as a postcoital contraceptive, the copper-containing IUD has shown much promise. In one study of 42 women, the Copper-7® IUD was inserted up to five days after unprotected intercourse, and no pregnancies occurred. In 15 (36%) of these women, hormonal studies indicated that fertilization had occurred. In another study involving 299 women, no pregnancies were reported after unprotected intercourse and postcoital insertion of a copper-containing IUD up to seven days after intercourse.

HOW AN IUD PREVENTS PREGNANCY IF INSERTED AFTER INTERCOURSE

It is believed that insertion of a copper-containing IUD prevents pregnancy by retarding implantation of a fertilized egg. Implantation usually takes place several (4 to 7) days after ovulation. If a copper-containing IUD can be inserted shortly after unprotected intercourse, the risk of pregnancy may be greatly reduced. The sooner it is inserted after unprotected intercourse, the better.

Evidence suggests that unmedicated IUDs may take days to weeks to reach maximal effectiveness and, therefore, may be substantially less effective than copper-containing IUDs if inserted as a postcoital contraceptive. Also, a copper-containing IUD is easier to insert into a nulliparous (no previous pregnancy) uterus than an unmedicated (inert) IUD.

Side effects from insertion of an IUD do not, as a rule, appear to be as frequent or severe as some of those seen with postcoital DES use. Also, once an IUD has been inserted, it provides protection against future pregnancies. All precautions, warnings, and contraindications relative to IUD use that are presented in Chapter 2 must be observed, however.

BREAST-FEEDING AS BIRTH CONTROL

Breast-feeding does decrease fertility somewhat but it, in itself, *is not* an effective means of birth control. To prevent pregnancy when nursing, one *must* use a reliable contraceptive method when intercourse is resumed. Once the baby is weaned, the full range of birth control options may be considered.

CONCLUSION

Of the "high-risk" contraceptive methods presented in this chapter, the various rhythm methods are most widely used. Douching should not be considered a contraceptive method. Utilization of withdrawal as a contraceptive method is strongly discouraged. Effective postcoital approaches to contraception are available, but should only be employed under selected circumstances.

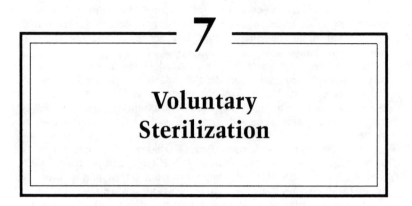

7

Voluntary
Sterilization

INTRODUCTION

Male and female sterilization techniques, first developed in the later part of the 19th century, were not employed to any appreciable extent until the 1930s. Since 1970, the use of voluntary sterilization as a practical approach to contraception has increased rapidly and achieved global popularity. Voluntary surgical sterilization of males and females is probably the most widely used contraceptive method in the world. Approximately 80 million couples worldwide used surgical sterilization methods to control fertility in 1978; by 1987 this number was estimated to be well over 150 million. Over one million voluntary sterilization procedures are performed for contraceptive purposes in the U.S. each year.

Among *advantages* of voluntary surgical sterilization as a contraceptive method are the following:

1. It is the most effective contraceptive method available.
2. It is well suited for couples desiring no more children. Each voluntary sterilization is estimated to prevent 1.5 to 2.5 live births.
3. A single decision is required, that being whether or not to have the sterilization procedure performed. No sustained

attention and motivation concerning proper use, check-ups at regular intervals, or expenditures for contraceptive supplies are required.
4. Sterilization procedures can be performed on men or women.
5. Risk of complications or death from the sterilization procedure is slight if the procedure is performed by qualified medical personnel in a proper environment.
6. Cost is minimal if amortized over the typical period of fertility. With voluntary sterilization, there is no need for further purchase of contraceptive drugs or devices, and no follow-up visits are required. Costs vary with the sterilization procedure chosen.
7. Once successfully performed, there is virtually no risk of side effects or complications from this method of contraception.

If requesting sterilization, you should understand that the resulting infertility is considered permanent, even though procedures are currently available which may reverse male and female infertility in some cases. The permanency of sterilization is regarded by most as a significant advantage.

Over three in 10 married couples in the U.S. have opted for male or female sterilization. Also, it is estimated that by 1978 over two million unmarried U.S. citizens had undergone voluntary sterilization. Voluntary sterilization appears to be the most popular contraceptive method among U.S. couples married 10 or more years; its popularity is increasing among younger couples.

Selection of male or female sterilization is a highly individualized matter. One cannot say what is best for another individual or couple, whether the male or female should undergo the procedure, or which procedure to employ in achieving infertility if choices of method are available, as with female sterilization. What is best is what is determined to be best by the sexually active couple. This chapter will provide factual information that should assist you in decision-making.

The choice of either male or female sterilization for contraceptive purposes depends on a variety of factors. Among these factors are the following:

1. Age
2. Number and age of living children
3. Length of marriage
4. Socioeconomic status
5. Education
6. Previous contraceptive use

7. Cost of procedure
8. Moral, ethical, cultural, and religious beliefs
9. Perceived risk versus benefit
10. The collective feelings and attitudes of both spouses, or the individual if unmarried.

Surveys analyzing satisfaction with voluntary sterilization indicate that most males and females are satisfied with the results. Approximately 95 percent of men and women report their sexual pleasure to be increased or unimpaired by sterilization. Most who expressed dissatisfaction experienced a divorce or death of a child or spouse that was unforeseen at the time of sterilization.

Voluntary sterilization in the male involves only one practical procedure, vasectomy, which involves blocking the passage of sperm through the vas deferens. Vasectomy is a safe, simple, and effective procedure that can be performed on an outpatient basis under local anesthesia. Vasectomy rivals female sterilization in popularity in the U.S. The only other sterilization procedure for males is castration, and this method of sterilization is totally unacceptable as a voluntary approach to fertility control.

Several approaches to voluntary sterilization are available to females. All female sterilization methods currently involve either cutting or blocking (with clips, bands, or electrocoagulation) both fallopian tubes so the egg released by the ovaries cannot be fertilized by sperm.

The five major operative techniques commonly used for female sterilization are:

1. Laparotomy (a procedure involving a large abdominal incision of approximately four inches or 10 cm).
2. Laparoscopy (tubal ligation [blocking] through a small abdominal incision).
3. Minilaparotomy (tubal ligation through a small abdominal incision of about one inch or 2.5 cm).
4. Colpotomy (tubal ligation requiring a small incision in the vagina).
5. Culdoscopy (tubal ligation via a small vaginal incision).

Laparotomy is a major operation requiring general anesthesia. Sterilization utilizing laparoscopy, minilaparotomy, colpotomy, or culdoscopy may be performed under local anesthesia on an outpatient basis. One of these less invasive procedures is generally preferred over laparotomy. Hysterectomy, involving removal of the uterus (subtotal hysterectomy) or uterus and ovaries (total hysterectomy), is no longer considered a viable approach to voluntary sterilization because of higher health risks associated with the operative procedure.

LEGAL ASPECTS OF VOLUNTARY STERILIZATION

Legal barriers to the free choice of sterilization as a contraceptive method are diminishing throughout the world. Voluntary sterilization as a means of contraception is now rarely associated with antiquated criminal codes developed to prevent mayhem, castration, and various other forms of corporal injury or mutilations that rendered men less able to perform their feudal obligations to a monarch. Contemporary court rulings, new legislation, government statements, and ministerial regulations in developed and developing countries are increasingly leaving the decision on whether to be sterilized to the individual, rather than to medical authorities or government officials. With few exceptions, the world now views voluntary sterilization as a legitimate medical procedure and holds to the belief that individuals and couples have the basic human right to determine the size of their families and spacing of their children.

The current legal status of voluntary sterilization can be divided into four categories. These are included below:

1. Countries where legislation explicitly declares that voluntary sterilization is legal.
2. Countries where voluntary sterilization is legal because no law prohibits it.
3. Countries where voluntary sterilization is a criminal offense.
4. Countries where the legal status of voluntary sterilization is unclear.

In the U.S., the states of Connecticut, Oregon, Georgia, North Carolina, Virginia, and West Virginia recognize by statute the right of adults to decide whether to be sterilized. In the remaining states, where no specific law prohibits or recognizes voluntary sterilization, the legality of voluntary sterilization has been confirmed by numerous court decisions, opinions of state attorneys general, inclusion of sterilization services in state-funded health care services, and the existence of statutory regulation of different aspects of the procedure that suggests legality. Contraceptive sterilization is generally legal in any area where the legal system is based on English law, which holds that any act not declared illegal is, therefore, legal.

Because voluntary sterilization is generally considered irreversible, physicians, lawyers, and public policymakers have identified several key issues that should be considered as voluntary sterilization laws are developed and revised. Among these issues are considerations related to personal choice, sterilization for therapeutic reasons, informed consent and voluntarism, and sterilization of minors, incompetents, and institutionalized persons.

The principle of *personal choice* implies that you have the right to choice of contraception; you establish your own criteria for reaching that decision; you reach the decision voluntarily; no governmental or medical body reviews your decision; spousal consent is not required; no special age, parity, or other standards exist; and the procedure is generally available. Few laws deal with all these issues. Common sense suggests that you consult with your marriage partner before seeking sterilization. Regarding age, most countries that allow sterilization on request attempt to limit the procedure to mature individuals at or above the age of majority, which is variably defined throughout the world but ranges from 18 to 35 years of age. Some countries specify that a person must have a certain number of children before voluntary sterilization can occur; no such requirement exists in the U.S.

Therapeutic considerations are often the criteria under which sterilization of women is allowed in countries that otherwise prohibit the procedure. If the purpose is to protect the health of a woman, the legal question of what is therapeutic inevitably arises. The medicolegal trend is to adopt a broad definition of health. Health is defined by the World Health Organization as "a state of complete mental, physical, and social well-being, not merely the absence of disease or infirmity." Under this definition, a woman who considers sterilization necessary for her mental health or social welfare could seek the procedure.

Informed consent is essential to any surgical procedure under medical law. Consent is considered informed if given after obtaining substantial information on the operative procedure, risks, possibility of failure, and other potential consequences, and alternatives to the operative procedure under consideration. The key consideration with voluntary sterilization is that you understand that the procedure should be considered irreversible, although with some potential for reversal. Benefits, as well as risks, should also be discussed in the dialogue associated with informed consent. You will be expected to sign a form stating that you understand the risk and benefit implications of the operative procedure.

Sterilization of minors, incompetents, and institutionalized patients is often complicated by questions about the ability or freedom to make an informed decision. The authoritarian atmosphere of mental, correctional, or other involuntary confinement environments may retard objective decision-making. Third-party consent for sterilization of minors or the mentally incompetent raises serious moral, ethical, philosophical, and legal questions. This area of consent is poorly defined and highly variable from state to state and country to country.

Recent reforms in laws on voluntary sterilization have succeeded in removing this operation from criminal codes and incorporating it into the fabric of health law and family planning programs. Such reforms are very sensitive to human rights issues and the necessity of informed personal consent.

MALE STERILIZATION

VASECTOMY

Vasectomy and Its Popularity as a Contraceptive Measure

Vasectomy is a surgical sterilization procedure for men. The procedure involves making one or two small incisions in the scrotum and severing both of the vas deferens (see Figure 24). This surgical step prevents the passage of sperm from the testes, where it is formed, into the systems of ducts and tubes of the male reproductive

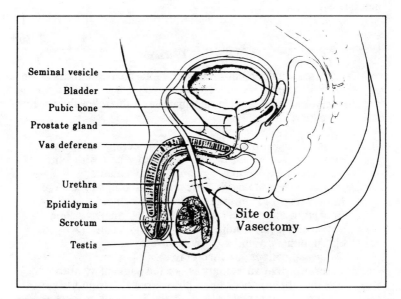

FIGURE 24

Male reproductive system showing the site of vasectomy

tract, and ultimately into the female reproductive system. Several methods of sealing the ends of the severed vas deferens are available.

The skepticism, fear, and misinformation concerning vasectomy is no longer widespread in the U.S. Public education efforts have convinced most men that vasectomy is in no way related to castration and does not cause ill effects such as impotence, decreased libido (sexual desire), inability to ejaculate, impaired virility, hair loss, premature aging and wrinkling, skin disease, high-pitched voice, heart disease, multiple sclerosis, or cancer. Some men, however, regardless of the facts, equate masculinity with fertility and find vasectomy unacceptable. However, a growing number of men feel, quite appropriately, that birth control is as much the man's responsibility as the woman's.

Some women oppose vasectomy out of fear that the operation will make their husbands physically weak and impotent. Other women feel that a vasectomy will free husbands to engage in extramarital affairs.

Testimony to the popularity of vasectomy in the U.S. is the fact that vasectomy is almost as frequently employed as female sterilization as a voluntary means of contraception. An estimated 500,000 U.S. men undergo a vasectomy each year. Vasectomy is one of the safest, simplest, most effective, and least expensive contraceptive methods available.

The Vasectomy Procedure

Careful and accurate counseling and informed consent is essential before you undergo a vasectomy. If you are a candidate for a vasectomy, you should receive information on the following aspects of the procedure:

1. Benefits, risks, failure rates, possible complications and side effects associated with vasectomy and with other permanent and temporary contraceptive methods
2. Permanence and possible irreversibility of the procedure
3. Importance of continuing some other means of contraception after vasectomy until semen analysis shows absence of sperm, until you have had at least 15 to 20 ejaculations, or until six weeks have passed
4. Contraindications to vasectomy
5. Assurance that vasectomy is not the same as castration and that there is no known physiological reason for vasectomy to adversely affect sexual behavior or performance

6. Assurance that withholding or withdrawing consent at any time before vasectomy will not prejudice future care

Preoperative care requires little preparation. A simple medical history should be obtained and a physical exam conducted. To minimize the chance of infection, the scrotum is usually shaved, or the hair clipped, and a local antiseptic is applied. The doctor scrubs thoroughly, wears surgical gloves, and uses sterile instruments. The area of the scrotal incision(s) is injected with a small amount of local anesthetic. If you are extremely anxious or nervous, you may ask for, or may be given, a mild tranquilizer about one hour before the procedure.

The operative procedure generally takes 15 minutes or less and is most often performed in the physician's office. Most vasectomies in the U.S. are performed by urologists, but general surgeons, internists, and family practitioners also perform this procedure. The physician makes either a single incision in the middle of the scrotum or an incision on each side of the scrotum. The most common procedure is to make two incisions, one over each vas. The incision is generally less than one inch in length. Each of the vas deferentia is located, pulled out through the incision, and severed completely. Some physicians remove about one centimeter (less than one-half inch) of each vas deferens to decrease the likelihood that it will grow back together.

The ends of the vas deferens are then sealed by ligation (tying the ends with sutures), coagulation with electricity (electrocoagulation or fulguration) or heat (thermocoagulation), or by using clips. After the ends of each of the severed vas deferens are sealed, the sheath covering each vas is closed, and the scrotal incision is closed. Most physicians prefer to stitch the incision(s) with absorbable sutures that do not have to be removed; they simply disappear as healing occurs. Nonabsorbable sutures are more frequently associated with minor infection and have to be removed a few days after surgery.

Postoperative care is not complex. You should have someone drive you home, and you should rest, lying down, for several hours. You should avoid strenuous exercise or activity for about a week. Wearing an athletic supporter will provide scrotal support and aid in preventing pain and swelling in the area. Mild pain medication (such as aspirin, acetaminophen, Empirin® with Codeine, Tylenol® with Codeine, or Darvon®) may relieve the minor pain and discomfort which may occur and persist for one or two days after the surgery. A small dressing should be kept over the incision for several days, with the dressing changed every two days. Report swelling or tenderness that persists and/or pus at the site of incision to your physician.

Onset of Infertility with Vasectomy

Vasectomy does not result in immediate infertility. Although you may resume protected intercourse about seven days after surgery, stored sperm must be expelled before one becomes infertile. You and your sexual partner(s) must employ alternate methods of contraception for several weeks after surgery.

It is estimated that it may take anywhere from eight to 20 ejaculations to completely eliminate all active sperm. Some investigators report complete expulsion of sperm one week after surgery, while others report that 10 or more weeks are required, depending on the frequency of ejaculation. There is no accepted standard of how many ejaculations or weeks after vasectomy are required before infertility is achieved. The most conservative approach, and one that is highly recommended, is to have the physician's laboratory analyze a sample of sperm after eight to 10 ejaculations, and than analyze a second sample following another series of ejaculations. You may consider yourself sterile after two consecutive reports of no sperm in the ejaculate.

Effectiveness of Vasectomy

Vasectomy is one of the most effective methods of contraception. Vasectomy is as effective as, and probably more effective than, the combination (estrogen-progestin) oral contraceptive tablet ("the pill"), with no apparent risk of systemic adverse effects due to chemically induced changes in body chemistry. Pregnancy rates are substantially less than one per 100 woman-years if the operation is properly conducted and you observe appropriate precautions in the immediate postoperative period. Although failure of the procedure is rare, reasons for failure are listed below:

1. Engaging in unprotected intercourse before the reproductive tract is completely void of sperm. This is the most common reason for pregnancy after vasectomy.
2. The vas deferens rejoins in some manner. This "growing back together" usually follows formation of a sperm granuloma (benign tumor) which forms as an inflammatory response to sperm that leak from the vas. Narrow channels may develop within the granuloma, and these channels can reconnect the two ends of the severed vas or form a duct between them. This may allow sperm to pass into the ejaculate. This event is extremely rare and is a function largely of the quality of the operative procedure and how the vas deferentia were sealed.

3. Operating on the wrong structure. Hardened lymphatic ducts or thrombosed veins may be mistaken for the vas deferens by the inexperienced surgeon. Choose experienced surgeons who perform vasectomies frequently; such individuals should have little or no difficulty in distinguishing the vas deferens from other structures in the spermatic cord and scrotal sac.
4. Very rarely a birth defect may result in duplication of one vas deferens (or both). If the physician operates on only two, contraceptive failure may result. This congenital defect is most likely to be detected by physicians experienced in performing vasectomies.

Conditions Where Vasectomy Should Not Be Performed

There are few contraindications to vasectomy. Local skin infections of the scrotum or infections of the genital tract should be successfully treated before the operation. Certain conditions exist which are not absolute contraindications, but may require hospitalization where better equipment and postoperative monitoring and care are available. Medical conditions which may make the operation difficult or dangerous include the presence of an inguinal hernia, history of previous hernia surgery, an undescended testicle, a hydrocele (collection of fluid around a testicle), varicocele (a varicose enlargement of the veins of the spermatic cord), scar tissue from previous surgery, diseases of the blood that may interfere with normal clotting of the blood, coronary artery disease, and diabetes. If you believe that vasectomy will cure sexual dysfunction, you will probably be discouraged from undergoing the procedure. A history of serious marital, sexual, or psychological instability should be considered a possible contraindication to vasectomy, since such men are more likely to report side effects from vasectomy. Reports of vasectomy-related side effects by such individuals are often (but not always) psychosomatic (imagined) and not reflective of true physiological complications.

Safety of Vasectomy

Vasectomy is among the safest contraceptive procedures. Short-term or postoperative side effects are usually minor, and most disappear within a week or two. The most common complaints after surgery are pain and swelling around the incision. The area will appear bruised and will be sensitive due to unavoidable local trauma of the procedure. About half of men who have had a vasectomy report local pain, swelling, and bruising.

A hematoma (mass of clotted blood) may occur in one to three percent of men who receive a vasectomy. This complication can often be prevented by avoiding heavy straining and physical activity and by wearing an athletic supporter for at least one week after surgery. Ice packs and mild pain relievers help relieve the symptoms. Most hematomas dissolve and are resorbed with no medical intervention.

Other complications of vasectomy are extremely rare and include epididymitis, swelling and tenderness of testicles, hydrocele (collection of fluid around testes), granulomas (benign tumors), adhesions (scarring of the vas deferens that may produce some pain), and infection. Infection may be the complication of greatest potential consequence, but this occurs in less than one percent of vasectomies.

Most infectious complications are superficial skin infections that occur around the site of the incision or sutures within three to four days after surgery. Since most of these infections are due to nonabsorbable sutures (stitches), absorbable sutures are preferred. Deep infections of the vas deferens or epididymis are extremely rare. Both superficial and deep infections may require antibiotic therapy. There have been no deaths reported in the U.S. from complications of vasectomy surgery.

Studies of the long-term psychological effects of vasectomy indicate that over 95 percent report no psychological problems. The great majority of men report they have no regrets and would recommend the operation to others. Most vasectomized men, and their wives, report either no change or improved marital happiness and sexual satisfaction. Psychological problems and complaints do occur in one to five percent of vasectomized men. Complaints include weakness, depression, insomnia, decreased libido, decreased ability to work, nervousness, headache, uneasiness, weight loss, and general worsening of health. Such complaints are generally thought to be manifestations of a behavioral disturbance that is independent of vasectomy. There are no known biological, biochemical, or physiological reasons why such symptoms should be attributable to vasectomy.

Reversal of the Contraceptive Effect of a Vasectomy

As stated previously, vasectomy should be considered irreversible, although experienced surgeons have reported restoring fertility in approximately 50 percent of cases. Demand for vasectomy reversal is not high (about two per 1000 vasectomized men in the U.S.). The most frequent reasons given for desiring a vasectomy reversal are remarriage after divorce or death of a spouse, death of one or more children, desire for more children as finances improve, and psychological problems with infertility.

Unlike vasectomy, reversal of vasectomy is a very complex and expensive procedure requiring sophisticated surgical expertise, hospitalization, a fully equipped and staffed surgical suite, and 1.5 to 3 hours of surgery. The surgical technique most commonly employed is performed using an operating microscope (microsurgery). The scarred ends of the vas deferens are removed and the two ends then rejoined. Side effects from the reversal surgery are infrequent. Pregnancy rates among wives of men who have had reversals are variable. Functional success (pregnancy) depends on sperm producing capacity of the male, reversal technique and skill of the surgeon, and fertility of the wife.

Cost of a Vasectomy

When performed in a doctor's office or clinic, a vasectomy generally costs $250 to $400. If performed in a hospital, the cost is much higher as there are physician's fees plus charges for anesthesia, laboratory tests, operating room, and other ancillary charges. Reversal surgery costs several thousand dollars.

CASTRATION

Male castration involves surgical removal of the testes and produces male infertility. It is *never* a legitimate approach to contraception. Male castration is seldom indicated to treat medical disorders and is most often thought of as a primitive form of punishment.

FEMALE STERILIZATION

TUBAL STERILIZATION

History of Tubal Sterilization in Females

Female sterilization typically involves blocking the fallopian tubes of the reproductive tract so the released ovum (egg) cannot be reached by sperm. Various operative procedures and techniques may be employed to occlude (block) the fallopian tubes. These methods are highly effective and relatively safe. Approximately 500,000 U.S. women undergo tubal sterilization each year.

Female sterilization by tubal ligation (blocking by tying) was first performed in London in 1823. In the 19th and early 20th century, this was a hazardous operation as it involved all the risks of abdominal surgery and required days of hospitalization and weeks of convalescence. Female sterilization by blocking fallopian tubes was rarely performed until the 1930s when new procedures were employed. Today tubal sterilization is popular and readily available. You may choose from five operative techniques: laparotomy, laparoscopy, minilaparotomy, colpotomy, and culdoscopy. Some of these procedures may be conducted on an outpatient basis.

Factors to Consider in Making the Decision to Undergo Tubal Sterilization

As with vasectomy in men, you should consider tubal sterilization to be irreversible. Even though the incidence of success in restoring fertility through microsurgery is increasing, the success of such procedures is variable and unpredictable. Abdominal surgery and careful rejoining of the fallopian tubes is required.

You may request tubal sterilization after childbirth. Tubal sterilization immediately after delivery, and while still hospitalized, certainly has economic advantages. Also, there are few medical reasons which would prevent tubal sterilization immediately after giving birth. One significant disadvantage of timing sterilization with delivery is that some major congenital defects or acquired diseases or infections of the infant may not be recognized during the first several hours after birth.

Tubal sterilization may be performed immediately after abortion. There are few clinical reasons why this cannot be done; this is often, however, a time of great emotional turmoil. It may be best to delay sterilization in such instances.

Operative Procedures Employed in Tubal Sterilization

Five operative procedures are currently employed in tubal sterilization: laparotomy (requiring a large abdominal incision), laparoscopy and minilaparotomy (requiring a small abdominal incision), and colpotomy and culdoscopy (requiring a small vaginal incision). These approaches permit tubal occlusion of any part of the fallopian tubes. The choice of method depends on your preference, your physician's recommendations regarding safety and effectiveness of the various methods, and your physician's training and degree of skill. Factors which may influence selection of operative method are included in Table 18.

TABLE 18
SELECTED CHARACTERISTICS OF TUBAL STERILIZATION METHODS

	Conventional Abdominal Laparotomy	Laparoscopy	Minilaparotomy	Colpotomy	Culdoscopy
Advantages	convenient immediately after childbirth; easily learned by physician	low complication rate; little discomfort; small scar; short recovery period	may be done on outpatient basis with local anesthesia; little discomfort; small scar; short recovery period; easy for physician to learn; relatively low cost; low complication rate	no visible scar; little discomfort; relatively inexpensive; brief procedure; not used postpartum	no visible scar; little discomfort; brief procedure; not used postpartum
Disadvantages	visible scar; long recovery time; cost associated with hospitalization	requires high degree of physician training and skill	difficult in obese women	higher complication rate (such as infection)	requires high degree of physician training and skill
Failure Rate	0 to 2%	0.1 to 2.0%	0.2 to 0.6%	0 to 0.055%	0 to 0.055%
Reversibility	10 to 50%	10 to 50%	10 to 50%	10 to 50%	10 to 50%
Complications	0 to 7.4%	0.1 to 7%	0 to 6.5%	1.6 to 13%	1.6 to 13%
Anesthesia	general or local	general or local	local (usually)	general or local	general or local
Facility	operating room	operating room or outpatient	outpatient (usually)	operating room or outpatient	operating room or outpatient
Recovery Time	2 to 5 days	1 to 5 days	1 to 5 days	1 to 14 days	1 to 14 days

149

Once an abdominal or vaginal incision has been made, the entire contents of the peritoneal cavity and pelvic area may be visualized by placing a narrow telescopic instrument through the incision in the abdominal or vaginal wall. The light source inserted through the abdominal wall is called a laparoscope, and the light source inserted through the vaginal wall in a culdoscopy or colpotomy is called a culdoscope. These are telescopic instruments which provide very intense light and give off no heat. The diameter of these light sources is approximately that of a drinking straw or pencil. Specially designed instruments may be passed through these devices to accomplish tubal sterilization, or a second incision may be made for insertion of instruments for occluding the fallopian tubes.

Tubal sterilization via laparotomy is not a popular procedure today. Among the factors which account for the lack of popularity of this operative approach are cost, pain, prolonged recovery time, scarring, and required hospitalization.

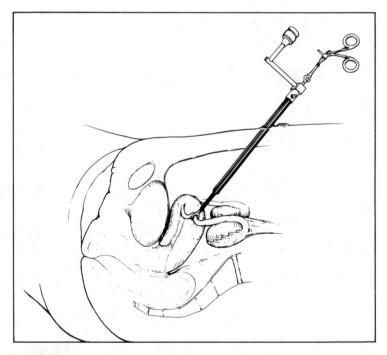

FIGURE 25

Grasping a fallopian tube through an operating laparoscope inserted through an incision near the navel

The two most popular abdominal operative procedures are laparoscopy and minilaparotomy. Both of these procedures require use of the laparoscope viewing instrument, involve one or two small abdominal incisions, produce little scarring and little discomfort after surgery, may be performed on an outpatient basis, may not require general anesthesia, are highly effective, and have a low complication rate.

Laparoscopy or laparoscopic tubal ligation, also called "band-aid sterilization" due to the small incision, has become increasingly popular (see Figure 25). In the laparoscopic procedure, you are positioned on the operating table in a manner similar to that for a pelvic examination. The abdominal area is thoroughly cleaned with an antiseptic solution. A local anesthetic is injected under the skin and into the underlying tissue surrounding the navel. If general anesthesia is employed, an intravenous, ultra-short-acting barbiturate may be used before the anesthesiologist administers an anesthetic gas by mask. Some physicians employ spinal or epidural anesthesia.

After anesthesia is administered, a small (one inch or less) incision is made at the lower border of the navel. A long metal instrument, called a trocar, is inserted through the incision. The trocar is surrounded by a sleeve, and once in place, the trocar is removed and the sleeve left in place. The laparoscope, which contains a light source, and forceps are then inserted through the sleeve. Some physicians prefer to use a two-incision technique in which a second incision is made in the lower abdomen and used as an entry for the forceps.

The fallopian tube is then grasped with the forceps. The special forceps, called electrocoagulation forceps, are connected to an electrical current. When the physician presses a foot pedal, an electrical current passes through the electrocoagulation forceps and burns the fallopian tubes. Some physicians burn the fallopian tubes in several places. Others burn the tubes in one place, apply upward traction at the point of the burn, and break the fallopian tube in half.

After both tubes are coagulated (burned), the physician checks for bleeding. Instruments are then removed and the incision or incisions closed with one or more absorbable sutures, and a sterile dressing is applied.

Most women leave the hospital or clinic within six to 10 hours. Arrangements should be made to have someone drive you home, however, because residual lethargy, drowsiness, and impaired coordination may last for several more hours. Minor discomfort due to the incision(s) may last for several hours, but can be managed well with mild analgesics such as aspirin or Tylenol®. If the incision is red and/or producing a watery fluid, warm water soaks should be applied three or four times daily. If redness or local inflammation persists, an infection may be present. Under this rare circumstance, consult your physician.

Minilaparotomy or "minilap" is a very popular tubal sterilization procedure. Preparation of the operative site is the same as with laparoscopy, and local anesthesia is almost always employed. In this operative procedure, an instrument is inserted into the cervix of the uterus and the uterus is pushed up against the abdominal wall. A small incision is then made directly over the top of the elevated uterus near the top of the pubic-hairline. The fallopian tubes are then brought up to and through the incision with forceps. The tubes may then be tied, burned, cut, clipped, banded, or plugged. Postsurgical care is the same as with laparoscopy.

The two operative procedures for tubal sterilization which utilize the vaginal approach are culdoscopy and colpotomy. Both procedures may be conducted under local or general anesthesia. Electrocoagulation is rarely used to occlude the fallopian tubes when the vaginal approach is employed. As is obvious from Table 18, the complication rate from the vaginal approach to tubal sterilization is about twice as high as with the abdominal approach.

In culdoscopy the pelvic cavity is viewed through an optical instrument (culdoscope), which is inserted through a small vaginal incision. A second instrument is used to bring the fallopian tubes through the incision, where they are blocked by mechanical means. In culdoscopy there is no visible scar. Culdoscopy is a very brief and simple procedure which produces little postsurgical discomfort.

Colpotomy requires a vaginal incision just behind the cervix. The lower portion of the abdominal cavity may be entered through this incision. As with culdoscopy, the fallopian tubes are brought out through the incision and occluded (blocked) by one of various means. The fallopian tubes are replaced and the incision stitched.

Blocking of the Fallopian Tubes

Once the abdominal cavity has been entered and the fallopian tubes located, there are several methods by which the physician may occlude (block) the tubes. Tubal ligation, or tying of the fallopian tubes with nonabsorbable, nonreactive thread, is the oldest and simplest approach to tubal occlusion. It is seldom used today because of the higher failure rate. Another approach involves ligation and crushing. In this method, the tube is picked up to form a loop, and the base of the loop is crushed with a clamp and tied with a nonabsorbable suture material. Like simple ligation, this method is associated with an unacceptably high failure rate. Division, ligation, and burial involve severing (cutting) each fallopian tube, tying each end with a special thread, and burying the stumps in surrounding tissue. Procedures involving resection (removal of a segment of each fallopian tube) and ligation of the stumps are easier to perform than burying the severed ends of the tubes and are very effective.

Fulguration (burning of a segment or segments of each fallopian tube) is used frequently today. The electrical current applied through special forceps produces heat, which dehydrates and chars the tubes. Some physicians may choose to not only electrocoagulate the tubes, but also sever them. The probability of recanalization (reopening) of a fallopian tube after this procedure is extremely remote. Fulguration is a highly effective and quick procedure.

Clips and bands have been investigated as means to occlude the fallopian tubes. They are relatively easy to apply, effects are potentially reversible when removed, and they are not expensive. Disadvantages appear to be an unacceptably high failure rate, and the possibility of an increased risk of ectopic pregnancy.

Chemicals (such as quinacrine, silver nitrate, and adhesive chemicals) have been evaluated for their ability to occlude the tubes. They hold little promise as useful methods as they are often highly toxic to surrounding tissue, require special instruments for administration, and are often ineffective after a single administration.

Solid plugs are being investigated. Such devices may allow for reversal of sterilization when removed from the fallopian tubes. Dacron®, Teflon®, Nylon®, ceramic, silicone, and polyethylene plugs have been or are now being evaluated. The ultimate role of such removable plugs in tubal sterilization has not yet been determined.

Use of a carbon dioxide laser is also being evaluated as a heat source to occlude fallopian tubes. The laser beam eliminates the need to touch the treated area. The expense of such technology may prevent its widespread use if it offers little advantage over existing methods relative to effectiveness, safety, and reversibility.

Onset of Infertility With Tubal Sterilization

Theoretically, tubal sterilization results in immediate infertility. There is a very unlikely probability that pregnancy could occur if intercourse occurred within 24 hours after surgery and an egg had been released the day of the surgery and passed the point of occlusion before the operative procedure. Few women would consider intercourse in the immediate postsurgical period (24 to 48 hours after the operative procedure), however.

Effectiveness of Tubal Sterilization

Tubal sterilization, along with vasectomy, is probably the most effective approach to contraception, excluding strict abstinence (see Table 18). What is surprising is that it is not 100 percent effective. On extremely rare occasions tubes may grow back together. Physician error may result in tying off, burning, or cutting a supporting ligament rather than a fallopian tube. You should utilize a physician experienced in performing specific tubal sterilization procedures to minimize the risk of failure, if you choose tubal sterilization.

Conditions Where Tubal Sterilization Should Not Be Performed

There are definite situations and conditions in which tubal sterilization should not be performed. Absolute contraindications to tubal sterilization via the abdominal route include any type of malignancy of organs and tissues of the abdominal cavity, any obstructive disorder of the intestines, and advanced pregnancy. There are numerous relative contraindications to abdominal tubal sterilization in which one must weigh the potential benefits of the operative procedure against potential risks. Most of these are included in Table 19.

Obesity, particularly if the fat is concentrated around the abdominal area rather than throughout the body, may make laparotomy, laparoscopy, and minilaparotomy more difficult. If a general anesthetic is employed and the obese patient also suffers from cardiovascular or respiratory disease, the benefits may not warrant the

TABLE 19
RELATIVE CONTRAINDICATIONS TO TUBAL STERILIZATION VIA THE ABDOMINAL ROUTE*

- previous abdominal surgery with extensive abdominal scarring and abdominal adhesions
- extreme obesity
- hernia (unrepaired)
- pelvic inflammatory disease (PID) or any other unresolved infection of organs or tissues of the abdominal cavity
- peritonitis (inflammation of the inner lining of the abdominal cavity)
- severe cardiovascular or respiratory disease

*excludes absolute contraindications

risk of an adverse cardiac or respiratory event. Hernias (umbilical, inguinal, and hiatal) create weakness of muscle wall and increase the chance that intestines may protrude into the operative field and be damaged by sterilization instruments. Any unresolved inflammatory and/or infectious process of the abdominal area should be effectively treated before abdominal tubal sterilization to minimize risks of spreading the infection.

All of the absolute and relative contraindications that apply in abdominal sterilization also apply in tubal sterilization via the vaginal route (that is, to culdoscopy and colpotomy). The physician may also consider local vaginal infections and benign uterine fibroids as relative contraindications. Tubal sterilization utilizing the vaginal route would seldom be utilized immediately after childbirth.

Safety of Tubal Sterilization

Tubal sterilization is considered a safe operative procedure, but is not without risk. Vasectomy is considered safer than any sterilization procedure performed on a woman.

As Table 18 indicates, the complication rates may vary from zero to 13 percent and tend to be higher with the vaginal operative procedures. The typical complication rate following abdominal tubal sterilization in the U.S. is two to four percent. Most complications from tubal sterilization are considered very minor and are related to superficial pain and discomfort associated with the incision. Deaths attributable to tubal sterilization are extremely rare. Over 5.0 million women underwent tubal sterilization in the 1970s; the fatality rate was only 3.6 per 100,000 procedures. Risk of death appears greater in women who received general anesthesia.

Reversal of the Contraceptive Effect of Tubal Sterilization

Tubal sterilization can be reversed in some cases, but the microsurgical procedure for restoring fertility is extremely complex, requires highly specialized surgical equipment and expertise, and is very expensive. The procedure involves rejoining portions of the fallopian tube that have been damaged or severed by a prior operation in such a way that egg and sperm may have an open passage and can ultimately unite.

The success of the microsurgery (that is, ultimately achieving pregnancy) depends on (1) the skill and experience of the surgeon, (2) the condition of the fallopian tubes prior to surgery, (3) the age, health, and fertility of the woman, and (4) the fertility of her partner.

Some forms of tubal sterilization are more reversible than others. The more the tube has been damaged during sterilization, the less likely the reversal surgery will succeed. Electrocoagulation (fulguration or burning) of tubes that destroys 4.0 or more cm of a tube is the most difficult to reverse. Clips, bands, plugs, and laser techniques may prove more reversible, although surgical rejoining of the tube is still required.

Only about one or two per 1000 women who have undergone tubal sterilization express the desire to undergo reversal surgery. If you undergo the reversal procedure, you should realize that the incidence of ectopic pregnancy appears to be at least 10 times higher when compared to women who have never undergone tubal surgery. The cost of reversal surgery, including physician fee, operating room charge, anesthesiologist fee, hospital room, and ancillary charges often exceeds $5000.

Cost of a Tubal Sterilization

Tubal sterilization, while not inexpensive, is not generally considered to be excessively expensive. Physician fees may range from $300 to $1000 for tubal sterilization via the abdominal or vaginal route. If hospitalized for one or two days and receiving general anesthesia, costs will escalate substantially. If tubal sterilization is conducted on an outpatient basis, charges of a few hundred dollars beyond that of the physician fee are typical. Comprehensive medical insurance policies cover most, if not all, charges associated with tubal sterilization. When one considers the cost of other contraceptive methods employed over a multiyear period of fertility, effectiveness, and overall safety, tubal sterilization is not so expensive. The difference is one payment versus a protracted series of payments.

Resumption of Intercourse After Tubal Sterilization

Contraceptive effectiveness is achieved on the day of tubal sterilization in most instances. Regardless of the operative method employed, however, you will typically experience some discomfort and anxiety about the procedure. Intercourse should be resumed whenever you feel comfortable with resumption of sexual activity. This is usually within a few (three to five) days after surgery. Resumption of sexual activity should be discussed with your physician.

HYSTERECTOMY

Hysterectomy involves surgical removal of uterus, fallopian tubes, and/or ovaries and produces female infertility. Sterilization is never a valid indication for hysterectomy, however, due to risk and expense.

A major controversy developed in the 1970s concerning abuse of this surgical procedure. It was found that an estimated 4,342,000 women between the ages of 15 and 44 underwent hysterectomy between 1970 and 1980 in the U.S. It is interesting to note that during this period twice as many hysterectomies were performed on insured women as on uninsured women. Hysterectomies were performed four times as often in the U.S. as in Sweden. Almost 35 percent of physicians practicing full-time gynecology in the 1970s were not certified by the American Board of Obstetrics and Gynecology, yet performed three times as many hysterectomies as certified specialists. Many hysterectomies were conducted for contraceptive purposes. Hysterectomy is only appropriate when a gynecological disease requires such a surgical procedure.

CONCLUSION

Numerous sterilization methods are available to the male and female. The choice of method is an individual matter. Informed choices are particularly critical with sterilization procedures because of implications for subsequent fertility.

8

Investigational Contraceptives

INTRODUCTION

Numerous new male and female contraceptive drugs and devices are being evaluated under experimental conditions. Items under investigation for use by the female include the cervical cap, long-acting injectable progestins, progestin-containing hormonal implants, progestin-releasing IUDs, hormone-releasing vaginal rings, once-a-month combination oral contraceptives, disposable diaphragms with controlled release spermicide, intracervical devices, intravaginal propranolol, an antipregnancy vaccine, and a contraceptive nasal spray. Male contraceptives being evaluated include a contraceptive nasal spray, long-acting hormones (androgen plus progestin), gossypol, chlorinated sugars, and sperm enzyme inhibitors. Some products hold more promise than others relative to safety and effectiveness, although all are discussed in this chapter.

CERVICAL CAP

PHYSICAL CHARACTERISTICS OF THE CERVICAL CAP

The cervical cap is a small, firm, cup-shaped rubber device that fits snugly over the cervix. Cervical caps have been used for birth control in Europe for decades, but their current level of popularity is not high. Widespread interest in the cervical cap has developed in the U.S. Cervical caps are not currently approved by the FDA for use in the U.S., however. Approximately 80 to 90 FDA-approved investigators are currently evaluating the cervical cap in U.S. women. Results of these studies will determine whether this contraceptive device is ultimately certified by the FDA as safe and effective and released to the market.

Three types of cervical caps are currently available in foreign countries (see Figure 26). The Prentif cavity-rim cap is the most commonly used. A thimble-shaped cap that fits snugly over the cervix, the Prentif cap is available in four sizes—22, 25, 28, and 31 mm inside rim diameter. The Dumas or vault cap is a shallow, bowl-shaped cap ranging in diameter from 50 to 75 mm. The Vimule cap is

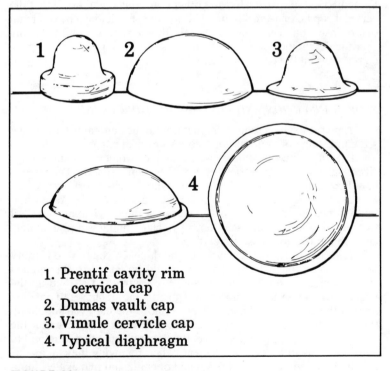

1. Prentif cavity rim
    cervical cap
2. Dumas vault cap
3. Vimule cervicle cap
4. Typical diaphragm

FIGURE 26

Size and shape of cervical caps (1-3)
in relationship to diaphragm (4)

a longer, bell-shaped cap with a flared rim for strength. The Vimule cap is available in three sizes—42, 48, and 54 mm. The Prentif cap covers the cervix only; the larger Dumas and Vimule caps cover the cervix and part of the upper vaginal vault. When compared to the diaphragm (see Figure 26), the cervical cap is deeper but smaller in diameter, usually more rigid, and held in place in part by suction rather than by spring tension in the rim.

HOW THE CERVICAL CAP WORKS

The cap works like the diaphragm to form a physical barrier over the cervix, thus preventing entry of viable sperm into the area harboring a fertilizable egg. Cervical caps are designed to be used with a vaginal spermicide. Most instructions accompanying caps sold in the United Kingdom, Australia, and other countries recommend that the cervical cap be one-third to one-half full of spermicidal jelly or cream before insertion. This amounts to less than one teaspoonful. Adding spermicide should increase effectiveness by killing sperm that may come between the cervix and cap.

PROPER INSERTION AND REMOVAL OF THE CERVICAL CAP

A pelvic exam is required to determine the general health status, size, and shape of your cervix before a cervical cap can be selected. The Prentif cavity-rim appears well suited for women with an average sized, relatively symmetrical cervix. The more shallow Dumas cap may be more appropriate for women who have a short cervix; the Vimule cap may be best for women with a long cervix. When correctly fitted, none of the caps should touch the cervical opening. All women should probably see their physician annually, and definitely after childbirth, for possible refitting.

Prior to insertion, the physician should teach you how to identify the cervix by touch. A spermicide should be added to the cupped side of the cap, and the cap slid into the vagina and pushed up the posterior vaginal wall as far as it will go and until it slips into position around the cervix (see Figure 27). To remove the cap, you should tip the cap with a finger to break the seal, then hook a finger under the rim of the cap and pull forward gently. Some women find it helpful to bear down, as in a bowel movement, when removing the cap as this brings the cervix closer to the vaginal opening and makes the rim of the cap easier to reach.

The cap plus spermicide must be in place prior to intercourse. Some physicians advise inserting the cap at least one-half hour

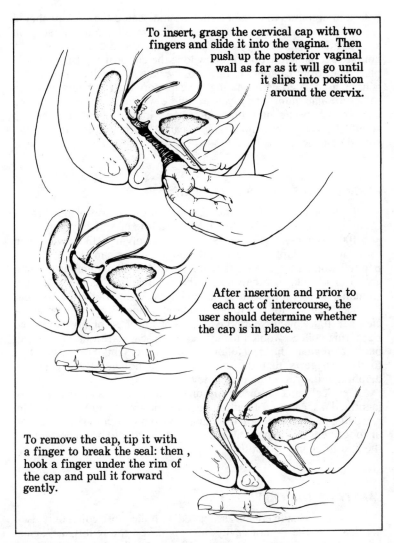

To insert, grasp the cervical cap with two fingers and slide it into the vagina. Then push up the posterior vaginal wall as far as it will go until it slips into position around the cervix.

After insertion and prior to each act of intercourse, the user should determine whether the cap is in place.

To remove the cap, tip it with a finger to break the seal: then , hook a finger under the rim of the cap and pull it forward gently.

FIGURE 27

Insertion and removal of cervical cap

before intercourse to enhance suction and secure the fit. You should leave the cap in place for at least six hours after intercourse. You should also check the position of the cap before each act of intercourse. Recommendations on how long the cervical cap can be left in place vary from 24 hours to three to five days. Offensive vaginal odor is often associated with wearing the cap more than 24 hours. In order to assure maximum safety, you would be well advised to remove the cap six to 24 hours after intercourse. As with the diaphragm, the cap should be gently but thoroughly cleaned after removal, dried, and stored in a cool place.

EFFECTIVENESS OF THE CERVICAL CAP

Preliminary results in the U.S. indicate that use of the Prentif cavity-rim cap is associated with a failure rate of 8 to 20 pregnancies per 100 woman-years. In a 1983 study involving 313 cervical cap users and 317 diaphragm users, the 6-month pregnancy rate was 5.7 per 100 women for cap users and 4.7 per 100 diaphragm users. In a group of 413 cervical cap users, the failure rate was eight per 100 woman-years. Another study involving 90 women advised to wear their cervical cap for two to three days at a time revealed 16 pregnancies per 100 woman-years. Over one-fourth of 34 highly motivated California college women using the Prentif cavity-rim or Vimule cap became pregnant during a follow-up period averaging 11 months. Data to date suggests that the cervical cap is not as effective as the diaphragm in preventing pregnancy.

Cervical caps fail primarily due to misuse. Reasons frequently identified as causes of failure include not using any spermicide, removing the cap too soon (less than six hours) after intercourse, and dislodgement due to poor fit. Failure rates appear to be highest during the first three months of use.

SAFETY OF THE CERVICAL CAP

No serious side effects associated with the more commonly used cervical cap, the Prentif cavity-rim cap, have been reported. Vaginal injury has been associated with the Vimule cap, however, perhaps due to the relatively sharp-edged rim. In a study of 50 cap users, half reported that vaginal odor was a problem, especially after two days of continuous wear. Heavy bacterial growth is often associated with odor. The role of cervical cap related increases in bacterial growth on incidence of pelvic inflammatory disease (PID), vaginal infection, toxic shock syndrome (TSS), and urinary tract infection has not yet been determined. Bacterial growth and odor can be minimized by wearing the cervical cap for 24 hours or less.

USE OF THE CERVICAL CAP

Not every woman can use a cervical cap. A U.S. investigator reported that only approximately 50 percent of women interested in using a Prentif cavity-rim cap are good candidates for use. Those who cannot use the cervical cap usually have a diseased cervix, abnormal cervical anatomy, or difficulty learning how to insert and remove a cap. Conditions which may prevent use of the cervical cap include the following:

1. Cervical erosion or laceration
2. Abnormal cervical shape
3. Cervical cysts
4. Inflammation of the cervix (cervicitis)
5. Inflammation of structures around the cervix such as ovaries, fallopian tubes, or uterus, which may be suggestive of pelvic inflammation and/or infection

ADVANTAGES AND DISADVANTAGES OF A CERVICAL CAP

The cervical cap has some advantages. In the United Kingdom and several other countries, the cervical cap is usually recommended as a barrier method only when the woman cannot be fitted for a diaphragm. Some feel the cap is more convenient than a diaphragm because:

1. A cap may be left in place longer than 24 hours
2. A cap may be inserted many hours or even a day or two before coitus
3. Small amounts of spermicide are used, therefore caps are less messy than diaphragms
4. Caps are less expensive than diaphragms
5. Caps may reduce the risk of acquiring sexually transmitted diseases by blocking the reproductive tract

Frequently reported disadvantages include:

1. Odor associated with use
2. Difficulty in insertion and removal
3. Discomfort during intercourse for the man and/or woman

4. Fear of dislodgement during intercourse
5. Local irritation
6. A relatively high accidental pregnancy rate
7. Need for consistent and very careful use with each act of intercourse

LONG-ACTING INJECTABLE PROGESTINS

In an effort to improve effectiveness, while decreasing the risk of adverse effects, new approaches to hormonal contraception continue to be evaluated. The long-acting injectable progestins offer both promise and problems. The progestin receiving the most attention as a long-acting injectable contraceptive is medroxyprogesterone (Depo-Provera®). Depo-Provera® is specially designed in a slow-release injectable dosage form. A single intramuscular injection of 150 mg is usually given and appears to be effective for three months. Another long-acting injectable progestin is norethindrone enanthate (Noristerat®). It is injected intramuscularly at a dose of 200 mg every eight weeks.

Neither of these drugs is approved for use as a contraceptive in the U.S., but both are used as contraceptives in over 100 other countries. Approval of long-acting injectable progestins as contraceptives in the U.S. has not been granted by the FDA because of controversial data concerning the cancer causing ability of Depo-Provera®.

EFFECTIVENESS OF LONG-ACTING INJECTABLE PROGESTINS

Both Depo-Provera® and Noristerat® are highly effective methods of contraception. Depo-Provera® doses of 150 mg injected every three months, or 200 mg of Noristerat® injected every two months, allows less than 1.0 pregnancy per 100 woman-years. These currently available injectable progestins appear to be as effective as the combination (estrogen-progestin) oral contraceptives and are more effective than the progestin-only "minipill."

HOW THE LONG-ACTING INJECTABLE PROGESTINS PREVENT PREGNANCY

Injectable progestins work in several ways to prevent pregnancy. Ovulation is prevented in most women as progestins prevent the surge of luteinizing hormone (LH) normally seen at midcycle and just prior to ovulation. They may also work by making the cervical mucus very thick, thus creating a barrier to passage of sperm. Injectable progestins also possess chemical activity that changes the nature of the endometrium. These chemically induced changes may impair implantation of a fertilized egg.

ADVANTAGES OF THE LONG-ACTING INJECTABLE PROGESTINS

Long-acting injectable progestins have many advantages associated with their use as a contraceptive. Among these advantages are the following:

1. High contraceptive effectiveness. Effectiveness is on a par with the combination (estrogen-progestin) oral contraceptive pill.
2. Use is independent of the act of intercourse.
3. Reversible contraceptive action since the effects of the drug wear off.
4. Simple to administer, requiring no daily routine.
5. Long acting. (Depo-Provera® may be injected intramuscularly every three months in 150 mg doses; Noristerat® should be injected every two months in 200 mg doses.)
6. Relatively low incidence of significant side effects, except for menstrual disturbances.
7. Some lactating women receiving injections of Depo-Provera® may experience an increased supply of breast milk. The drug does not significantly inhibit lactation.
8. Depo-Provera®, like oral contraceptives, appears to reduce the risk of pelvic inflammatory disease (PID).
9. Contains no estrogen, therefore, does not share some drawbacks of "the pill" (such as increased risk of blood clots, stroke, and heart attack).
10. Depo-Provera® may reduce the symptoms of sickle-cell disease in people of African descent.
11. Cost of Depo-Provera® and Noristerat® to international donor agencies and family planning organizations is $0.50 to $1.00 per dose. The injection fee is an additional charge.

DISADVANTAGES OF THE LONG-ACTING INJECTABLE PROGESTINS

Disadvantages associated with use of long-acting injectable progestins include the following:

1. A relatively high incidence of abnormal menstrual bleeding. Bleeding may be irregular and the menstrual period may not occur. Menstrual irregularities are the main reason for discontinuing use.
2. A typical delay of four to five months for fertility to return after discontinuing the drug. There is no evidence that fertility is permanently impaired, however.
3. Fear that development of benign and malignant breast tumors in beagle dogs and endometrial cancer in monkeys receiving long-acting injectable progestins in large doses might also occur in humans receiving such injections. Such fears related to the drugs' long-term cancer-causing potential in humans are the primary reason these drugs are not currently available in the U.S.
4. Effects cannot be quickly stopped as the drug is long-acting and is not physically removable.
5. Pain and discomfort of an injection.

ADVERSE EFFECTS ASSOCIATED WITH USE OF LONG-ACTING INJECTABLE PROGESTINS

Menstrual Cycle Disturbances

Most women using injectable progestins experience some menstrual cycle abnormalities. Symptoms vary from absence of bleeding (amenorrhea) to irregular bleeding, spotting, and changes in the frequency, duration, and amount of blood loss. Irregular bleeding and spotting may decrease with length of use. Depo-Provera® appears more likely to cause irregular bleeding, spotting, and amenorrhea than Noristerat®. Approximately six to 25 percent of women stop using injectable progestins in the first year because of menstrual irregularities.

Weight Gain

Most women utilizing injectable progestins gain weight. The addition of body weight appears to be due to increased body fat, not to fluid retention. It is theorized that progestins stimulate the appetite control center in the brain. The average weight gain ranges from less than two pounds up to 10 pounds in the first year of use. Some women gain considerably more. Weight gain may level off or continue to increase.

Cardiovascular Effects

Unlike the combination pill (estrogen-progestin), the progestin-only injection appears to have little or no effect on either blood pressure or blood clotting. Increased risk of blood clots is usually associated with estrogen therapy. The effect of progestin injections on high-density lipoproteins (HDL) and cholesterol levels in the blood is not clear. The apparent risk of cardiovascular complications from long-acting progestin injections appears slight.

Metabolic Effects

Depo-Provera® appears to alter carbohydrate metabolism in some individuals. Depo-Provera® may raise blood glucose levels in a small number of women. Precautions should be observed if you are diabetic or borderline diabetic. Slight adjustments in diet, doses of oral blood sugar lowering drugs, or insulin dosage may be required in diabetics. Injectable progestins are not contraindicated (prohibited) in diabetics, however.

Delayed Ovulation After Stopping the Drug

In most users of injectable progestins, fertility (ovulation) returns within four to five months after discontinuing use. Former users of Depo-Provera® usually require 1.5 to 3 months longer to conceive than former users of oral contraceptives or an IUD. The duration of infertility may depend on the rate of metabolism of the injected progestin and body weight.

Miscellaneous Side Effects

Other side effects include headache, abdominal distension, nausea, dizziness, nervousness, change in skin pigmentation, lessening of libido, diminished frequency of orgasm, and acne. The incidence of headache varies from one to 17 percent of users of long-acting injectable progestins, but is seldom given as a reason for discontinuing the drug. Other side effects occur rarely.

RELATIONSHIP BETWEEN LONG-ACTING INJECTABLE PROGESTINS AND BIRTH DEFECTS

In rare cases where pregnant women were exposed to a long-acting injectable progestin, no increase in malformations or prematurity have been noted. Likewise, there has been no reported increase in birth defects, stillbirths, multiple births, sex ratio (males to females), or birthweights of children of former injectable progestin contraceptive users.

RISKS TO NURSING INFANTS IF LACTATING MOTHERS RECEIVE CONTRACEPTIVE INJECTIONS OF LONG-ACTING PROGESTINS

Although little objective data is available, risks to nursing infants whose mothers receive long-acting progestin injections appear to be slight. Postpartum (after birth) injection of Depo-Provera® either improves breast-feeding performance (increased volume) or has no measurable effect. Depo-Provera® does not appear to adversely alter the composition of breast milk. The concentration of protein and fat in the breast milk of Depo-Provera® users is the same as or higher than in nonusers. Lactose content is unaffected.

When a breast-feeding woman uses any drug regularly, quantities of the drug may pass into breast milk and are consumed by the infant. The amount of contraceptive drug transmitted to the infant via breast milk is very small (probably less than 1/200th [0.5%] of the dose the mother took). The amount in the mother's milk is, as would be expected, highest immediately after an injection and declines thereafter.

HORMONAL IMPLANTS

HOW HORMONAL IMPLANTS PREVENT PREGNANCY

Contraceptive implants are usually made of a flexible, non-biodegradable substance known as polydimethylsiloxane (Silastic®). This polymer may be shaped into a hollow capsule and filled with a hormone or molded into solid rods impregnated with a hormone. The Population Council favors levonorgestrel as the contraceptive hormone for implantation. Levonorgestrel is preferable over many other progestins because it diffuses slowly through the Silastic® carrier into the bloodstream and is highly effective in small amounts.

Progestin-containing implants prevent pregnancy by the same mechanism(s) as long-acting injectable progestins. The investigational rods or capsules are usually 2.0 to 4.0 cm (0.8 to 1.6 inches) in length and approximately 2.4 mm in diameter, and are placed just under the skin with a large hypodermic needle. Implants are usually placed in the inner side of the upper arm so they are less visible than if implanted on the inside of the forearm. Although the presence of the implant may be vaguely detectable visually, this does not deter most users.

Placement of the inserts requires the expertise of a specially trained health worker. Local anesthesia is required, and the entire procedure usually takes 10 to 15 minutes. If properly placed, removal is a simple process. During removal, the area is anesthetized and a tiny incision (approximately 5 mm) made in the skin over each implant. Implants may be removed at any time.

The amount of hormone released by the implant can vary, depending on the following factors:

1. Type of hormone. Some hormones diffuse out of the Silastic® more rapidly than others. With all hormones, the rate of release decreases over time, but most implants currently being evaluated retain adequate contraceptive effectiveness for at least three years, and often longer.
2. The surface area of the rod or capsule. The greater the surface area of the implant the greater the rate of progestin release.
3. The type of implant. Rods have a release rate three to four times greater than capsules because in rods the hormone travels a shorter distance to reach the surface of the implant.
4. The number of rods or capsules used. From one to 12 rod or capsule implants have been tested.
5. Sterilization of the implant. Some rods and capsules should not be sterilized by irradiation as this may reduce the rate of release of the contraceptive hormone.
6. Characteristics of individual users. In some women, dense, fibrous tissue forms around implants and may slow release of contraceptive hormone, although apparently not seriously enough to increase pregnancy rates. Physical activity, amount of body fat, and local blood supply may influence the rate at which the hormone enters the blood stream.

The Population Council is involved in testing two implant systems. The Norplant® system consists of six capsules, each containing 36 mg of levonorgestrel. It is estimated that the effective life of this system is at least five years. The Norplant® system is being compared with the Norplant II® system. The Norplant II® system consists of two capsules, each containing 70 mg of levonorgestrel. Two rather than six implants will facilitate insertion and removal, and may prove preferable.

HOW EFFECTIVE ARE HORMONAL IMPLANTS?

The contraceptive effectiveness of levonorgestrel-containing contraceptive implants (Norplant®, Norplant II®) rivals the combination oral contraceptives. First year pregnancy rates are consistently and substantially below 1.0 pregnancy per 100 woman-years. The

Norplant® system of implant generally produces pregnancy rates between 0.2 and 0.6 pregnancies per 100 woman-years. Data suggests that pregnancy rates may increase somewhat during the 4th and 5th years of use. Even if the optimally effective life is three years, rather than five, one clinic visit can provide over 1,000 days of contraception. Many women would find such convenience and security very appealing.

ADVANTAGES OF CONTRACEPTIVE HORMONAL IMPLANTS

The contraceptive hormonal implant offers numerous advantages over other contraceptive drugs and devices. Among advantages of this investigational product are the following:

1. Effectiveness. The capsule and rod implants carrying the progestin levonorgestrel appear to be as effective as the oral contraceptive pill. Rods and capsules containing levonorgestrel appear to be equally effective.
2. Length of action. Certain contraceptive hormonal implants have been shown to be very effective for three to five years.
3. Reversibility. Contraceptive effects are reversible upon removal of the hormonal implants. Of 53 women who wanted to conceive, 77 percent were pregnant within one year after removal of the hormonal implant.
4. Use is independent of the act of intercourse. No interruption is associated with its use.
5. Safety. These implants contain no estrogen, therefore, adverse effects associated with estrogen (as seen with the combination oral contraceptives) are avoided.
6. Rapid onset of contraceptive action. Levonorgestrel reaches an optimal level in the bloodstream soon after implantation.
7. Ease of insertion and removal. Insertion and removal is usually a simple office procedure utilizing local anesthesia.
8. Patient acceptability. Continuation rates are very high. Most trials reveal a continuation rate of 75 to 85 percent after one year of use. In one study of hormonal implant users, 80 to 85 percent of women recommended the implants to friends and relatives.
9. Cost. If approved by the FDA, hormonal implants will sell for approximately $30–$35 plus the cost of insertion and ultimate removal. This compares with a 5-year cost

of approximately $600 if an oral contraceptive is employed.

DISADVANTAGES OF CONTRACEPTIVE HORMONAL IMPLANTS

As with all contraceptive drugs and devices, there are disadvantages associated with contraceptive implant use including:

1. Adverse effects. The progestin contained in the implant may disrupt the menstrual cycle. Numerous other side effects have been reported.
2. Pain on insertion and removal. Approximately 30 percent of users found removal painful. Fewer complaints are associated with insertion.
3. Awareness of presence during use. Approximately 10 to 12 percent of users reported minor irritation or annoyance during use of implants. Some implants are slightly visible under the skin. Approximately seven percent of users considered the detectable presence of the implant to be the feature they most disliked. Use of the inner side of the upper arm rather than the underside of the forearm as the site of implantation should eliminate most of the cosmetic objections.

ADVERSE EFFECTS ASSOCIATED WITH USE OF HORMONAL IMPLANTS

As mentioned previously, progestin-containing implants may disrupt the menstrual cycle. Irregular and prolonged bleeding is the most common complaint. Amenorrhea may also occur. In two studies evaluating discontinuation rates, Norplant® capsules were discontinued by seven percent of one group and 9.5 percent of another group at the end of one year because of irregular menstrual cycles. This adverse effect accounts for approximately half of all first year discontinuations. Bleeding disturbances do, however, decrease over time. Use of implants with higher daily release rates of levonorgestrel appears to reduce irregular or prolonged bleeding and increase amenorrhea. In spite of bleeding disorders, anemia is an unlikely event.

Numerous other adverse effects may be associated with progestin-containing hormonal implants. A slight weight gain (between three and six pounds) occurs in some first-year users. Some androgenic adverse effects, such as hair growth and acne, have occurred

172 / SEXCARE

in up to 15 percent of women, but rarely require removal of the implant. Headache, nervousness, and mental depression have been reported in 15 to 33 percent of Norplant® users. Whether these are events induced primarily by the implant is not clear. Signs of inflammation in the implant area occur in fewer than one in 100 users.

PROGESTIN-RELEASING INTRAUTERINE DEVICES

Natural and synthetic progestins were first added to IUDs in the early 1970s. The only progestin-releasing IUD on the market today is the T-shaped Progestasert®, which contains 38 mg of natural progesterone released at a constant rate of approximately 65 mcg per day for one year. Numerous facts and figures on Progestasert® are presented in Chapter 2 (The Intrauterine Device).

T-shaped IUDs that release other progestins are being investigated. The World Health Organization (WHO) is testing a T-shaped device that releases levonorgestrel, a synthetic progestin. The Population Council is also conducting research on levonorgestrel-containing IUDs. Among the objectives of such research is to increase the duration of action over that of Progestasert® (one year), increase effectiveness, avoid or minimize systemic adverse effects and minimize the probability of ectopic pregnancy in IUD users. Further research is required before levonorgestrel-containing IUDs are approved for use in the U.S. Preliminary research has provided some promising findings.

HORMONE-RELEASING VAGINAL RINGS

A hormone-releasing vaginal ring is a doughnut-shaped circular ring of Silastic® polymer, approximately two inches (50 to 60 mm) in diameter, containing a progestin or an estrogen-progestin combination. The device is inserted into the vagina near the cervix (see Figure 28). As with hormonal implants, the active hormonal agent slowly and continuously diffuses out of the polymer. The hormone is then absorbed through the vagina, enters the bloodstream, and exerts its contraceptive effect.

Unlike diaphragms, vaginal rings do not have to be precisely fitted since they do not act as barriers to sperm. If the rings are expelled, they should be quickly reinserted; such action will prevent any loss of contraceptive effectiveness. Both sexual partners may be aware of the presence of the ring during intercourse. It may produce discomfort for the female during intercourse and may be an annoyance for some males. The vaginal ring should not be removed during intercourse, however.

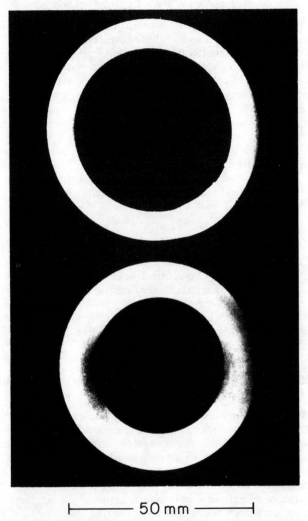

├───── 50 mm ─────┤

FIGURE 28

Hormone releasing vaginal rings

PREVENTION OF PREGNANCY BY VAGINAL RINGS

The combination ring that contains both estrogen and progestin is designed to release enough of these hormones to prevent ovulation. This ring is used intermittently. The recommended usage pattern is to leave the ring in the vagina continuously for three weeks followed by removal for one week. The estrogenic component minimizes the chance of breakthrough bleeding. The estrogen-progestin ring may be used for up to six months, and longer acting rings are being developed.

The ring that contains the progestin levonorgestrel only does not suppress ovulation, but exerts its contraceptive action through effects on the endometrium and cervical mucus. The progestin-only ring under investigation can be worn continuously for three months and should then be discarded. It should not be removed monthly.

EFFECTIVENESS OF HORMONE RELEASING VAGINAL RINGS

Early studies evaluating the estrogen-progestin vaginal ring suggest that this device may be as effective as low-dose combination oral contraceptives. Pregnancy rates were 1.8 per 100 woman-years using a 50 mm ring and 0.7 per 100 woman-years using the 58 mm ring. Sufficient data to adequately assess the effectiveness of the progestin-only vaginal ring is not currently available, however.

ADVERSE EFFECTS ASSOCIATED WITH USE OF THE HORMONE RELEASING VAGINAL RING

The combination estrogen-progestin ring produces vaginal discharge and associated inflammation and discomfort which causes five to seven percent of ring-users to stop using the method. Breakthrough bleeding accounts for seven to eight percent of women discontinuing use; only about four percent of combination oral contraceptive users discontinue the drug because of breakthrough bleeding. Side effects such as headache, nausea, and dizziness appear less common among users of the vaginal ring than among oral contraceptive users. Long-term effects are unknown.

With the progestin-only ring, normal ovulation and menstrual bleeding appears to be only slightly disrupted. Further research is required before the true nature of incidence and severity of side effects induced by this device will be apparent.

ONCE-A-MONTH COMBINED PILLS

Several oral contraceptives taken only once each month are currently utilized in China. Almost all once-a-month combined pills contain the estrogen quinestrol, which is stored in body fat and released slowly over time. The most widely used Chinese once-a-month pill contains 3.0 mg of quinestrol (an estrogen) and 12 mg of norgestrel (a progestin). The first pill is taken on the 5th day of the menstrual cycle and the second pill is taken 20 days later. Thereafter the user takes one pill every four weeks. Many safety and effectiveness questions remain unanswered, and general availability of such a product is unlikely in the foreseeable future.

MALE CONTRACEPTION

INTRODUCTION

There are three events that lend themselves to contraceptive intervention in the male—sperm passage, sperm motility, and sperm production. The condom and vasectomy interfere with the passage of sperm. As discussed earlier, withdrawal is highly ineffective. Research today is focusing on sperm motility and sperm production. Investigators are searching for the male contraceptive that is highly effective, nontoxic, reversible, self-administered, intercourse-independent, and inexpensive. The most promising male contraceptives under investigation are long-acting hormones that suppress sperm production, gossypol (a cottonseed derivative), which decreases sperm motility and possibly sperm production, and chlorinated sugars that appear to suppress sperm motility.

Regarding suppression of sperm production, it is not absolutely clear just how far sperm production must fall to prevent conception. The standard figure for male subfertility is 20 million sperm or less per ml of semen ejaculate. A recent report indicates that nine women became pregnant by men whose sperm counts were below 10 million per ml, and in five of these men, sperm counts were below one million per ml. This data clearly suggests that for complete effectiveness, any male contraceptive that relies on the mechanism of suppressing sperm counts must stop sperm production entirely.

LONG-ACTING HORMONES

Most research on a male contraceptive utilizing long-acting hormones combine an androgen and a progestin. Both suppress production of follicle stimulating hormone (FSH) and luteinizing hormone (LH), which are essential for sperm production. Various progestins have been evaluated. The only androgen evaluated has been testosterone.

Use of either an androgen or progestin alone will prevent sperm production, but contraceptive doses of either drug given alone are so high they produce intolerable adverse effects. According to one prominent investigator, the "most effective and practical combination" tested is medroxyprogesterone acetate and testosterone. Without testosterone (an androgen), the contraceptive doses of medroxyprogesterone acetate (a progestin) would produce intolerable loss of libido, impotence, and breast enlargement in some men. Studies utilizing monthly injections of this combination at various dosage levels reveal declines in sperm production to less than 10 million sperm per ml of semen in over 75 percent of men. Complete suppression of sperm count is not achievable at doses that do not produce serious toxicity, however. Because of this fact, and the unpredictability of effectiveness with anything less than complete suppression of sperm, the long-acting hormones as a male contraceptive may never reach the marketplace.

GOSSYPOL

Gossypol, an orally active chemical, was discovered in China when it was noted that this constituent of uncooked cottonseed oil was responsible for an epidemic of infertility in men. Gossypol appears to have two effects on the male reproductive system. The motility of stored sperm declines sharply within a few days after the start of treatment. After approximately three weeks of oral gossypol therapy, the ejaculate contains mostly immotile sperm. Continued treatment slows or stops the production of sperm.

In tests performed in China between 1974 and 1978, the usual gossypol regimen was 20 mg per day for three months followed by 50 mg per week for maintenance. The mechanism by which the orally administered gossypol slows sperm motility and retards sperm production is not known. An attractive feature of gossypol is that it does not suppress hormone production of the testes, thus libido is not reduced and androgen (testosterone) therapy is not required.

Chinese scientists claim to have administered gossypol pills for at least six months to 4,000 men and demonstrated a contraceptive effectiveness rate of 99 percent. Some of the men were on the gossypol pill for more than six years. Fertility generally returns to normal within about three months of termination of use in most men. Some men experience lengthy delays in return of fertility, however. Cases of irreversible infertility (sterility) induced by gossypol have been reported. Gossypol has also been implicated in causing serious electrolyte imbalances in male users. Plasma potassium levels are particularly likely to be reduced.

Findings relative to the role of gossypol as a male oral contraceptive are intriguing, but effectiveness data is not conclusive. Well controlled clinical trials are needed. Additionally, fundamental issues of safety and reversibility of this method need clarification. Numerous gossypol derivatives are being tested to see if they possess advantages over the parent compound. Availability of gossypol or its derivatives as a male oral contraceptive is years away from the market, even if questions of effectiveness and safety are answered favorably.

CHLORINATED SUGARS

In an effort to arrive at new and more powerful artificial sweeteners, certain hydroxyl groups on glucose and sucrose were replaced with one to five chloride atoms. It was found that such changes in the basic sucrose molecule increased sweetness by 2,000 to 4,000 times. During routine toxicity testing, it was found, however, that some of the compounds inhibited male fertility by suppressing sperm motility.

Chlorinated sugars do not appear to have any adverse effect on libido, formation of sperm, or weight of testes when evaluated in rats. Functional androgen status does not appear to be impaired. Offspring of female rats mated with male rats who received chlorinated sugars were normally developed. Contraceptive effects of chlorinated sugars appear to be reversible when treatment is terminated.

The mechanism by which chlorinated sugars appear to impair sperm motility is based on their interference with carbohydrate metabolism in sperm. Sperm from animals treated with chlorinated sugars do not metabolize glucose properly and appear unable to produce the energy required for sperm motility and other essential processes of fertility.

ANTIPREGNANCY VACCINE

Human chorionic gonadotropin (HCG) is a hormone released by a freshly fertilized ovum that signals the body to release the hormone progesterone, preventing menstruation and preparation of the endometrium for implantation of the fertilized egg and development of the placenta. An Indian physician isolated part of the complex HCG molecule and produced a vaccine which stimulates the formation of HCG antibodies by the body. These antibodies neutralize HCG and block its signal to release progesterone. As a result, the next menses occurs and the ovum is washed out. Implantation of a fertilized ovum would not be possible.

Such a vaccine could be effective for several years, but the effects would not be reversible until the body's antibody count decreased greatly. If one desired to continue contraception, booster injections could be administered in the final months of the effective period.

Numerous theoretical advantages of a contraceptive vaccine exist. Several potential risks are also apparent. Years of study and evaluation will be needed to answer many of the questions of safety and effectiveness associated with such a vaccine contraceptive.

CONTRACEPTIVE NASAL SPRAYS

A promising new contraceptive method is the use of nasal sprays containing chemical cousins of the brain hormone, luteinizing hormone-releasing hormone (LHRH). These chemicals have been shown to temporarily inhibit sperm production in males and ovulation in females.

Much work remains in the development of such a contraceptive, which may be most effective when utilized by the male. Compounds similar to LHRH may interfere with the production of luteinizing hormone (LH) and follicle-stimulating hormone (FSH), thus suppressing the production of sperm by impairing testosterone production in the testes. Supplemental androgens would be required to maintain the male libido. Chronic use of androgens raises questions of safety. Effectiveness data is not available to date. LHRH-like chemicals are very unstable and lose most of their potency when taken orally. Daily injection of such a drug is impractical. The once or twice daily use of a nasal spray has been suggested, but reliability and patient acceptability of this delivery mode has not been evaluated.

OTHER INVESTIGATIONAL METHODS

DISPOSABLE DIAPHRAGM WITH CONTROLLED-RELEASE SPERMICIDE

A disposable diaphragm made of a synthetic elastomer with a nonmetallic reinforcement with the spermicide nonoxynol-9 premixed into the elastomer has been developed, and clinical testing began in 1984. The disposable diaphragm is stronger than traditional diaphragms made of latex. The nonoxynol-9 spermicide diffuses out of the diaphragm in a controlled fashion after insertion. The diaphragm, as currently designed, can be worn and is expected to be effective for up to 24 hours. The time-release feature eliminates the need for additional applications of spermicide if intercourse is repeated.

The disposable diaphragm with controlled-release spermicide would be fitted by a physician. Additional diaphragms would be purchased by a refillable prescription.

SPERM ENZYME INHIBITORS

Research is continuing in the area of sperm enzyme inhibitors. One European manufacturer is already marketing a vaginal suppository (A-Gen 53®) which contains a sperm enzyme inhibitor. Sperm enzyme inhibitors act either by immobilizing sperm or by preventing them from penetrating the ovum. In a clinical test involving 103 women, A-Gen 53® proved nontoxic, and the failure rate was only 1.1 pregnancies per 100 woman-years. No sperm enzyme inhibitors are currently available in the U.S., but researchers are optimistic about future use.

INTRACERVICAL DEVICES

Several intracervical devices (ICDs) that fit in the cervix of the uterus and release drugs continuously have been evaluated. Progestins or estrogens, or both, may be incorporated into the device.

Clinical trials have not shown any particular advantages of the ICD over the hormone-releasing IUD. The World Health Organization has discontinued research on ICDs because they do not appear to offer any contraceptive advantage over existing products.

PROPRANOLOL

Propranolol (Inderal®), one of the wonder drugs of the 1970s, which is used to treat high blood pressure, angina, migraine headache, irregular heart rhythm, and heart attack victims, may also have value as a contraceptive. Preliminary data suggests an 80 mg tablet inserted daily into the vagina may have substantial contraceptive effectiveness. A single 80 mg propranolol tablet was inserted intravaginally each evening from the last day of the menstrual cycle until the first day of the next menstrual cycle in 198 sexually active, nonlactating women over an 11-month period. The calculated pregnancy rate was 3.4 per 100 woman-years, comparable to the effectiveness of existing vaginal spermicides. No adverse effects were encountered.

Further studies are required to fully evaluate the safety and effectiveness of intravaginal propranolol as a contraceptive. Individuals should not use this contraceptive method until further testing is conducted.

CONCLUSION

A great deal of innovation in contraceptive methodology is occurring. Safety and effectiveness considerations are paramount. Some of the products presented in this chapter will likely reach the U.S. marketplace in the 1990s.

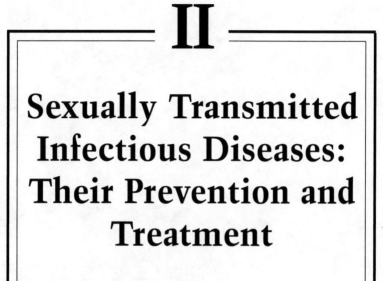

II

Sexually Transmitted Infectious Diseases: Their Prevention and Treatment

9

Gonorrhea

INTRODUCTION

Despite widespread and often sensational press coverage of genital herpes and acquired immune deficiency syndrome (AIDS), gonorrhea remains pervasive and one of the most serious of the sexually transmitted diseases. Gonorrhea is an infectious disease that can produce severe symptoms and, in some cases, severe complications if not treated appropriately.

References to a sexually transmitted infection, which was probably gonorrhea, are present in Biblical and ancient Chinese writings. It was Hippocrates who described some of the first scientific observations of gonococcal urethritis. Despite early references to the disease, it was not until 1879 that Albert Neisser isolated the bacteria responsible, *Neisseria gonorrhoeae*.

Gonorrhea, which is also known as "clap," "a dose," "strain," "gleet," "G.C.," "morning drop," and "the whites," affects only humans. Infection occurs when the microorganism *Neisseria gonorrhoeae* attaches itself to the walls of various tissues of the body, including the urethra, cervix, pharynx (throat), and rectum.

PREVALENCE OF GONORRHEA

Gonorrhea is one of the most frequently reported bacterial communicable diseases. Its prevalence (the number of people who are

183

infected at any given point in time) varies widely among different segments of the population. Nationally, about 2 percent of women seen by private physicians and 5 percent of women seen in gynecology clinics are reported to be infected. Approximately 1.3 to 1.8 million new cases of gonorrhea are reported in the United States each year, but the actual incidence rate is estimated to be nearer 2.5 million per year because many cases are not reported. Gonorrhea occurs at least 10 to 20 times more frequently than syphilis. The incidence of gonorrhea in the United States increased dramatically between the 1950s and the late 1970s, then leveled off and even decreased slightly. Some have suggested that this slight decline in incidence may be due to a reduction in the average number of sexual partners or increased use of barrier contraceptives due to fear of developing genital herpes or AIDS.

Gonorrhea affects both men and women, with a 1.5:1 male to female ratio. Persons between the ages of 16 and 24 are most frequently affected, and 85 percent of patients with gonorrhea are 30 years of age or younger. The disease is more prevalent in urban areas, nonwhite populations, persons of low socioeconomic status, those with multiple sexual partners, females using intrauterine devices (IUDs), and among single persons living alone. Persons living in rural areas, those with higher socioeconomic status, married individuals, and those using barrier forms of contraception (condoms, diaphragms) have lower than average prevalence rates.

CAUSES OF GONORRHEA

Gonorrhea occurs when *Neisseria gonorrhoeae* is transmitted from an infected individual to a noninfected person. In order for transmission to take place and cause an infection, the bacteria must attach itself to the wall of mucous tissue and begin to grow and reproduce. The most frequently affected tissues are the urethra (the canal carrying urine from the bladder to the outside), cervix, pharynx (throat), and rectum.

SPREAD OF GONORRHEA

The bacteria responsible for gonorrhea die upon drying. Although it is conceivable that the disease could be spread by touching contaminated inanimate objects, gonorrhea is almost exclusively spread through sexual contact. One of the major problems in controlling gonorrhea is that many infected people have minor symptoms or no symptoms at all. Because of the lack of symptoms, these persons do not realize they have the disease and unknowingly transmit it to their sexual partners. These asymptomatic persons do not seek treatment and accumulate in the population. It is estimated that 80 percent of females, and 50 to 70 percent of males, with gonorrhea have minor or no symptoms; these individuals are the primary transmitters of the disease. It is important to realize that individuals with no symptoms are just as infectious as those who have obvious symptoms.

The type of sexual contact is important in determining the likelihood of infection. For instance, it is estimated that 60 to 80 percent of females having intercourse with a male with urethral gonorrhea will develop the disease, whereas only approximately 30 to 35 percent of males having sex with an infected female will develop gonorrhea after a single exposure. Oral-genital sex with an infected male creates a high probability of producing a gonococcal infection of the throat (pharyngeal gonorrhea) while oral-genital contact with an infected female will rarely result in pharyngeal gonorrhea in the sexual partner. Homosexual contact between males frequently results in the spread of gonorrhea; however, contact between homosexual females results in a much lower incidence of transmission.

Although young adults are most frequently affected by gonorrhea, infants and children are also victimized by the disease. The gonococcal organism may infect the thin membrane covering the eyes (conjunctiva), throat (pharynx), lungs, or anal canal of a baby during childbirth if the mother has gonorrhea. In female children from one year of age to puberty, vulvovaginal gonorrhea occasionally occurs due to sexual molestation, usually by an infected relative.

SYMPTOMS OF GONORRHEA

As mentioned previously, gonorrhea may produce a broad spectrum of clinical effects ranging from no symptoms at all to severe disease affecting several different parts of the body at one time (see Table 20). In males, one of the most common manifestations is infection of the urethra, known as gonococcal urethritis. Symptoms usually occur after a two-day to two-week incubation period. Symptoms may include a clear or milky discharge, painful and frequent urination, and redness of the tip of the penis. Symptoms may be so mild that there is only a slight tingling or an unusual sensation in the penis on urination. There may also be a few drops of clear discharge prior to urination in the morning ("morning drop"). Rarely, the gonococcus may spread from the urethra to the epididymis or prostate gland and cause infection. Many men who develop gonococcal urethritis will experience at least mild symptoms and discharge. Some seek treatment, but others never have, or ignore, symptoms and transmit the infection to others.

TABLE 20
EARLY SYMPTOMS OF GONORRHEA*

Sex	Area of Involvement	Symptoms
Male	Urethra (canal carrying urine from the bladder to the outside)	Urethral discharge (clear or milky; 2 to 14 days after infection)
		Frequent urination
		Painful urination
		Slight redness at end of penis
	Anorectal Region	Rectal mucous discharge
		Slight bleeding
		Burning and itching
	Pharyngeal Region	Local inflammation such as sore throat, enlarged tonsils, or swollen lymph nodes
Female	Cervix	Frequent and painful urination
		Increased vaginal discharge
		Abnormal menstrual bleeding
		Lower abdominal pain
	Anorectal Region	Rectal mucous discharge
		Slight bleeding
		Burning and itching
	Pharyngeal Region	Local inflammation such as sore throat, enlarged tonsils, or swollen lymph nodes

*Approximately 80 percent of females and 50 to 70 percent of males with gonorrhea will have no symptoms or minor symptoms that generally are not recognized.

In females, the most frequent manifestation of gonorrhea is inflammation of the cervix of the uterus. Symptoms of this infection may include painful and frequent urination (which may be misinterpreted as a sign of a bladder infection), increased vaginal discharge, abnormal menstrual bleeding, anorectal discomfort, and low abdominal pain. If untreated, the gonococcus may spread to the fallopian tubes and cause pelvic inflammatory disease (PID), which occurs in approximately 15 percent of women with gonococcal infection of the cervix. Vaginitis is rare, except in children who have been sexually abused.

The throat and anorectal regions may be affected in both men and women. Anorectal infection is usually seen in women (as an extension of cervical involvement) and homosexual men. This form of infection often produces no symptoms, but affected individuals may notice a mucous rectal discharge, slight bleeding, anal burning or itching, and constipation. Pharyngeal infection occurs in 20 percent of homosexual men and 20 percent of women who regularly engage in fellatio. It occurs in only 5 percent of heterosexual men with gonorrhea, and is transmitted by cunnilingus. Pharyngeal involvement usually produces no symptoms, although tonsillitis and local inflammation may occur.

A less frequent, but more serious, manifestation of the disease is disseminated gonorrhea, also known as the arthritis-dermatitis syndrome. This is caused when the gonococcus enters the bloodstream and is spread throughout the body. Patients with disseminated gonorrhea usually do not have symptoms of urethral, cervical, pharyngeal, or anorectal infection. The onset of this syndrome is characterized by fever, painful joints, and skin lesions. Several joints are usually affected, with the wrists, fingers, knees, and ankles most often involved. The skin lesions usually occur on the arms, wrists, hands, ankles, and feet. They begin as red patches which progress to small blisters and then pustules. As the sores develop, their centers become gray in color. Eventually, the skin lesions fade leaving no scar. The arthritis-dermatitis syndrome may spontaneously resolve within a week, or it may progress to a potentially severe arthritis (septic arthritis). One or more joints may become painful and swollen with accumulation of fluid in the joint space. If untreated, progressive destruction of the joint may occur. In addition to septic arthritis, disseminated gonococcal infection may rarely affect the heart (endocarditis) or the brain (meningitis).

ADDITIONAL COMPLICATIONS OF GONORRHEA

In both sexes, untreated gonorrhea may lead to numerous complications, including disseminated disease as described above and its complications of severe septic arthritis, meningitis, and endocarditis (see Table 21). In males, recurrent urethral infections may lead to an extension of the infection to the epididymis or to urethral stricture (narrowing). Females are particularly at risk for developing complications secondary to gonorrhea. In addition to the potential for disseminated disease, females may develop pelvic inflammatory disease (PID). This is caused by the spread of *Neisseria gonorrhoeae* from the cervix to the endometrium, fallopian tubes, and ovaries. It is

TABLE 21
POTENTIAL COMPLICATIONS OF UNTREATED GONORRHEA

Sex	Complication
Male	Epididymitis (inflammation of the epididymis) Prostatitis (inflammation of the prostate gland) Seminal vesiculitis (inflammation of the seminal vesicle) Periurethral abscess (a localized pus-containing infection in the area of the urethra) Cystitis (inflammation of the bladder) Arthritis-dermatitis syndrome (characterized by fever, painful joints and skin lesions; occurs only if gonococcus is disseminated throughout the bloodstream) Sterility (secondary to scarring in the male reproductive tract) Endocarditis (rare; occurs only if gonorrhea is disseminated throughout bloodstream) Meningitis (rare; occurs only if gonorrhea is disseminated throughout bloodstream)
Female	Involvement of Skene's and Bartholin's glands (which may become infected and inflamed due to their location external to the vaginal opening) Parametritis (inflammation of the uterus) Cystitis (inflammation of the bladder) Proctitis (inflammation of the rectum) Pelvic Inflammatory Disease: • salpingitis (inflammation of the fallopian tube(s)) • pelvic abscess (a localized, pus containing infection in the pelvic region) • pyosalpinx (fallopian tube swollen with pus) • adhesions (scar tissue) • peritonitis (inflammation of tissue lining the abdominal cavity) Sterility (secondary to scarring in the fallopian tubes) Endocarditis (rare; occurs only if gonorrhea is disseminated throughout bloodstream) Meningitis (rare; occurs only if gonorrhea is disseminated throughout bloodstream)

estimated that the incidence of PID due to all causes in the United States is in considerable excess of one million cases per year, with 20 to 50 percent of the cases due to gonorrhea. Ten to 15 percent of these cases result in infertility (sterility) due to blockage of the fallopian tubes.

DIAGNOSIS OF GONORRHEA

A positive diagnosis of gonorrhea is made by identifying *Neisseria gonorrhoeae* in the urethral or cervical discharge or any site of sexual contact. Nonprescription (over-the-counter) home specimen kits for gonorrhea detection have been marketed recently. The manufacturer claims 95 percent accuracy if a good specimen is obtained. The kit includes a sterile swab, slide, slide case, laboratory instruction, and a code number to maintain confidentiality when reporting results. The test is self-administered, mailed to a laboratory, and analyzed, and results are available by toll-free telephone number. The diagnosis should be confirmed by a physician prior to initiation of treatment.

TREATMENT OF GONORRHEA

Fortunately, most strains of *Neisseria gonorrhoeae* are susceptible to a large number of antibiotics including penicillins, cephalosporins, tetracyclines, and erythromycin. The site of infection, severity of disease, and likelihood of patient compliance with therapy are all important factors in choosing appropriate treatment. See Table 22 for treatment guidelines of uncomplicated gonorrhea infections.

For uncomplicated infections of the urethra or cervix, penicillins or tetracyclines are most often used. The penicillins, including intramuscular injection of procaine penicillin G or oral ampicillin or amoxicillin, are usually given as a single dose with probenecid. Probenecid decreases the elimination of penicillin through the kidneys and results in higher concentrations of penicillin. Advantages of the penicillins are their low cost, high cure rate, relative safety during pregnancy, and high compliance rate due to the need for only a single dose. Disadvantages are the risk of penicillin allergy and the potential emergence of postgonococcal (chlamydial) urethritis after treatment. The syndrome of postgonococcal urethritis usually becomes apparent two to three weeks after treatment of gonorrhea. It is due to infection of the urethra by *Chlamydia trachomatis*. This organism may infect a person at the same time as the gonococcus, but is not

TABLE 22
COMMONLY EMPLOYED TREATMENT OF UNCOMPLICATED GONORRHEA INVOLVING THE URETHRA, CERVIX, PHARYNX, OR RECTUM IN THE ADULT

Site of Infection	Drug	Comments (See legend on next page)
Urethra[1]/ Cervix	*Treatments of Choice* (not in order of preference)	
	Oral amoxicillin 3.0 gm plus oral probenecid 1 gm (one dose)	2,3
	Oral ampicillin 3.5 gm plus oral probenecid 1 gm (one dose)	2,3
	Procaine penicillin G 4.8 million units intramuscularly (i.m.) plus oral probenecid 1 gm (one dose)	2,3,4
	Combined regimen of oral amoxicillin or ampicillin at the above doses followed by oral tetracycline 500 mg four times daily for 7 days or oral doxycycline 100 mg 2 times a day for 7 days.	8
	Alternative Treatments (not in order of preference)	
	Oral tetracycline 500 mg 4 times a day for 7 days	5,6,7,8
	Oral doxycycline 100 mg 2 times a day for 7 days	5,6,7,8
	Spectinomycin 2 gm i.m. (one dose) if resistant to penicillins	2,4,5
	Cefoxitin 2 gm i.m. plus oral probenecid 1 gm (one dose)	2,4,5
Pharyngeal (area of the throat)	Procaine penicillin G 4.8 million units i.m. plus oral probenecid 1 gm (one dose)	2,4
	Oral tetracycline 500 mg 4 times a day for 7 days	5,6,7
	Oral doxycycline 100 mg 2 times a day for 7 days	5,6,7

Anorectal (rectal area)	Procaine penicillin G 4.8 million units i.m. plus oral probenecid 1 gm (one dose)	2,4
	Spectinomycin 2 gm i.m. (one dose)	2,4,5
	Cefoxitin 2 gm i.m. plus oral probenecid 1 gm (one dose)	2,4,5

[1] Urethra of male and female
[2] Single dose treatment
[3] Will not treat postgonococcal urethritis
[4] Requires injection
[5] Acceptable alternative if patient is allergic to penicillin
[6] Do not use in pregnancy
[7] Requires strict patient compliance
[8] Will also treat postgonococcal urethritis due to chlamydial infection

adequately treated by penicillin or a cephalosporin antibiotic. Postgonococcal urethritis due to *Chlamydia trachomatis* can usually be effectively treated with tetracycline or doxycycline.

Tetracyclines are relatively safe and effective alternatives to penicillin, and may eliminate the possibility of postgonococcal urethritis since they act against both *Neisseria gonorrhoeae* and *Chlamydia trachomatis*. However, they must be taken for seven days and should not be used in pregnant women. If a pregnant woman is allergic to penicillin, then ceftriaxone, spectinomycin, or erythromycin are good alternatives. Treated individuals should return to the physician four to seven days after treatment to verify they are cured.

For those with anorectal or pharyngeal infections, intramuscular procaine penicillin G plus probenecid is effective. However, oral penicillins such as ampicillin and amoxicillin have high failure rates. Tetracyclines are effective therapy for pharyngeal infections, but ineffective if there is anorectal involvement. In those with anorectal gonorrhea who are allergic to penicillin, spectinomycin is an effective alternative.

Disseminated gonorrhea usually requires hospitalization and intravenous antibiotic therapy. Penicillin G, ampicillin, or amoxicillin are usually administered intravenously until clinical improvement occurs, followed by seven to ten days of oral therapy. Alternatively, certain intravenous cephalosporins may be utilized (such as cefoxitin, cefotaxime, or ceftriaxone). Meningitis and endocarditis are usually treated with high doses of intravenous penicillin or selected cephalosporins.

Since 1980, there have been increased outbreaks of penicillin-resistant *Neisseria gonorrhoeae,* especially in large cities, including New York, San Diego, and Miami. Until recently, resistant organisms were usually encountered in persons who contracted the disease in Southeast Asia or the Philippines. Resistance to penicillin and the tetracyclines is a result of the production of an enzyme (penicillinase) by the bacteria. These resistant organisms are commonly referred to as penicillinase-producing *Neisseria gonorrhoeae* (PPNG). Over 10 percent of the reported cases of gonorrhea are due to PPNG, but the incidence is certain to increase. Eventually, penicillins and tetracyclines may not be effective for many cases, and alternative antibiotic therapy must be sought. Agents including spectinomycin, sulfamethoxazole-trimethoprim, and ceftriaxone have been used effectively to treat resistant cases. At present, PPNG need only be suspected if gonorrhea is contracted overseas or if appropriate therapy with a penicillin or tetracycline fails to produce a cure.

Because gonorrhea often produces no symptoms, it is extremely important that all recent sexual partners of an infected individual be traced and receive treatment so as not to unknowingly transmit the infection to others. Treatment of all sexual partners is also essential in order to avoid a "ping-pong effect," which occurs when a person who contracts gonorrhea transmits the infection to a previously unin-fected sexual partner. Subsequently, the gonorrhea victim is treated, but the asymptomatic partner is not. When sexual contact is re-sumed, the person is quickly reinfected by his or her partner.

PREVENTION OF GONORRHEA

The only absolute way to prevent gonorrhea is to abstain from sexual contact. Condoms are relatively effective in preventing trans-mission, and condoms plus contraceptive spermicides are even more effective. Douching by females and urination after intercourse are not reliable preventive measures. Researchers are attempting to produce a vaccine against gonorrhea, but it is not yet available. It is a common misconception that once a person has had gonorrhea he or she is immune to further infections. A person can become infected repeat-edly through contact with an infected sexual partner, regardless of whether or not they have been previously infected.

CONCLUSION

Gonorrhea may be a very serious disease, particularly if not diagnosed promptly and treated effectively. Complications of untreated gonorrhea can severely impair the quality of life—and may be fatal. Situations complicating treatment of gonorrhea are the emergence of resistant strains of the bacteria causing gonorrhea, failure of some victims to demonstrate symptoms early in the disease, a casual public attitude about the importance of treatment, and failure to identify and treat all sexual partners of infected individuals. Better control of this prevalent, but highly treatable, disease cannot occur until victims become more conscientious and informed about how gonorrhea is spread, its symptoms and complications, the importance of prompt and effective treatment, and steps which may be taken to prevent the disease.

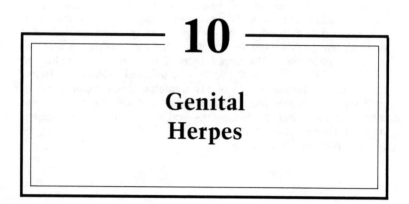

10

Genital
Herpes

INTRODUCTION

Genital herpes has become a major health problem in the United States, reaching epidemic proportions over the last two decades. Many people are terrified of herpes because they are aware that it is an incurable disease. Although genital herpes is generating a great deal of public concern, it is important to realize that except in severe cases the disease is far from being a life-threatening condition.

Genital herpes is a disease associated with a great deal of confusion and anxiety. Facts about genital herpes include:

1. Genital herpes affects both males and females.
2. Approximately 30 percent of those who develop genital herpes never suffer another attack of lesions.
3. Only 5 to 10 percent of those with genital herpes will suffer from frequent, recurrent attacks (more than six episodes per year).
4. Except for the developing fetus, the newborn, and those with an immune system deficiency, genital herpes is *not* a life-threatening condition.
5. Although no cure is available for genital herpes, new drugs have been developed which reduce or minimize the frequency and severity of genital herpes attacks.

Derived from the Greek term "herpein" meaning "to creep," the term herpes has been used throughout the centuries to describe a number of spreading lesions that appear on the skin. The disease was familiar to ancient Romans, who attempted to rid themselves of herpes by placing a ban on kissing. During the 1700s, Parisians witnessed a near epidemic of genital herpes.

It was not until 1814 that Thomas Bateman applied the term "herpes" to lesions appearing on the genitals. In the late 19th century, researchers surmised that genital herpes was in some way related to sexual intercourse. In 1912, a particular type of herpes, called herpes simplex virus (HSV) was discovered. In 1946 HSV was isolated in the laboratory from a human being. Since that time, herpes has progressed from being a relatively obscure microorganism to being the causative agent of one of the most widely feared diseases affecting men and women.

PREVALENCE OF GENITAL HERPES

As many as 20 million people in the U.S. harbor HSV-1 or HSV-2 (the two strains of the virus). Since 1966 there has been a 10-fold increase in the number of reported cases, with 300,000 to 500,000 new cases occurring each year. Only two other sexually transmitted diseases (gonorrhea and nongonococcal urethritis) occur more often than genital herpes. At a given time, however, herpes is present in a larger number of people since it is incurable.

Although social, economic, and racial status are not factors in determining who develops genital herpes, certain groups of people are more likely to get the disease based on sexual practices. Persons most likely to develop genital herpes begin to have sex at an early age, have multiple partners, and engage in sex frequently. Individuals between 15 to 41 years are in the group most often infected by genital herpes. Another development contributing to the rise of genital herpes is the widespread use of contraceptive methods, such as oral contraceptives (birth control pills) and intrauterine devices (IUDs), that offer little or no protection against sexually transmitted diseases.

TYPES OF HERPES VIRUS

Cold sores, chickenpox, and shingles all have one thing in common—each is caused by a herpes virus. There are about 50 different types of herpes virus, but only the following five are known to affect humans:

1. Herpes Simplex Virus Type 1 (HSV-1)
2. Herpes Simplex Virus Type 2 (HSV-2)
3. Varicella-Zoster Virus (VZV)
4. Epstein-Barr Virus
5. Cytomegalovirus (CMV)

Of these five viruses, the herpes simplex varieties (HSV-1 and HSV-2) cause what is known as genital herpes. The HSV-1 variety of herpes simplex is the primary cause of cold sores. Varicella-Zoster (also called herpes zoster) is best known as chickenpox, and reappears later in adult years in some persons in the form of shingles. The Epstein-Barr virus is otherwise known as mononucleosis (also "mono" or "kissing disease"). Cytomegalovirus (CMV) occasionally causes hepatitis or mononucleosis.

GENITAL HERPES AND HOW IT IS SPREAD

Genital herpes is caused by the herpes simplex virus (HSV), which is generally transmitted by direct contact with an active lesion located on the skin or mucous membranes (mouth, lips, labia, vagina, urethra, or penis). After exposure, the virus migrates along nerve fibers to the junctions of the nerves located next to the spinal cord called sensory nerve ganglia. The virus may remain in the nerve cells for life in a latent (inactive) stage. Several weeks, months, or years later it may return along the nerve fibers to reappear on the surface of the skin or mucous membranes to cause another infection (see Figure 29).

Until the last two decades, the two types of herpes simplex viruses were fairly easy to distinguish, not from appearance (both types produce lesions that look about the same), but from where they appeared on the body. Herpes simplex virus type 1 (HSV-1) was traditionally responsible for infections above the waist, particularly involving the mouth, lips, throat, eyes, brain, and joints (arthritis). Most people recognize HSV-1 lesions as common cold sores.

Because of the increasing variety of sexual practices, genital herpes can be spread in several ways. The practice of oral-genital, anal-genital, and oral-anal sex has weakened the traditional boundaries that seemed to confine genital herpes in the past. The incidence of HSV-2 occurring in the mouth or throat, and HSV-1 appearing in the genital or rectal area has increased steadily over the last two decades. The highest incidence of herpes appearing in nontraditional locations occurs in 18 to 24 year olds, reflecting this group's lack of knowledge and/or more liberal attitude toward sexual practices. Nonetheless, herpes simplex virus type 2 (HSV-2) is the virus re-

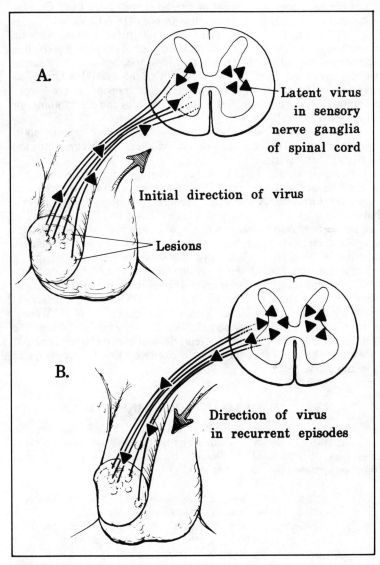

FIGURE 29

Pathway of herpes virus infection in initial genital herpes episode (A) and in recurrent episodes (B)

sponsible for about 85 percent of genital herpes infections. On rare occasion, some people are infected with both HSV-1 and HSV-2.

Genital herpes is most often transmitted by contact with an active lesion or fluid from a lesion during sexual contact. Rarely, it is transmitted by the hands. Hands that have touched an active lesion are the major cause of herpes infection of the eye (also known as herpes keratitis or ocular herpes). The risk of transmission of herpes by contact with contaminated surfaces (such as towels, clothing, or toilet seats) is small, but real.

The saliva of an individual with active lesions may be contagious. Approximately 10 percent of those infected have a high concentration of virus in their saliva.

The question has been raised concerning the possible transmission of herpes simplex virus (HSV) via water from hot tubs and accessory furniture. A group of researchers collected water from a hot tub in a health spa and found no evidence of HSV virus in the sample tested. Additionally, when spa water was added to herpes simplex samples kept on hand in a lab, the virus was immediately inactivated. However, when HSV lab samples were placed in tap water and distilled water, the virus survived for up to 4.5 hours. Since HSV lab samples survived for several hours in tap and distilled water, there may be a chance, although slight, that HSV can be transmitted via avenues other than human contact. Transmission of HSV from water at a public swimming pool, however, is very unlikely due to the high chlorine and/or bromine content. Several experts have noted that rubbing of the skin or even rubbing broken skin may be necessary to transmit HSV.

TYPES OF GENITAL HERPES INFECTIONS

Herpes simplex virus (HSV) infections are classified according to whether or not the individual has experienced a previous infection of either type of virus. The following are the classifications of genital infections caused by the herpes simplex virus:

1. *Primary initial* is when an individual has had no previous exposure to infection by herpes simplex virus.
2. *Nonprimary initial* is when an individual has been previously exposed to infection by herpes simplex virus.
3. *Recurrent* or *reactivated* is subsequent flareup of HSV when an individual has experienced a previous episode of primary or nonprimary infection due to herpes simplex virus.

Clinicians determine the type of initial genital herpes infection an individual has by testing for herpes simplex virus antibodies circulating in the blood. Lack of antibodies in the blood signifies no previous exposure to HSV; therefore, the individual is said to have a primary genital herpes infection.

If antibodies for herpes simplex virus are found, the infection is considered nonprimary initial herpes. Antibodies circulating in the blood indicate that the individual has experienced a previous herpes simplex virus infection. At least 80 percent of adults possess antibodies to HSV-1 by age 25 (see Figure 30). The prevalence of HSV-2 antibodies increases during adolescence through young adulthood, which coincides with increasing sexual activity in these age groups.

With most other infectious diseases the presence of antibodies in the blood may signify that the individual has developed a degree of protection (immunity) to the organism. Herpes simplex virus antibodies are unable to enter the nervous system where the virus is free to reproduce. Only when the herpes simplex virus (HSV) leaves the nervous system can circulating antibodies have any beneficial effect. Although the herpes antibodies in the blood may protect the individual from widespread internal herpes infection, they cannot prevent a

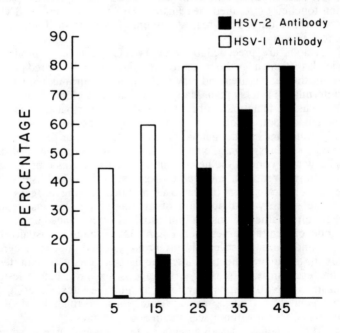

FIGURE 30

Percent of individuals in U.S. with HSV antibodies

recurrent herpes episode due to their inability to eliminate the virus from the sensory nerve ganglia of the central nervous system.

The presence of HSV-1 antibodies suggests that the individual may have the ability to form antibodies to HSV-2. If the initial infection was caused by HSV-1, instead of HSV-2, the individual is less likely to suffer a recurrent episode of genital herpes.

Approximately 5 to 10 million cases of recurrent genital herpes infections occur annually in the United States. About two-thirds of these had an initial genital herpes infection caused by HSV-2. Less than 10 percent of those infected initially with HSV-1 have recurrent genital herpes attacks.

SIGNS AND SYMPTOMS OF GENITAL HERPES

Although the name may indicate otherwise, genital herpes affects a wide variety of areas in and on the body. The most visible sign of genital herpes is the appearance of a small, soft, blisterlike area (vesicle), which ruptures to form genital sores (ulcers) that are painful when touched or scraped (see Figure 31). Active lesions shed virus for about five days. The greatest amount of virus is shed during day number two of an attack.

Lesions are preceded by what is referred to as a prodrome, which lasts from a few hours up to a few days. Vesicles or red patches form in the genital area and may cause itching, burning, tenderness, or intermittent prickly pain. Many individuals experience fever, headache, tension, facial pain, and/or pain of the lower back, groin, buttock, leg, or foot. Throughout the infection, a generalized swelling of the lymph glands in the genital area may occur. Four to seven days (average six days) from the appearance of initial symptoms, blisters appear which contain the herpes simplex virus. At this time, general discomfort is reduced, and the prodrome subsides. The blisters then break open, drain, crust or scab over, and heal leaving no scars.

The severity and duration of genital herpes lesions depend largely on whether or not the individual has experienced a previous episode of genital herpes (see Figure 32). Symptoms usually last longer and are more severe during primary initial attacks of herpes virus. In a primary infection, after the herpes virus is transmitted it incubates from two to 20 days (average is six days) before lesions appear. Up to 20 lesions may form at multiple sites, covering the entire genital area during primary infections. Fortunately, HSV lesions usually heal without scarring in about 14 days.

Primary genital herpes infections may involve large areas and often form lesions on both sides of the genitals. The most common site for lesions to appear in males is on the shaft and glans (head) of the penis. In females, lesions appear most often on the cervix. Cer-

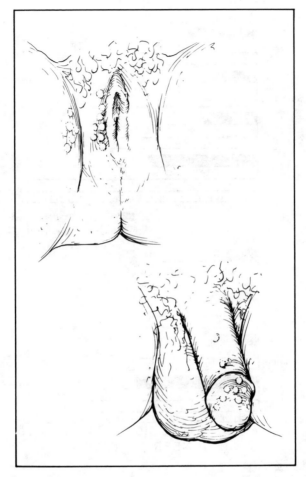

FIGURE 31
Typical genital herpes lesions

vical lesions are much harder to detect and more difficult to treat, which may attest at least partially to why herpes infections are more severe and last longer in women than in men. In women, lesions in an initial genital herpes infection remain active about 10 days and may take up to 20 days to heal. In men, lesions last only about half as long. Figure 32 reveals the course of the disease and the longer duration of symptoms that women experience.

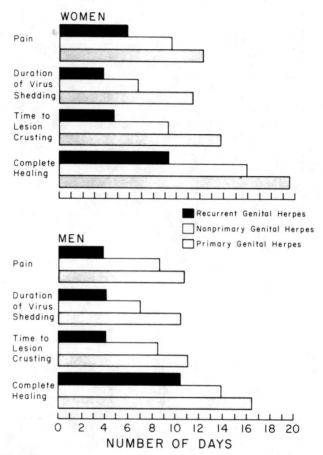

FIGURE 32

Genital herpes infections and duration of selected signs and symptoms between women and men

Only approximately one-half of those with primary genital herpes experience internal (systemic) symptoms such as headache, stiff neck, difficult or painful urination, and mild intolerance to light. Abdominal pain accompanies genital lesions in most women. Fortunately, only approximately one in three individuals with genital herpes suffer recurring attacks. A large number of those experiencing recurrent attacks report that frequency and severity of symptoms are reduced with the passage of time.

Symptoms are less severe and of shorter duration in a nonprimary initial infection. Many times, less than three lesions appear. Those having a nonprimary episode also have milder recurrent attacks.

Recurrent episodes of genital herpes may be triggered by emotional stress, physical stress, sunlight and/or ultraviolet light exposure, lack of sleep, poor diet, infection, fever, menstruation, wearing tight jeans or leotards, and consumption of drugs that compromise the immune system.

In a recurrent infection, 30 percent of women report only one lesion. Three out of four women experience three lesions or less. Recurrent infections last the fewest days (average is five to 10) and often produce only mild symptoms.

Genital herpes can be confused with other sexually transmitted diseases (STDs) that cause genital lesions (sores). Chancroid, another cause of genital lesions, is similar in appearance to genital herpes. Syphilis sores (chancres) may also be mistaken for genital herpes lesions. Symptoms of genital herpes, such as swollen genital lymph glands, are also mimicked in chlamydia infections.

Although a cure for genital herpes does not yet exist, you should seek medical advice if a herpes-like genital lesion appears, because treatments to reduce spreading and alleviate symptoms are available. It is unwise to self-diagnose herpes lesions, especially since the disease can be so easily mistaken for another condition which is curable. It is essential to notify the physician at the first sign of a genital lesion. The physician must perform tests in order to confirm the exact cause of a genital lesion.

COMPLICATIONS OF GENITAL HERPES

Although the disease can be very uncomfortable, genital herpes does not represent a serious or life-threatening condition for most people. However, in a few cases genital herpes can be devastating, especially to unborn children, newborns, and immune deficient patients.

GENITAL HERPES INFECTION DURING PREGNANCY

One of the most tragic consequences of genital herpes is transmitting the infection to a newborn (neonatal herpes). The rate at which neonatal herpes is increasing coincides with the overall rate of increase of genital herpes infections in adults. In one study, the rate of herpes infection seen in newborns more than quadrupled between 1966 and 1981 (from 2.6 to 11.9 cases per 100,000 births). The trans-

---

TABLE 23
PRECAUTIONS FOR PREGNANT AND NURSING WOMEN

1. The physician should be informed if a previous episode of genital lesions has ever occurred because genital herpes infection is not apparent in 50 to 70 percent of expectant mothers.
2. The physician should be informed if any past or present sexual partner of the mother-to-be has ever had a genital herpes infection.
3. Avoid sex during the last months of pregnancy, so as not to activate a latent infection—especially if a sexual partner has a history of genital herpes.
4. Mothers with active genital herpes should wear sterile gowns and wash hands frequently with a mild soap when attending the newborn.
5. A mother with active genital herpes can breast-feed an infant as long as no herpes lesions are present on the breast.

---

mission of either HSV-1 or HSV-2 to a newborn infant as it passes through an infected birth canal is fatal in a majority of cases.

Approximately three out of five infants die within hours after vaginal delivery if the mother is infected with genital herpes. Surviving infants often suffer blindness and serious central nervous system damage.

HSV-2 is the cause of the majority of herpes virus infections of newborns. The risk to newborns is greatest if active herpes infection is present in women prior to vaginal delivery or membranes ruptured more than four hours prior to vaginal delivery. The chance of infection is greatly reduced if the infant is delivered by cesarian section within four hours after the rupture of membranes.

Fifty to 70 percent of expectant mothers with genital herpes infection have no symptoms of the disease. Although only one percent of infected mothers have active, contagious lesions at the time of birth, by one estimate infection of newborns with herpes causes over 500 infant deaths a year. Pregnant women should inform the obstetrician of any prior occurrence or exposure to genital herpes. It may very well save the life of the unborn child. Other precautions to be observed by the pregnant or nursing woman are included in Table 23. If an expectant mother or sexual partner has ever had a genital herpes infection, the physician may recommend a weekly laboratory test beginning in the 36th week of pregnancy.

GENITAL HERPES AND CANCER IN FEMALES

Evidence is accumulating which suggests a relationship between cervical cancer and herpes virus infections. Cervical cancer in women that have also had genital herpes often occurs at the same site on the cervix as where herpes lesions appeared. A similar association between genital herpes and cancer of the external genitalia in women (vulval cancer) has also been noted. Although the link between herpes infection and female genital cancer is strong, it remains unproven that herpes is the actual causal agent. Females with genital herpes should have a Pap smear at least twice annually.

OTHER COMPLICATIONS

Herpes pharyngitis (infection in the throat) can be caused by HSV-1 or HSV-2 and occurs in about 10 percent of those affected by genital herpes. The incidence of vaginitis (inflammation of the vagina) caused by HSV-2 has increased dramatically in the last decade. Other than gonorrhea, herpes simplex virus infection is the most common cause of proctitis (inflammation and infection of the rectum) in homosexual men. As mentioned previously, immune deficient patients are at high risk for developing disseminated herpes infection that may cause serious and possibly fatal consequences. Genital herpes strikes patients whose immune system, for reasons such as surgery, long-term illness, cancer, or chemotherapy for cancer, has become weakened. Genital herpes infections are more frequently reported in homosexual men having AIDS (Acquired Immune Deficiency Syndrome).

Viral meningitis (herpes infection of the brain and/or spinal cord of the central nervous system) occurs in four to eight percent of initial herpes infections, and is usually an uncomfortable, but rarely severe infection. In contrast, herpetic encephalitis (inflammation of the brain) is ultimately fatal in approximately 80 percent of those who experience this complication.

If a lesion is scratched or pricked, a secondary bacterial infection may occur. On occasion, fungal infections develop in the vagina, characteristically during the second week after herpes lesions appear.

TREATMENT OF GENITAL HERPES

Since no current treatment will completely eliminate either HSV-1 or HSV-2 from the body, genital herpes is an incurable infectious disease. Since an immediate cure and prevention of spread has eluded pharmaceutical research, treatment of genital herpes is aimed primarily at reducing discomfort of the symptoms. This is done in two ways. First, drugs are used to prevent the spread of herpes simplex virus near the site of the lesion and throughout the body (antiviral therapy). Second, other drugs and methods are used to reduce the symptoms of the disease such as pain, fever, and general discomfort (supportive therapy).

The following are the goals of treating the most common symptom, genital lesions:

1. Faster healing
2. Less pain during healing
3. Reduction of viral shedding time
4. Shorter period in which lesions are contagious
5. Fewer recurrences

Some of the newer antiviral agents fulfill some of the goals listed above.

MODERN ANTIVIRAL THERAPY

The following four drugs are approved for use against herpes infections:

1. Acyclovir (ACV)
2. Idoxuridine (IDU)
3. Trifluridine
4. Vidarabine

The mainstay of modern drug therapy for treatment of genital lesions caused by HSV-1 or HSV-2 is acyclovir (Zovirax®). Acyclovir (ACV) is the first drug to show enhanced antiviral action without significant toxicity. To date, acyclovir is the only compound approved by the FDA that has demonstrated effectiveness in treatment of the primary initial episode of genital herpes simplex virus infection.

Acyclovir works by inhibiting the formation of DNA in the virus-infected cell without interfering with DNA formation in normal human cells. In laboratory tests, acyclovir has proven to be an effective antiviral agent against both HSV-1 and HSV-2. It has also shown potential for use against Varicella-Zoster Virus (VZV), Epstein-Barr virus, and ocular herpes.

ACV comes in ointment, oral, and intravenous forms. Lesions in a primary infection disappear more rapidly, and the length of time they are contagious is shortened significantly when ACV is utilized.

ACV as a 5 percent ointment is effective in reducing the duration and severity of the symptoms in primary initial genital herpes infection (see Figure 33). Other than reducing the duration of viral shedding, the ointment is of little benefit when applied to lesions during recurrent attacks, and is not generally recommended in recurrent

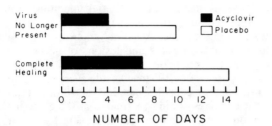

FIGURE 33

Comparison of treatment of initial herpes lesion with acyclovir and placebo*

*Patients experienced initial infection for up to 6 days before beginning therapy.

attacks because the duration of symptoms are short-lived. ACV ointment is seldom effective if therapy is not started immediately after symptoms develop. Applying ACV ointment to recurrent lesions may be more helpful to men than women. This is perhaps due to a greater number of external, therefore, more noticeable lesions that appear in males, which may allow earlier application of ACV ointment. Even then, ACV ointment may only be useful when large areas are affected by herpes lesions.

Best results are obtained when ACV ointment is applied to all genital herpes lesions every three hours, six times a day for seven days. The ointment should be applied with a rubber finger protector or rubber glove to avoid spreading the infection to other parts of the body. ACV ointment should be applied for no more and no less than the full seven-day course, regardless of how lesions have healed. If an application is missed, apply ointment as soon as possible, but not if it is almost time for the next application. Apply ACV ointment to the entire affected area, not just on the lesion(s). If no improvement is noted after one week, call your physician. ACV ointment is available at pharmacies with a prescription. A one-half inch ribbon of ointment will cover an area approximately four inches square. The cost of a 15-gram (one-half ounce) tube varies from $20 to $30.

Mild pain with slight burning or stinging may occur in about one-fourth of those applying ACV to herpes lesions. About four percent of users report mild itching. A rash may develop in approximately one in 300 users. Safe use in pregnancy and lactation has not been established. ACV ointment should not be used chronically to prevent recurrences of herpes lesions.

Oral ACV speeds healing of the initial infection, reduces the chance of sufferers spreading the disease, and reduces the frequency of recurrences in some people. A five-day course of oral ACV reduced the duration of symptoms and lesions of initial episodes of genital herpes by 50 percent in one study. The usual dose for an initial genital herpes infection is one 200 mg capsule every four hours, while awake, for a total of five capsules per day for 10 days (50 capsules total). Recurrent episodes should be treated at the earliest sign of a recurrence at a dose of one 200 mg capsule every four hours, while awake, for a total of five capsules per day for five days (25 capsules total).

Long-term use of oral ACV to prevent recurrent attacks of genital herpes has been studied. Several studies using oral ACV as a preventive agent have shown a significant reduction in the number of recurrences of genital herpes when the recurrence rate was high (more than six episodes per year). When ACV is given orally at the first sign of recurring symptoms, less virus may be given off and lesions may heal faster. Like the ointment, the oral form works best in those who begin therapy immediately after symptoms of a new infectious attack appear. If one waits a day or two after symptoms begin, the oral form does not work as well. Also, oral acyclovir is not as effective in preventing recurrences in those whose recurrence rate is low. The recommended dose for long-term suppressive therapy is one 200 mg capsule three times daily (or up to one 200 mg capsule five times daily) for up to six months.

Adverse effects from oral ACV are relatively minor and infrequent when taken for five to 10 days. Long-term use increases the incidence of adverse effects (see Table 24).

Intravenous ACV may be used to treat initial and recurrent mucosal and cutaneous HSV-1 and HSV-2 infections in immunocompromised adults and children and for extremely severe initial episodes of genital herpes in those who are not immunocompromised. Although the injectable ACV would be helpful in treatment of most initial or recurrent episodes, the need for hospitalization to receive i.v. acyclovir and the short duration of recurrent attacks make it impractical to use this dosage form except in the most severe cases.

Idoxuridine, the first agent used effectively to treat herpes keratitis (ocular herpes), was investigated for possible use against genital herpes. When used alone, idoxuridine exhibited little or no benefit when applied to genital herpes lesions. However, when dissolved in the solvent DMSO (dimethylsulfoxide), idoxuridine was superior to placebo in healing lesions more rapidly, while reducing the duration of viral shedding. As it does with other drugs, DMSO apparently enhanced the absorption of idoxuridine to make it more effective. Unfortunately, because of idoxuridine's potential to mutate cells and

TABLE 24
ADVERSE EFFECTS ASSOCIATED WITH SHORT-TERM AND LONG-TERM USE OF ORAL ACYCLOVIR (ZOVIRAX®)*

	Short-term Administration	*Long-term Administration*
Gastrointestinal	Nausea/vomiting (2.7%); diarrhea (0.3%)	Nausea/vomiting (8%); diarrhea (8.8%)
Central Nervous System	Headache (0.6%); fatigue (0.3%); dizziness	Headache (13.1%); vertigo (3.6%); insomnia, fatigue, irritability, depression (less than 3%)
Dermatologic	Skin rash (0.3%)	Skin rash, acne, accelerated hair loss (less than 3%)
Other	Loss of appetite, edema, leg pain, medication taste, sore throat (0.3%)	Joint pain (3.6%); fever, palpitations, sore throat, muscle cramps, menstrual abnormality (less than 3%)

Adapted with permission from *Facts and Comparisons Drug Information* (1987).

---

*The safety of using any form of acyclovir in pregnancy and in nursing mothers has not been established.

damage nerve fibers, the enhanced absorption brought on by DMSO may be less than desirable.

Trifluridine (Viroptic®) shows significant benefit for the initial treatment of ocular herpes, producing a cure rate of more than 95 percent. Viroptic® also has a low potential to produce toxic side effects.

Vidarabine (Vira-A®) has also proved useful in treating ocular herpes. Vira-A® is also utilized in treating herpes encephalitis and neonatal herpes. It inhibits DNA synthesis in cells infected with herpes virus in much the same way as acyclovir (ACV). Vidarabine is poorly absorbed through the skin, and therefore is not effective for external application to herpes lesions. It is used as an alternative to intravenous ACV in severe herpes infections.

Discovered in 1957, interferons have gained widespread public recognition for their potential role in cancer therapy. Additionally, they have shown promise as antiviral agents. Interferons appear to have an indirect antiviral activity by increasing production of enzymes that block viral reproduction. They may also exhibit antiviral activity by stimulating the immune system, which may inhibit the herpes virus. Clinical experience with interferons as antiviral agents is limited. They are presently being investigated as possible therapy in primary and recurrent genital herpes, varicella-zoster (chickenpox), herpes zoster (shingles), and cytomegalovirus (CMV) infections. A new approach to herpes therapy, which combines interferons with acyclovir, is also being investigated.

TREATMENT OF NEONATAL HERPES

Vidarabine (Vira-A®) has been used with some success in treating neonatal herpes. In one study, vidarabine reduced the number of deaths from over seven out of ten to less than four out of ten infants born with herpes simplex virus infection. Current studies are being conducted comparing ACV and vidarabine in treatment of neonatal herpes.

SUPPORTIVE TREATMENT OF GENITAL HERPES

The basic supportive therapy of genital herpes, in addition to use of an antiviral drug, is as follows:

1. Good hygiene
2. Adequate rest
3. Frequent soaks
4. Analgesic/anti-inflammatory therapy
5. Topical anesthetic therapy

Good hygiene involves keeping herpes lesions as dry as possible in order to promote crusting and faster healing of lesions. The first step is to wash the affected area with warm soapy water, rinse the area thoroughly, and carefully pat dry, making sure not to dry non-affected areas with the same towel. Povidone-iodine (Betadine®) helps relieve uncomfortable symptoms and protect the lesions from becoming infected with bacteria. Drying agents (astringents) may relieve some pain. Warm air from a hand-held dryer may help keep lesions dry and relieve surface discomfort.

Adequate rest during a genital herpes infection is encouraged. Genital herpes sufferers may experience a vague feeling of discomfort, which can be at least partially relieved with adequate rest. Since genital herpes lesions require frequent attention, one may want to stay home from school or work during very severe attacks.

Pain and fever are common symptoms of genital herpes. They can often be relieved by taking aspirin or acetaminophen. Motrin®, the commonly used prescription analgesic ibuprofen, that is now available without a prescription under the name of Advil® or Nuprin®, can be used as an alternative to aspirin or acetaminophen. Naprosyn®, a prescription anti-inflammatory drug, may be requested from the physician to relieve pain.

Symptoms such as painful urination may be reduced by urinating while soaking the genital area in a warm sitz bath or while under a warm shower. As herpes simplex virus may remain alive in tap water for up to 4.5 hours, soaking in a warm tub may transfer the infection to noninfected areas of the body and is not recommended.

Topical anesthetics, such as lidocaine or benzocaine, may be used for severe itching. These agents may be applied directly to the lesion, but should be used with caution as they may cause inflammation or a hypersensitivity (allergic) reaction in some individuals. Xylocaine Ointment®, Unguentine Spray®, Americaine First Aid Spray®, aero CAINE®, or Americaine Anesthetic Aerosol® may be used because they have a high concentration of anesthetic but do not contain menthol, a possible irritant. Additionally, these products contain alcohol or water, which are less likely to keep lesions moist and delay healing.

DRUGS THAT CAN PREVENT GENITAL HERPES

Researchers are working to develop a vaccine which will prevent genital herpes infection. A vaccine would hopefully induce the body to produce antibodies which would prevent the herpes simplex virus from ever reaching the nerve cells. If such a vaccine is developed, it would protect those who never had the disease. However, some vaccines might also have the potential to help those who already have the disease by lessening the severity of recurrent attacks.

QUACK REMEDIES

The fact that herpes affects approximately 20 million people in the United States assures a large market for fraudulent remedies. The incurable status of the disease gives many individuals a feeling of helplessness, which makes them susceptible to quack peddlers offering miracle cures. As mentioned previously, symptoms of recurrent herpes infections go away about six days after symptoms first appear. The uninformed consumer may attribute the disappearance of a herpes flareup to the use of a so-called miracle cure, rather than acknowledging the disappearance of symptoms as being the result of the natural course of the disease.

A number of products making claims of effectiveness have appeared. They are promoted mainly in newspapers and magazines and are invariably more sensational than helpful. These questionable products include:

1. LSO-1—lithium succinate ointment
2. Herpitex—butylated hydroxytoluene, a food additive
3. Lysine tablets—an amino acid
4. Zinc
5. Vitamin C—ascorbic acid

In 1983 the FDA, in a regulatory letter, charged the manufacturers of LSO-1 and Herpitex with marketing a drug for an "unapproved" use. They were requested to cease marketing these preparations as a cure for genital herpes or face possible litigation. The letter further added that lysine tablets are also not approved as a cure for the disease. Although in most cases lysine tablets do not carry labeling with medical claims, they are promoted in many health food stores as a treatment or preventive measure against genital herpes.

Consumers are bombarded with reports about amazing remedies and disease-preventing therapies. For example, articles recommending a lysine-rich diet for treatment and prevention of genital herpes have appeared as feature stories in numerous consumer publications, yet two properly conducted studies have shown lysine to be ineffective in treating oral HSV infection. No well controlled study has proved lysine is effective in treating genital herpes. Zinc and vitamin C therapy for treatment of genital herpes lesions have not undergone scientific evaluation, although this combination has been purported in the lay press to reduce formation of resistant strains of herpes simplex virus.

LIVING WITH GENITAL HERPES

The manner in which genital herpes has been handled by the press has probably contributed to the anxiety that genital herpes sufferers often experience. The incurable status of genital herpes has been sensationalized. The focus is often on the serious effects the disease has on newborns and patients with an immune system deficiency, but these complications rarely occur.

The social stigma of having herpes is overwhelming for some individuals. There have been several reports of persons contemplating suicide after learning of their herpes infection. Any disease acquired from sexual activity is likely to cause some sufferers a certain amount of guilt and anxiety. A feeling of helplessness and lack of control due to the recurrent nature of herpes only serves to worsen the anxiety and strengthen the feeling of guilt.

Genital herpes occurs most often in 15 to 41 year olds. For many of these individuals, herpes represents their first long-term illness. Even though herpes is discomforting and distressing, one must put things in proper perspective and realize that genital herpes is survivable and minimally disruptive of a normal life-style. In fact, for most people herpes flare-ups are only an occasional annoyance. Only approximately 10 percent of those affected suffer from frequent, recurrent attacks.

Not all HSV-2 infections are sexually transmitted. Although not very common, herpes can be transferred by indirect contact, such as from shaking a hand that has just rubbed an active oral or genital lesion. Kissing a person with an active oral lesion is another means of acquiring herpes.

Herpes can be acquired and exist in the body in an inactive form for many years before it actually appears as an infection. At the time of exposure, the virus may not have produced noticeable lesions. If symptoms other than lesions occur, the initial infection may well have been attributed to some other condition. Having genital herpes doesn't necessarily mean marital infidelity.

Herpes sufferers do, however, have a responsibility to current or potential sex partners to inform them of the condition. Many who now have herpes no doubt wish that a past sexual partner with herpes had informed them of the fact in advance. On the other hand, it is probably not generally appropriate to tell friends and associates with whom sex is unlikely that you have genital herpes. Most people are not fully aware of the facts about herpes and may overreact, resulting in social rejection.

To minimize the chance of transmitting herpes infection to a sexual partner, avoid intercourse while pain or lesions exist (see Table 25). One study revealed that 60 percent of new infections were acquired during sexual contact with a partner who had lesions. The apparent lack of knowledge about signs and symptoms, and the periods when transmission of the disease is most likely, is strong evidence that public education about genital herpes should be enhanced. Control of genital herpes infection is complicated by the fact that some people unknowingly shed virus for several days after lesions have healed. Others, especially women, may not even be aware they have an infection since active virus may be present in the absence of lesions and other symptoms.

CONCLUSION

Although herpes viruses have been infecting people for thousands of years, only recently has this infection received widespread attention. The growing variety of sexual practices will certainly make

---

TABLE 25
ADVICE FOR PERSONS WITH GENITAL HERPES

1. At the first sign of a genital lesion see a physician.
2. Avoid sexual contact (including kissing) during periods when lesions are visible, especially during the blistering stage when infection is most contagious.
3. Keep genital area clean. Dry genital area carefully and thoroughly.
4. Apply acyclovir ointment, or any other medication, with a finger protector or rubber glove to prevent infecting another part of the body.
5. Wear only 100 percent cotton underwear and loose-fitting clothing during periods when lesions are visible. Women should avoid pantyhose with nylon crotch inserts.
6. In heterosexual and homosexual couples where one or both partners has had a genital herpes infection, the use of barrier methods such as condoms or spermicide (containing nonoxynol-9) should be considered to reduce the risk of transmission during a flare-up of genital herpes.
7. If lesions have occurred on the cervix, the female should use a diaphragm, even when lesions do not appear on the external genital area. The use of a vaginal contraceptive sponge impregnated with spermicide (nonoxynol-9) may serve as a physical and chemical barrier against cervical herpes lesions.
8. Smear spermicide on outer genitalia. This will not assure freedom from infection but, in theory, it may offer added protection.
9. Sexually active women of childbearing age who have had genital herpes infections should get a Pap smear every six months to improve the chances for early detection of cervical cancer.
10. Avoid wearing wet clothing (such as bathing suits) for extended periods as this tends to aggravate and spread lesions.

---

the differences between HSV-1 and HSV-2 infections more difficult to distinguish. It should be remembered that the herpes virus is no respecter of wealth, upbringing, social position, or status. Antiviral agents represent a major step in conquering genital herpes. If antiviral research follows the route of success in developing antibiotics to treat bacteria, drugs that may drastically reduce the symptoms of genital herpes, or even cure the disease, may not be far away. Development of a safe and effective vaccine could result in the isolation or possible elimination of HSV infections within one or two generations. Until that time, genital herpes sufferers should realize the disease is not as serious as some have been led to believe. Not only is it possible to live with the disease, but also, with a few restrictions, an affected individual can continue to lead a normal, sexually active life.

11

Acquired Immunodeficiency Syndrome (AIDS)

INTRODUCTION

Acquired immunodeficiency syndrome (AIDS) has a short but bitter history. No disease since the "Black Death" of 14th-century Europe has so intensely occupied the mind of the public. The reaction of American society to AIDS has ranged from hysteria and panic to ostracism and discrimination. AIDS remains incurable, and the incidence rate is rapidly accelerating. This fact contributes to a paranoid mentality in which many people believe they live intimately with death. AIDS may indeed result in a medical holocaust if dramatic measures are not taken to prevent the spread of the disease and if effective treatment is not developed soon.

The degree to which infected individuals appear contagious is widely misunderstood. This misunderstanding contributes to feelings of fear, panic, and paranoia. Individuals living outside the high-risk groups appear to have less than one chance in a million (one in 1,000,000) of developing AIDS. That compares favorably with the probability you will die in an automobile accident (one in 5,000), be murdered (one in 10,000), or be struck by lightning (one in 600,000). This chapter emphasizes behavioral measures which can be taken to minimize risk.

Precautions must be observed to diminish the spread of AIDS. The virus is adaptable and may continue to mutate in such a way that new pathways of infection may develop. There is no answer to the haunting question of what directions the disease will take in the future. Increased public education and awareness are the best strategies currently for isolating the disease and slowing its spread.

A basic step in understanding AIDS is to recognize the difference between infection by the AIDS virus (HTLV-III), AIDS-Related Complex(ARC), and AIDS itself (see Table 26). The 1 million to 2 million Americans infected with the AIDS virus will not necessarily develop AIDS-Related Complex (ARC) or AIDS, but they may infect other people. Recent studies suggest that 30 to 60 percent of those infected by the AIDS virus may ultimately develop AIDS. AIDS-Related Complex (ARC) is less serious than AIDS (see Table 26). AIDS is a progression from AIDS-Related Complex (ARC), and AIDS represents the incontrovertible threat to life.

TABLE 26
GLOSSARY OF FREQUENTLY USED TERMS

HTLV-III	The virus which causes AIDS (*H*uman *T*-*L*ymphotrophic *V*irus-type III). The virus may also be referred to as LAV (*L*ymphadenopathy-*a*ssociated *v*irus) or as the AIDS virus or HIV (Human Immunodeficiency Virus)
AIDS-Related Complex (ARC)	A constellation of symptoms experienced by some with a positive blood test for the AIDS virus. Symptoms include tiredness, swollen lymph glands (especially of neck, armpit, and groin region), recurrent fever, diarrhea, weight loss, and night sweats. ARC does not necessarily progress on to AIDS, although it does in many instances.
AIDS	AIDS is a progression from AIDS-Related Complex (ARC) in which the immune system is severely depressed and in which severe, life-threatening infections and certain types of cancer develop.
High-Risk Group	A group with a high incidence of AIDS or AIDS-Related Complex (ARC) relative to the general

	population. Examples of high-risk groups are (a) homosexual and bisexual men, (b) i.v. drug abusers who share contaminated needles and other injection paraphernalia, (c) those who have sex with a homosexual or bisexual man or i.v. drug abuser, and (d) prostitutes (at least 50 percent of "street" prostitutes are infected with the AIDS virus).
High-Risk Sex	Sex in which body fluids are exchanged via oral-genital, oral-rectal, or penile-rectal contact. Unprotected penile-vaginal heterosexual contact may evolve as high-risk in the U.S., as it is in certain portions of central Africa.
Casual Contact	Nonsexual physical contact (such as touching, embracing, sitting together, hand shaking, sharing clothing, coughing, sneezing, breathing common air).

PREVALENCE OF AIDS

In June 1981 the Centers for Disease Control (CDC) published reports of the unusual development of five cases of *Pneumocystis carinii* pneumonia among five previously healthy male homosexuals in Los Angeles. Shortly thereafter came equally surprising reports of an aggressive form of cancer known as Kaposi's sarcoma among gay men in New York and California. Additional cases were traced back to 1978. Until 1981, *Pneumocystis carinii* pneumonia had been seen primarily in individuals with a severely impaired immune system. Other opportunistic organisms known to infect AIDS patients include various types of fungus, cytomegalovirus (CMV), herpes, and toxoplasma. Kaposi's sarcoma, until the development of AIDS, had been a rare type of skin cancer seen primarily in elderly men.

Early cases provided a glimpse of a disease that is today producing stark statistics; tremendous physical, psychological, moral, ethical, and social suffering; and one of the great medical challenges and dilemmas of all time. From 1981 through 1986, over 30,000 cases of AIDS were reported in the U.S. It is estimated that 5.0 to 10 million people are infected by the AIDS virus worldwide. Over 1.0 million worldwide were experiencing the AIDS-Related Complex (ARC) in 1986. Some 100,000 individuals, worldwide, were believed to be suffering from the fatal illness in 1986. Approximately 53 percent of all victims to date have died. Survival after diagnosis varies from weeks to several months. Approximately 75 percent of AIDS victims are dead within two years after the onset of the disease. Most will die from six months to five years after developing AIDS.

Approximately 15,000 new cases were diagnosed in the U.S. in 1986. The number of cases is doubling every 11 to 12 months. The U.S. Public Health Service estimates that AIDS will multiply more than 10 times between 1986 and 1991. Some believe that up to 2 million Americans have been infected by the AIDS virus, but have no symptoms. Up to 20 to 30 percent of these could develop AIDS over the next few years. Approximately 270,000 cases of fully developed AIDS are expected in the U.S. by 1991; the cumulative death toll from AIDS could reach 179,000 by 1991. Approximately 54,000 U.S. citizens could lose their lives to AIDS in 1991 alone. By 1991 the number of people infected by the AIDS virus worldwide could reach 100 million; up to 3.0 million AIDS cases could exist by 1991.

AIDS has been reported from all 50 states and the District of Columbia. There have been no significant changes in age, race, and sex distribution. AIDS is 14 times more prevalent in men than women; over 90 percent of AIDS victims are males. Men are more likely to infect women than vice versa. Approximately 89 percent of all cases have occurred in the 20 to 49 year age group. In 1986, 60 percent of AIDS victims were white, 25 percent were black, and 14 percent were Hispanic. Approximately 30 percent of AIDS cases have occurred in New York, 23 percent in California, seven percent in Florida, six percent in New Jersey, and five percent in Texas. New York City and San Francisco accounted for 40 percent of all AIDS cases in 1986. By 1991 it is expected that 80 percent of cases will occur in other localities.

Most AIDS cases occur in high-risk populations (see Table 26). The majority (over 70 percent) of AIDS cases in the U.S. are reported in homosexual or bisexual men. Intravenous drug abusers utilizing contaminated needles and other injection paraphernalia account for about 20 percent of cases. One percent of cases occurs in individuals with hemophilia or similar disorders; 4 percent occur through heterosexual contact with an individual infected by the AIDS virus. Five percent of cases either occur by other means or the method of transmission is not verifiable. Over 300 children had developed AIDS by 1986. For selected facts about AIDS, see Table 27.

THE CAUSE OF AIDS

What is the origin of AIDS? Why has this lethal, bizarre killer been unleashed upon the world? The scenario is like science fiction; the virus is viewed by many as some unbelievable "Andromeda strain." AIDS is a very real, human, here-and-now threat, however.

Prevalence of the AIDS virus in central Africa has led to speculation that the disease originated on that continent. The initial carrier of the AIDS virus, or one closely related, was probably the green monkey of central Africa. This monkey may have harbored a harmless virus in its bloodstream for many years. No more than 10 to 15 years ago, nature apparently altered the genetic code of the virus through a natural, random, evolutionary mutation. The result was apparently the lethal HTLV-III strain of the virus.

Recent studies indicate that approximately 70 percent of African green monkeys are infected with a virus similar to HTLV-III. The virus does not harm the monkeys. The AIDS virus (HTLV-III) has crossed the boundary from animal to man. The AIDS virus is unique because it is the only virus known which specifically attacks the immune system.

The crossover from animal to man is not difficult to understand. African green monkeys often live in close association with people; bites are not uncommon. Factors which may have promoted the spread of AIDS in Africa include poor sanitation, contaminated water supplies, use and reuse of unsterilized needles in small clinics, and local rituals involving scarification and exchange of blood. High-risk sexual practices and the mobility of the world's population assured the spread of AIDS to other continents.

HOW THE AIDS VIRUS (HTLV-III) DAMAGES THE HUMAN IMMUNE SYSTEM

HTLV-III, which produces AIDS, is a virulent scourge of the human immune system. The body's immune system is comprised of several lines of chemical defenders that constantly wage war on bacteria, viruses, fungi, protozoa, cancer cells, and other invaders. Of the body's 100 trillion cells, one in every 100 has a protective function.

HOW THE IMMUNE SYSTEM NORMALLY WORKS

The human body possesses a remarkable array of internal protectors. Among the most powerful defenders of the body are three

---

TABLE 27
SELECTED FACTS ABOUT AIDS

- AIDS is caused by a virus (HTLV-III).

- The virus may create a defect in the body's immune system and result in AIDS.

- There is no specific treatment or cure for AIDS, and there have been no reports of the immune defect spontaneously resolving.

- AIDS is always fatal. It is, in effect, a death sentence.

- Approximately 75 percent of AIDS victims die within two years of developing symptoms of AIDS.

- From 1 to 2 million Americans are believed to be infected with the AIDS virus (HTLV-III).

- The AIDS virus probably remains in the body for life.

- Not all of those infected appear to develop AIDS-Related Complex (ARC) and a smaller proportion develop AIDS.

- The percentage of individuals infected with HTLV-III who will develop AIDS is not known, but may be as high as 30 to 60 percent, or higher, in some high-risk groups.

- The virus may smolder in the body for six months to five years, or even longer, before symptoms occur.

- Some people infected with the AIDS virus develop the less serious AIDS-Related Complex (see Table 26).

- People who are infected with the AIDS virus, but do not have symptoms of AIDS or ARC, may infect other people.

- Homosexual and bisexual men account for over 70 percent of AIDS cases.

- Sexual transmission appears to require intimate sexual contact and exchange of body fluids. Semen is most likely to transmit the disease during sexual intimacy.

- A simple blood test is available at clinics, health departments, and doctor's office which can detect antibodies to HTLV-III in your blood and thus tell you if you are infected by HTLV-III.

- People infected with the AIDS virus who are conscientious about their health appear to have a better chance of never developing AIDS.

- No one knows for sure how long the AIDS virus can live outside the body and on inanimate objects such as toilet seats, table tops, bed linens, towels, dishes, eating utensils, doorknobs, telephones, office equipment, furniture, or in swimming pools or hot tubs. The AIDS virus can live up to 15 days in infected blood which has been removed from the body and properly stored in a blood bank. Infection from surface contact is unlikely as the virus would have to enter the bloodstream to be infectious.

- Condoms reduce (but do not entirely eliminate) the chance of spreading the virus in semen.
- The AIDS virus can be spread in a single sexual encounter with an infected person. Risk is increased with multiple sexual partners.
- There is *no* risk of becoming infected by the AIDS virus when donating blood.
- Blood transfusions are not absolutely safe, but the screening tests are approximately 99.5 percent reliable. Blood from an infected donor is not used in transfusions.
- There is no test for AIDS itself, just for infection by HTLV-III.

---

types of white blood cells produced in the bone marrow. These are *macrophages,* three types of *T cells* (also known as T lymphocytes), and *B cells.* Each contributes uniquely to the body's defense against invaders.

Macrophages are the scavenger cells of the body. They surround, engulf, and generally attempt to consume anything they find in the bloodstream, tissue, or lymph fluid which they perceive as foreign to the body. When a macrophage captures a piece of protein, called an antigen, from an invading microorganism, it alerts a highly specialized group of white blood cells, helper T cells (T lymphocytes), to join the fight.

Helper T cells recognize the foreign antigen and, although they do not attack chemical invaders themselves, play the vital role of sending urgent chemical signals to killer T cells telling them to multiply rapidly. Helper T cells also stimulate the production of more macrophages and the B cells.

Killer T cells recognize the invaders, reproduce quickly, and trigger a chemical reaction that destroys the cell wall of microorganisms or destroys infected cells before the virus inside has time to multiply.

B cells of the spleen and lymph nodes produce chemical weapons called antibodies. Antibodies attach themselves to the antigen of foreign cells, thus killing them or slowing them down. When antibody attacks foreign antigen, the foreign cells become easy prey for macrophages.

Once invading cells are diminished, the *suppressor T cells* take over to call off the attack by slowing production of other T cells and B cells. Macrophages persist until the litter of dead cells and by-products of metabolism of the foreign agents are removed from the body.

Memory cells are thought to be formed during an initial infection. They appear to circulate in the blood or lymph fluid for years. Through their presence, the body's response to similar attacks in the future should be more swift and specific.

HOW AIDS AFFECTS THE IMMUNE SYSTEM

If the body's immune system protects us from a host of bacterial, fungal, protozoal, and viral invaders, why then is HTLV-III so deadly? Of all the enemies of the body, viruses are the simplest and most devious. HTLV-III is the most devious and deadly of all viruses. HTLV-III, like many other viruses, is simply a bundle of genes with a protein coat. The genes contain information for making more copies of the virus. Because a virus is too simple to reproduce itself on its own, it reproduces inside a normal cell. The AIDS virus enters the human body like Greeks inside the Trojan horse, concealed inside a helper T cell from an infected host. It is typically carried into the body via infected blood or semen.

The helper T cells of the new victim recognize the foreign helper T cells which contain the AIDS virus as foreign, *but* when the two helper T cells meet, the AIDS virus slips through the cell membrane into the defending cell. Before the defending helper T cell can signal killer T cells, B cells, and macrophages to multiply and join the fight, the helper T cell is "turned off" by HTLV-III. The critical initiator of the body's immune system response (the helper T cell) is inactivated as a lymphocyte.

The helper T cell is then "turned on" again, but this time it is as an "AIDS virus factory." The genetic information of the AIDS virus works inside the helper T cell to produce more AIDS virus. HTLV-III appears to have a unique genetic component which allows it to reproduce itself hundreds of times faster than other types of virus. Eventually the AIDS virus will rupture the host cell, killing it, and infecting other normal helper T cells. As this process repeats itself, the body's immune system may be weakened on a very large scale.

Because of the profound immune system suppression, a person infected by the AIDS virus may be unable to effectively combat what would normally be trivial infections or to prevent Kaposi's sarcoma. The AIDS virus is like a time bomb in the body. When, or if, it will produce life-threatening suppression of the immune system cannot be predicted.

IDENTIFICATION OF THOSE INFECTED WITH THE AIDS VIRUS (HTLV-III)

THE AIDS-SCREENING TEST

Once HTLV-III was identified as the agent responsible for producing AIDS, it became possible to develop an effective screening test which could detect antibodies formed by the body in response to the presence of the virus. The HTLV-III antibody test was licensed in March 1985. The test is highly sensitive. The goal of the test is to screen HTLV-III positive blood out of the nation's blood supply. This purpose has been served with over 99 percent efficiency. Any blood or plasma tested positive for the AIDS antibody is discarded. The U.S. Public Health Service also recommends that the HTLV-III antibody test be used to screen blood and serum from donors of organs, tissue, or sperm intended for human use. The HTLV-III antibody test has been administered to all 2.3 million members of the U.S. armed forces.

The HTLV-III antibody test seldom fails to detect antibodies to the AIDS virus when they are present, but there have been several reports of false-positive test results. A false-positive result indicates that antibodies to the AIDS virus are present when they are not. A second test to confirm a positive result may be advisable. Less expensive and more specific and sensitive tests are being developed.

LIMITATIONS OF THE HTLV-III ANTIBODY TEST

The primary value of the HTLV-III antibody test has been in assuring the quality of the nation's blood supply. Because the full implications of antibodies to the AIDS virus in the bloodstream is not known, this test is used for limited purposes only. There are certain things the HTLV-III antibody test cannot do, including the following:

1. It cannot diagnose AIDS.
2. It cannot predict future illness due to AIDS-Related Complex (ARC) or AIDS.
3. It cannot determine immunity to, or protection from, the virus.
4. It cannot determine one's ability to infect other people.

A person with a positive test result has probably been infected with HTLV-III, or a similar virus, at some time in the past. A person with a negative result has probably not been infected with HTLV-III, but if tested soon after exposure to the AIDS virus, antibodies to the virus may not be detectable, yet the test may be positive at a later date.

The U.S. Public Health Service has recommended that all Americans in the high-risk group for developing AIDS have the HTLV-III antibody test performed periodically. If you are worried that you may be infected because of a previous sexual experience, blood transfusion, organ transplant, accidental puncture with a contaminated needle, i.v. drug use, casual contact with an infected person, or for any other reason, you may wish to have the test to reassure yourself. Local, county, and state health departments, clinics, and local physicians can conduct the test for you. A woman considering pregnancy who has a positive HTLV-III antibody test or who is at risk for becoming infected may wish to defer pregnancy until more is known about risk to the developing fetus.

The U.S. Public Health Service and the American Medical Association have recommended follow-up testing of all patients who have a positive HTLV-III antibody test. Aspects of confidentiality should be discussed with the agency or individual conducting the test. Confidentiality of results should be protected to the greatest extent compatible with the best interest of the public health and consistent with an individual's civil rights.

SYMPTOMS OF AIDS-RELATED COMPLEX (ARC) AND AIDS

HEALTHY CARRIER STATE

Most who are infected by HTLV-III are presently in a healthy carrier state. Such individuals have no symptoms and are in good general health. Many of these individuals will develop AIDS-Related Complex (ARC), and some will develop AIDS. The incubation period of the AIDS virus may be five years or longer. If, when, or under what conditions one may develop symptoms of ARC or AIDS is not predictable.

AIDS-RELATED COMPLEX (ARC)

AIDS-Related Complex (ARC) is also known as chronic lymphadenopathy syndrome. Symptoms, in addition to those included in the definition of ARC (see Table 26), include a decrease in the white blood cell count, anemia, decrease in thrombocytes (which assist in blood clotting), and fungal infections in the mouth. Some people with ARC develop a life-threatening infection or a malignancy. When this happens, the person is classified as having AIDS.

Only a minority of those infected by HTLV-III eventually develop AIDS. Percentages may change, but current projections suggest that up to 20 percent of those with ARC will ultimately develop AIDS. This percentage may be considerably higher in certain high-risk groups, such as promiscuous homosexuals engaging in indiscriminate sexual practices.

AIDS

The symptoms of AIDS are the symptoms associated with the disorders which occur as complications of the HTLV-III induced suppression of the body's immune system.

The most common infection in AIDS is still *Pneumocystis carinii* pneumonia (PCP). The percentage of AIDS victims who experience PCP is approximately 60 percent. The most commonly associated malignancy is Kaposi's sarcoma (KS). About 19 percent experience KS alone. Approximately six percent experience both PCP and KS. The remaining 15 percent succumb to other opportunistic infections or malignancies.

The onset of *Pneumocystis carinii* pneumonia is often mild with fever, cough, and labored breathing. The pneumonia eventually overwhelms the lungs and leads to death. *Pneumocystis carinii* has also been reported to invade the eye and central nervous system in AIDS victims. Eye involvement may lead to blindness. Central nervous system involvement may result in meningitis.

Fungal infections, ranging from infection of the mouth to meningitis, occur in 80 to 90 percent of AIDS cases. Herpes infections in AIDS victims may lead to encephalitis, and cytomegalovirus (CMV) may produce symptoms ranging from a mononucleosis-like syndrome to blindness and life-threatening pneumonia and encephalitis. Mycobacteria may infect the lungs, bone marrow, kidneys, liver, gastrointestinal tract, lymph nodes, and spleen. Toxoplasmosis may cause encephalitis and brain abscess, which may rapidly progress to death. Numerous bacteria and protozoa produce profuse diarrhea, abdominal pain and cramping, fluid and electrolyte depletion, muscle weakness, and low blood pressure.

Kaposi's sarcoma, a malignant disorder, is very aggressive in the AIDS victim. Initially a single, oval-shaped, nodular, purple-brown lesion may develop. The invasive lesions spread over the torso, head, neck, and arms. The malignancy progresses rapidly to the lungs, liver, spleen, lymph nodes, testes, and gastrointestinal tract in 70 percent of cases. Other malignancies identified in AIDS victims include

Hodgkin's disease, Burkitt's lymphoma, lymphoblastic lymphoma, and cerebral lymphoma.

One case of AIDS, in which both *Pneumocystis carinii* pneumonia and Kaposi's sarcoma existed, was described as follows:

> Jack first noticed dark purple spots on his leg. He had no other symptoms. The cancer spread quickly. Fungal infections took hold in his mouth and throat. Pneumonia choked his lungs. He became weak, and wasted away before my eyes. The cancer blocked lymph glands, and fluid did not drain normally from his body. His legs and arms swelled grotesquely. Movement was difficult. Breathing was labored. Talking was impossible. Death was a tender mercy.

The catastrophic, apocalyptic episode described above is vivid evidence of the urgency needed in addressing AIDS. Social discipline, public education, preventive measures, and resources to fund research to identify a viable treatment must be given an extremely high priority by the public and private sector.

HOW AIDS IS SPREAD (RISK FACTORS)

AIDS is spread primarily by direct entry of HTLV-III into the bloodstream. The most common ways in which AIDS is spread are as follows:

1. *Intimate sexual contact with an infected person.* Semen is one of the primary carriers of HTLV-III. Penile-rectal, oral-genital, and oral-rectal exchange of body fluids are most likely to lead to AIDS. Anal (penile-rectal) intercourse appears to be associated with a high risk of infection as tears in rectal tissue frequently occur; this allows infected semen to enter the bloodstream of a male or female sexual partner. Oral lesions increase the likelihood that oral-genital and oral-rectal sex may lead to infection by HTLV-III. Remember, over 70 percent of cases of AIDS occurs in homosexual or bisexual men.
2. *Using contaminated needles and other injection paraphernalia used by an infected person.* Blood remains in contaminated needles and injection paraphernalia. This allows direct inoculation of HTLV-III into the bloodstream. Remember, approximately 20 percent of AIDS cases occur in intravenous drug abusers who use "dirty" needles or injection equipment.

3. *Injection of infected blood or blood products.* As the nation's blood supply is screened for antibodies to HTLV-III, development of AIDS by this mechanism has declined.
4. *Infection of newborns by an infected mother.* The mother's contaminated blood may infect a developing child in the uterus or at birth.

HTLV-III has been found in various body fluids and tissues including blood, semen, bone marrow, tears, saliva, urine, cerebrospinal fluid, lymph nodes, feces, vaginal secretions, the spleen, brain tissue, and nerve tissue. The question has been raised concerning the possibility that biting insects (such as mosquitoes and lice) may transmit HTLV-III. Biting insects do not appear to be a contributor to the spread of AIDS.

Much concern has been expressed by those who may come in contact with various body fluids of individuals infected by HTLV-III (such as schoolteachers, day care center personnel, nurses, physicians, hospital orderlies, dentists, dental hygienists, undertakers, opticians, contact lens fitters, actors and actresses asked to engage in open-mouth kissing, those who pierce ears, prisoners, and many others). Casual contact (see Table 26) does not appear to increase the risk of acquiring AIDS. Almost all AIDS cases involve contact with infected semen or blood. Contact with other contaminated body fluids may emerge as a problem, and precautions are recommended to minimize the risks of those exposed to any contaminated body fluid, but contact with infected body fluids (other than blood or semen) is not recognized as a common means of becoming infected.

PREVENTING THE SPREAD OF AIDS

French and African researchers began human-testing of an AIDS vaccine in 1986, but no effective vaccine or drug to treat AIDS is expected before the early to mid 1990s, if then. *The best approach to managing AIDS is to prevent its spread.* Although AIDS cannot be stopped, it can be slowed. That is possible through mass education, individual counseling, and observation of the necessary precautions. *To avoid AIDS, you must practice living defensively, particularly as life pertains to sexual activity.* Prevention is fairly simple. *You have the power to protect yourself more than medical science can protect you.* Remember, when you make love to someone who is sexually casual, irresponsible, or promiscuous and has a history of multiple sexual partners, you are, in effect, having a sexual relationship with those sexual partners if they are/were infected by the AIDS virus or another sexually transmitted disease.

The U.S. Public Health Service has issued the following recommendations on *"safe sex"*:

1. Do not have sexual contact with persons who are known to have, or are suspected of having, AIDS; who are known to be, or are suspected of being, carriers of the virus; or who have a positive result on the HTLV-III antibody test.
2. Do not have sex with multiple partners, or with persons who have had multiple partners (including prostitutes). The more partners you have, the greater your risk of contracting AIDS. A permanent, monogamous sexual relationship is encouraged.
3. Do not have sex with people who inject drugs (including prostitutes).
4. Protect yourself and your partner during sexual activity. If you suspect that you or your partner have been exposed to the HTLV-III virus, then use condoms to reduce the possibility of transmitting the virus, avoid oral-genital contact, avoid sexual practices that may cause injury or rips in tissue, avoid open-mouthed, intimate kissing, and avoid contact with any body fluids (semen, blood, feces, or urine).

Other steps which can be taken to prevent the spread of AIDS are as follows:

1. Do not inject street drugs. If you inject drugs, your risk may be lessened by not sharing needles or syringes.
2. Do not attempt to donate blood if you are in one of the high-risk groups for AIDS.
3. Do not donate blood, plasma, body organs, other tissue, or sperm if you (male) have had sex with another man since 1977.
4. Do not attempt to breast-feed your baby if you (female) have a positive HTLV-III antibody test.
5. Avoid practices such as being shaved, tattooed, having ears pierced, or undergoing acupuncture in places where sterilization of equipment is not assured.
6. Do not share toothbrushes, razors, or other devices that could be contaminated with blood.

Health care personnel, family members, and friends should observe certain precautions when ministering to the needs of known or suspected AIDS victims. Precautions which can protect the helper, while preventing the spread of AIDS, are as follows:

1. Avoid direct contact with blood, any body fluid, mucous membranes, secretions, or excretions from known or suspected AIDS victims. Gloves should be worn routinely, and other appropriate barriers, such as masks, gowns, and eye coverings, should be used when needed.
2. Avoid accidental exposure of your open wounds (including minor scratches and rashes) to any of the above substances from AIDS victims. Use of disposable gloves is advisable.
3. Wash hands thoroughly and immediately if contaminated with any body fluid from an AIDS victim.
4. Substances or instruments contaminated by blood, semen, or other body fluids of the AIDS victim should be properly disposed of or sterilized before reuse.
5. Blood spills must be cleaned promptly with full-strength sodium hypochlorite solution (Clorox®).
6. Careful handling and proper disposal of syringes, needles, and other sharp objects is essential in preventing work-related injuries and HTLV-III transmission.
7. Specimens from an AIDS victim must be properly labeled so as to alert health care personnel of the potential hazard and special handling required. Specimens should be transported in a container inside a container.

TREATMENT

As stated previously, no effective vaccine to prevent AIDS, or drug therapy to treat AIDS, is currently available. The best current approach to treatment is prevention of the spread of HTLV-III.

Numerous drugs are being evaluated for the treatment and cure of AIDS and restoration of the immune system. These drugs are in various stages of development. They may be years from the marketplace, and preliminary results indicate that the drugs do not alter the ultimate fatal course of AIDS.

A vaccine which will prevent AIDS will be difficult to develop. The proteins on the outer coat of HTLV-III act as antigens, but change rapidly to outsmart the immune-system antibodies, which may delay or slow down the virus. HTLV-III changes its "skin" like a chameleon. They trick their way past the body's immune system. A vaccine against one type of virus may not be protective against new variations of the virus.

Several antiviral drugs are currently being evaluated in the U.S. to determine their effectiveness in treating AIDS. These include suramin, azidothymidine (AZT), HP-23, foscarnet (trisodium phosphonoformate), CS-85, ribavirin, alpha-interferon, and ansamycin. Monoclonal antibody projects are underway to develop an antibody to neutralize HTLV-III early in the infection. Suramin, AZT, and HP-23 are further along in investigation than some of the other drugs. Preliminary results reveal reductions in amount of HTLV-III present in the blood, but the positive effect of the drug on the disease is often very short and poorly defined. Also, several of the antiviral drugs are very toxic.

Drugs under investigation that are designed to rebuild the weakened immune system of AIDS victims include interleukin-2 and gamma-interferon. Gamma-interferon produces a negligible clinical response and is prohibitively toxic. Interleukin-2 is the most promising immune system enhancer under investigation. High doses produce a short-lived enhancement of immune function and a minor improvement of Kaposi's sarcoma. No drug currently under investigation represents the much sought after "cure" for AIDS.

Symptoms of infections and malignancies, which occur as complications of AIDS, are treated with a host of drugs, but AIDS will eventually be fatal. The drugs employed, if utilized in individuals with an intact immune system, are more beneficial.

AIDS ISSUES AND CONTROVERSIES

AIDS presents serious social, ethical, moral, legal, and public health issues and controversies. Persons with AIDS often face social isolation, prejudice, breakdowns in confidentiality standards, loss of jobs, denial of insurance, eviction from housing, exclusion from public places, and second-class medical care. Some feel children with AIDS should not attend public schools. Undertakers have refused to embalm AIDS victims. In many minds, AIDS is a form of God's retribution for transgressions against His order.

As stated elsewhere in this chapter, HTLV-III is not readily contracted if one follows "safe sex" guidelines and other precautions recommended by the U.S. Public Health Service.

Some fear and concern by the public at large is appropriate. Many would prefer to err on the conservative side, not because of what we know about AIDS, but because of what we do not know. Fear should not give way to panic and irrational behavior, however. AIDS has only begun to touch the heterosexual population of the U.S. Children sneeze on one another, bloody one another's noses, drink after one another, swap food, bite each other, sit on toilets contaminated by urine, and yet, according to the American Academy of Pediatrics in a 1985 statement, "there has not been a single known case of one child infecting another child with AIDS." Reason, pragmatism, and vigilant concern should prevail on all sides of the AIDS issue.

What is the economic impact of AIDS? Who should pay? The average AIDS patient's hospital costs alone exceed $50,000. To this is added the cost of outpatient care, medication, loss of employment, reduced productivity, decreased life expectancy, and consumption of social and community support services. Psychological costs of AIDS to victims, family, friends, and business colleagues are untold.

Some large insurance carriers require the HTLV-III antibody screening test for large policy groups in high-risk states (California, New York, New Jersey, Florida, and Texas) and the District of Columbia. One national company no longer sells major medical insurance policies in New York due to the incidence of AIDS. By 1991, cost of medical care for U.S. AIDS victims is expected to be between $8 billion and $16 billion per year.

The physical and mental suffering, death rate, and economic threat associated with AIDS requires unprecedented action and a high national priority. The U.S. government has responded by significantly increasing appropriations to support AIDS research. The private sector has responded in a significant and positive way. The magnitude of the AIDS dilemma warrants a greater commitment of resources, however, so this malevolent threat may be diminished.

WHERE TO GET HELP

If you need help, there are several ways to get additional information. In addition to the resource centers included in Table 28, you may want to contact your local, county, or state health department or your physician for information and assistance.

TABLE 28
AIDS RESOURCE CENTERS

U.S. Public Health Service
AIDS Hotline
1-800-447-AIDS

National AIDS Hot Line
Centers for Disease Control
Atlanta, Georgia
1-800-342-AIDS

AIDS Task Force Hot Line
Albuquerque, New Mexico
505-266-8041

National Lesbian and Gay Health Foundation
P.O. Box 65472
Washington, DC 20035
202-797-3708

Whitman Walker Clinic
2335 18th St. NW
Washington, DC 20009
202-332-5295

National Gay Task Force
80 Fifth Avenue
New York City, New York 10011
1-800-221-7044

AIDS Resource Center
235 West 18th Street
New York City, New York 10011
212-206-1414

CONCLUSION

The incidence of AIDS will continue to increase for several years. AIDS and infection with HTLV-III will continue to carry a stigma, and infected persons will face social, as well as medical, problems. Public education should minimize panic and overzealous concern by the noninfected public.

Current modes of HTLV-III transmission will remain the predominant means by which HTLV-III is spread, although casual contact and heterosexual intercourse may result in a higher percentage of cases.

A continuing commitment to research is needed to develop a vaccine and effective drug therapy against HTLV-III. Control of AIDS and HTLV-III cannot await future research for a cure, however. Health professionals and a responsible society must work together to educate the public on how to prevent AIDS and care for its victims.

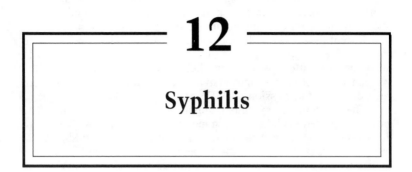

12

Syphilis

INTRODUCTION

It has been recognized since at least 1498 that syphilis is a sexually transmitted disease. Safe and effective treatment of syphilis at that time was nonexistent. Poisonous metals such as mercury were used initially for syphilis treatment, but with poor results. In 1907 an arsenic-containing compound appeared effective against syphilis. However, a year and one-half of treatment was required, severe adverse effects occurred, and treated patients often relapsed. Other chemical treatments were tried, but all were potentially dangerous, complicated to use, and not very effective. The successful use of penicillin to treat syphilis in 1943 proved to be the most important treatment breakthrough.

PREVALENCE OF SYPHILIS

Reported cases of syphilis in the United States reached a peak of approximately 85 cases per 100,000 people in 1946. The lowest number of reported cases (approximately 4 to 5 cases per 100,000 people) occurred in 1955. From 9.4 cases per 100,000 population in 1977, the incidence of syphilis in the U.S. increased to 14.6 cases per 100,000 population in 1982. This represents a total of 33,613 cases of primary or secondary syphilis in 1982. In 1983, the incidence of syphilis decreased by 3 percent compared to 1982. These figures only represent reported cases of syphilis. It has been estimated that for each reported case of syphilis, up to 5 cases may go unreported.

Recent decreases in the incidence rate of syphilis may be due to the effectiveness of public health programs in drawing attention to sexually transmitted diseases and their prevention. A decrease in the incidence rate of syphilis may also have resulted from public concern regarding the transmission of AIDS and/or genital herpes.

The incidence of syphilis is higher in men than in women. The ratio of reported syphilis cases in men and women in 1983 was 2.6 to 1. However, the overall incidence of syphilis decreased slightly in men but increased in women by 15 percent from 1981 to 1983. Cases of congenital syphilis (syphilis transmitted from the mother to the fetus, primarily during the second or third trimesters of pregnancy or during delivery) remained stable from 1981 to 1983. In a pregnant woman with untreated early syphilis, the risk of infecting the fetus is about 80 to 95 percent.

The incidence of syphilis is generally higher in nonwhite races than Caucasians, and in large urban areas. The higher incidence in nonwhite and urban areas may reflect more accurate case reporting by urban clinics.

CHARACTERISTICS OF SYPHILIS

Syphilis is a bacterial infectious disease that can be spread from person to person. Syphilis may be classified as either acquired or congenital. Congenital syphilis is transmitted from the mother to the fetus. This can occur via the mother's blood or during the passage of the fetus through the mother's infected birth canal. Although syphilis can be transmitted during any stage of pregnancy, the more recent the syphilis in the mother, and the farther along the pregnancy, the greater the risk of infecting the fetus. Acquired syphilis is transmitted from person to person through other means, the principal one being sexual intercourse.

Untreated syphilis is classified into stages that vary according to their time of onset (Table 29). Following exposure to the bacterium which causes syphilis, an incubation period of approximately 9 to 90 days occurs. During this period, the bacteria make their way through the lymph nodes, blood, and body tissues. Following the incubation period, a primary sore (also called a chancre) develops at the initial site of contact, generally the genital area. Whether the syphilis is treated or not, this primary lesion usually heals by itself within four to six weeks. Lesions of the secondary stage develop six weeks to several months after the initial exposure, but usually four to eight weeks after the chancre appears.

TABLE 29
CLASSIFICATION OF SYPHILIS

Stage	Time of Onset
Primary	9–90 days (Median = 21 days)
Secondary	6 weeks–several months (Usually 4–8 weeks following primary stage)
Latent	
Early	Less than 2 years
Late	Over 2 years
Tertiary (late)	3–20 years

Following the secondary stage, untreated syphilis enters the latent stage. In this stage, no symptoms of the disease are present. The latent stage is divided into two parts: the early stage, in which the syphilis is present for less than two years, and the late stage, in which the disease continues for more than two years. About 25 percent of those with syphilis in the early latent stage will develop relapses of the disease, with symptoms similar to the secondary stage.

The next stage, tertiary syphilis, is a slowly progressive stage of the disease that can affect almost any organ of the body. Signs and symptoms of tertiary syphilis can develop years after the initial exposure. About 25 percent of those with untreated syphilis die as a result of tertiary syphilis.

CAUSE OF SYPHILIS

Syphilis is caused by the bacterium *Treponema pallidum,* which only affects humans. *Treponema pallidum* is a thin, spiral-shaped microorganism that moves by bending like an accordion (see Figure 34). The organism is very difficult to grow in laboratories (outside of the body) and is readily killed by drying out, soap, heat, and cold temperatures.

TRANSMISSION OF SYPHILIS

Syphilis is transmitted by transfer of *Treponema pallidum* from person to person. Other than cases of congenital syphilis, most cases

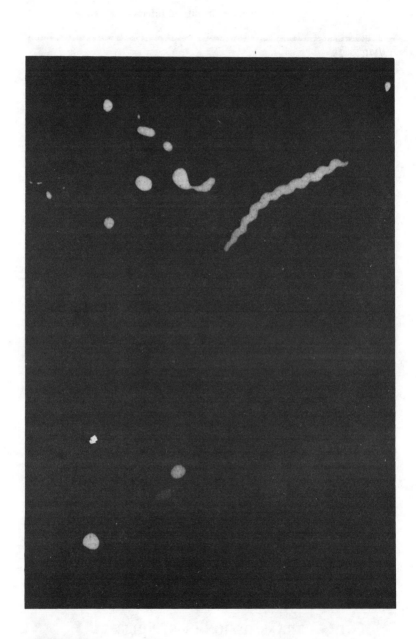

FIGURE 34
Appearance of *Treponema Pallidum* under a microscope

of acquired syphilis are spread through sexual contact. *Treponema pallidum* can easily infect and enter the body through mucous membranes of the mouth, vulva, vagina, anus, penis, and cut or scraped skin. Less commonly, syphilis can be transmitted from person to person through blood transfusions, if blood was donated by a person with syphilis in an infectious stage. Syphilis is rarely transmitted by handling infectious materials or through accidental needle pricks after a needle has been used in a person infected with syphilis. It is possible to spread syphilis through kissing if an infectious sore is present in the mouth.

Although direct sexual contact with a syphilis victim does not always result in transmission of the disease, about one out of two sexual encounters with a victim results in infection with syphilis. Syphilis victims are extremely contagious during the primary stage, when the chancre or initial lesion is present. The chancre contains thousands of *Treponema pallidum* organisms, and the disease is spread through intimate contact with the chancre. During the primary incubation period, the blood from a syphilis victim is also infectious.

During the secondary stage of syphilis, sores develop on the skin and mucous membranes. These lesions are contagious, especially those of the groin, mouth, and anus. In warm, moist, relatively enclosed areas such as the anus, groin, vulva, and scrotum, the lesions can combine and enlarge.

In the early latent stage of syphilis, syphilis victims are contagious during relapses. During the late latent and tertiary stages, they are generally not contagious. However, the blood may occasionally contain *Treponema pallidum* in the late latent stage, so pregnant women can still infect the fetus, and infection could still occur from a blood transfusion.

SIGNS, SYMPTOMS, AND COMPLICATIONS OF SYPHILIS

The signs and symptoms of syphilis depend on the stage that is present. Following contact with an infected person, the primary stage of syphilis develops. After the initial incubation period, a painless lesion (chancre) generally appears at the site of contact with *Treponema pallidum*. The chancre is most often found on the genitals, such as the penis in males and the labia and vulva in females. The lesion can also develop in the vagina or cervix and go unnoticed. The chancre can appear on the lips, tongue, or inside of the cheeks. In homosexual men, the chancre may appear on the anus, rectum, or inside the mouth. However, the primary lesion may occur on just about any area of the body. Although the chancre is usually painless, those with rectal syphilis may also complain of rectal discomfort or itching, pain with bowel movements, or some rectal bleeding.

Only one chancre usually develops, but more than one chancre can appear. The chancre starts as a reddish sore that eventually becomes ulcerated or indented, usually with hard firm edges. The ulcer is surrounded by a reddish area and may contain a yellow, pus-like material. The sore may also resemble a blister or pimple. Even if no treatment is given, the chancre will disappear in about two to 12 weeks, usually within four to six weeks.

In addition to the chancre, those with primary syphilis develop enlarged lymph nodes in the general area of the chancre. Since the chancre most commonly develops on the genitals, the lymph nodes in the groin area are often enlarged. This usually occurs within a week of the appearance of the sore. The lymph nodes become hard and enlarged and are also painless. Enlarged lymph nodes can remain for months after the chancre disappears.

If syphilis is untreated, the disease progresses into the second (secondary) stage, in which *Treponema pallidum* is present throughout many tissues and fluids in the body. Numerous signs and symptoms can be present in this stage. The areas most commonly involved (75 to 80 percent of cases) are the skin and mucous membranes. Sores or lesions generally appear fairly evenly on both sides of the body. The lesions most often appear as round, pale red or pink flat areas up to one-fourth to one-half inch in diameter that do not itch. They often appear on the back, chest, abdomen, shoulders, and arms, and can be confused with other types of skin conditions. Over a period of several weeks, other types of skin rashes can develop. Most commonly, raised reddish or copper-colored areas appear. These can appear on almost any part of the body, including the face and scalp. Lesions of the face and scalp can cause temporary, patchy loss of hair. The rash frequently occurs on the palms of the hands and soles of the feet. In warm, moist, partially enclosed areas such as the anal and rectal areas, the inner thighs, armpits, or the labia and vulva, the raised lesions can combine and enlarge to form masses called condylomata lata. The condylomata lata are pink or grayish in color.

About 30 percent of the time, lesions on the mucous membranes, also called mucous patches, occur along with the skin rashes. The lesions are flat, painless, silver-gray areas surrounded by a reddish coloration and can occur on areas such as the inner cheeks, lips, pharynx, vulva, vagina, and penis.

Other symptoms such as low fever, tiredness, loss of appetite, headache, sore throat, joint aches, or weight loss may occur with secondary syphilis. Enlargement of lymph nodes in many areas of the body occurs in 50 to 60 percent of patients. Less commonly (in less than 10 percent of patients) hepatitis, kidney problems, and inflammation of the eyes may occur. Meningitis has developed in about 1 to 2 percent of patients.

Even if untreated, the signs and symptoms of secondary syphilis disappear in roughly two to 12 weeks. This is then followed by the latent phase, which can continue for many years. In the latent phase, no symptoms of the disease are generally present. However, those in the early latent stage can experience relapses of syphilis, with the development of signs and symptoms similar to those in the secondary stage.

Up to 50 to 65 percent of those with latent syphilis never progress any further in terms of signs and symptoms of the disease. Even sensitive laboratory tests for syphilis may become negative during this time. Others go on to develop the tertiary (late) stage of the disease.

Tertiary syphilis has three major adverse effects: cardiovascular disease (affecting the heart and blood vessels), central nervous system disease, and the development of nodules or granules on almost any area of the body (also called granulomas or gummas). About 10 percent of those with untreated syphilis will develop cardiovascular disease, which can develop up to 40 years after the initial infection with syphilis. Signs and symptoms of cardiovascular disease include heart murmurs, inflammation of the aorta (the large artery leading from the left side of the heart out to the rest of the body), and the development of aneurysms. Aneurysms are caused by weakening of the wall lining an artery. This leads to an abnormal enlargement (ballooning) of the weakened area of the artery. This area continues to become larger and, depending on the location, can cause chest pain, cough, difficulty in swallowing, hoarseness, or shortness of breath. The aneurysm may eventually rupture, leading to massive bleeding and possibly death.

Another 10 percent of patients with untreated syphilis develop central nervous system disease, also called neurosyphilis, which often occurs within five to 30 years after the initial infection with *Treponema pallidum*. Neurosyphilis is more common in men than in women and in Caucasians than in blacks. In some cases, neurosyphilis is not associated with abnormal signs or symptoms and is diagnosed by laboratory examination of the spinal fluid. In other cases, meningitis develops, with headache being a primary symptom. Confusion, seizures, paralysis, and coma progressing to death may occur. The pupils of the eyes may be small and uneven in size. Ringing in the ears (tinnitus), a sensation of ear fullness, a spinning sensation (vertigo), or hearing loss can also occur. In still other cases of neurosyphilis, destruction of nerve cells in the brain occurs. Signs and symptoms of the progressive nerve destruction include irritability, memory and personality changes, delusions and hallucinations, insanity, speech problems, vision changes, greater than normal reflexes, and tremor of the hands, tongue, and lips.

Destruction of nerve cells along the spinal cord may also occur with neurosyphilis. This can result in abnormal sensations in the extremities, clumsy walking with the legs spread apart, incoordination, difficulties with urine control, impotence, sharp "lightning-like" pains in the legs, which either may come and go or may last for a few days, and pains in the stomach, rectal, or throat areas.

Approximately 15 percent of those with untreated syphilis will form gummas. Gummas are caused by inflammation and lead to the development of granules or nodules with dead cells in the center. Gummas most commonly affect the skin, bones, mouth, and upper respiratory tract. They generally occur singly. On the skin, gummas appear as painless areas or nodules that are reddish in color with darkened coloration around the outside. On bones, they can cause pain, tenderness, or fractures. In most cases, the gummas do not cause any complications and can heal on their own with scarring. However, gummas on the brain, heart, or liver can result in extensive damage which can lead to death.

Congenital syphilis is also classified into stages. Congenital syphilis is said to be early when signs and symptoms develop in children less than two years of age. After age two, the syphilis is classified as late. In most cases, signs and symptoms of syphilis are usually not present at birth and often develop within two to 10 weeks after birth.

Signs and symptoms of early congenital syphilis often resemble secondary syphilis in adults and include runny nose, rash, other skin and mucous membrane lesions that can occur over the entire body, and inflammation and structural changes affecting the growing parts of bones. Bone pain can be severe during the active disease. In this stage, the child is generally infectious. In addition, early congenital syphilis can affect other areas and organs of the body causing anemia, jaundice, enlarged lymph nodes, enlarged liver and spleen, kidney damage, pancreatitis (inflammation of the pancreas), growth retardation (while the fetus is still in the uterus), vision problems, and a type of pneumonia. In cases where signs and symptoms of syphilis are present in the infant at birth, the disease is usually severe, and the chances for survival are not good.

In almost two-thirds of cases of late congenital syphilis, no signs or symptoms are present. Signs and symptoms usually develop in the adolescent or preadolescent age groups and resemble many of the features of tertiary syphilis in adults. Signs and symptoms of late congenital syphilis include inflammation of the cornea of the eye (keratitis), light sensitivity, eye pain, and eventual scarring. Keratitis usually appears during the early teens and lasts for 18 to 24 months if untreated. It eventually disappears on its own. A complication of keratitis can be the development of glaucoma years later. Other signs and symptoms of late congenital syphilis include hearing loss, deafness, swelling and inflammation of the joints (especially the knees), and gummas. The heart, blood vessels, and central nervous system can also be affected. Central nervous system involvement can lead to slow mental functioning, seizures, or paralysis. Syphilis in children leads to characteristic changes in appearance. In at least 60 percent of cases of late congenital syphilis, the teeth are abnormally shaped, with notched, widely-spaced incisors (the front teeth on both the upper and lower jaws) and an extra cusp (upward ridge) on the first molars. In addition, abnormalities of the face are seen in at least 70 percent of infected children. Gummas can destroy the bridge of the nose, leading to collapse and a "saddlenose" appearance. A rounding or bulge of the forehead may be present. The top part of the shin on the leg may become curved outward (bow-shaped) and has been called "saber shins."

DEATH RATE FROM SYPHILIS

If adequate treatment is given during the primary, secondary, or latent stages of syphilis, cure will result. In tertiary syphilis, cardiovascular and nervous system complications are the most common causes of death. In one study, the death rate in untreated males with syphilis was approximately 15 percent, and in females the death rate was approximately 8 percent. In general, about one-fourth of patients with untreated syphilis die due to complications of tertiary syphilis.

The percentage of reported latent syphilis cases declined by 35 percent from 1969 to 1983. Since the number of latent syphilis cases and, therefore, the potential number of tertiary syphilis cases has decreased, then the number of deaths due to syphilis has probably also decreased as well.

TREATMENT OF SYPHILIS

Unlike other sexually transmitted diseases in which resistance to commonly used antibiotics may be a problem, syphilis remains extremely sensitive to penicillin, which consistently kills *Treponema pallidum*. The exact type and dose of treatment given depends on the stage of syphilis which is present. In general, penicillin G is the treatment of choice for syphilis. Although other antibiotics, such as cephalosporins, have been tested for syphilis treatment, penicillin remains the most effective and least expensive treatment.

For early syphilis of less than one year's duration (whether primary, secondary, or latent), the recommended treatment is a single dose of 2.4 million units of benzathine penicillin G, injected into the muscle. Benzathine penicillin G is a preparation of penicillin G in which the penicillin is slowly released from the muscle into the blood following intramuscular injection. This allows for prolonged, low concentrations of penicillin to be present in the body. Since *Treponema pallidum* is easily killed following prolonged exposure to penicillin G, benzathine penicillin G is an effective treatment for early syphilis. In patients allergic to penicillin, the antibiotic tetracycline, 500 mg four times daily by mouth for 15 days, can be given. In those who cannot take tetracycline and are allergic to penicillin, erythromycin, 500 mg four times daily by mouth for 15 days, can be given. Erythromycin is the least effective of the three antibiotics for syphilis treatment. Since both tetracycline and erythromycin must be taken for a prolonged period of time in order to be fully effective, it is extremely important that the drugs be taken regularly as directed.

For syphilis of longer than one year's duration at the time of diagnosis (except for neurosyphilis, which has its own special treatment), benzathine penicillin G, 2.4 million units intramuscularly, is given once a week for a total of three consecutive weeks.

In those with syphilis of longer than one year's duration who are allergic to penicillin, the effectiveness of other treatments has not been well established. However, tetracycline, 500 mg four times daily by mouth for 30 days, is given in such circumstances. The treatment duration is twice as long as the treatment duration for syphilis of less than one year's duration. In those who cannot take tetracycline and have definitely been shown to be allergic to penicillin, erythromycin, 500 mg four times daily by mouth for 30 days, should be given. Again, it is especially important that these drugs be taken strictly as directed in order to be fully effective against syphilis.

Individuals who have signs or symptoms of neurosyphilis, or those with late latent syphilis or syphilis of greater than one year's duration, should have a sample of the spinal fluid taken and tested for syphilis. If the spinal fluid is positive, treatment for neurosyphilis should begin immediately. In order for penicillin to be effective in treating neurosyphilis, the drug must enter the spinal fluid. Therefore, high doses of penicillin may be necessary. Treatments which can be used for neurosyphilis include: (1) aqueous crystalline penicillin G, 2 to 4 million units intravenously every four hours (12 to 24 million units per day) for 10 days, followed by benzathine penicillin G, 2.4 million units intramuscularly once weekly for three weeks; or (2) procaine penicillin G, 2.4 million units intramuscularly daily together with probenecid 500 mg by mouth four times daily for 10 days, followed by benzathine penicillin G, 2.4 million units intramuscularly once weekly for three weeks. Probenecid given with penicillin causes less penicillin to be eliminated from the body. In this way, the amount of penicillin available to fight the infection is increased. Alternatively, particularly if neurosyphilis is suspected but no symptoms exist, benzathine penicillin G, 2.4 million units intramuscularly once weekly for three weeks, can be given. If one has neurosyphilis and is allergic to penicillin, your doctor will probably consult a specialist in order to select the proper therapy.

Pregnant women with syphilis can be treated with penicillin G at the doses and dosing schedules described above, depending upon which stage of syphilis the mother has. In pregnant women with syphilis who are allergic to penicillin, erythromycin rather than tetracycline should be given. The appropriate dosing schedule for erythromycin varies, again depending on which stage of syphilis the mother has. Since erythromycin does not always enter the fetal blood in adequate concentrations, and is not always effective in these patients, the infant should receive benzathine penicillin G, 50,000 units per kilogram of body weight intramuscularly at birth. Since tetracycline may cause harmful effects in a developing fetus, tetracycline should not be given during pregnancy. If a woman with syphilis is treated before the 16th to 18th week of pregnancy, the fetus will generally not become infected.

Even if mothers receive appropriate penicillin therapy for syphilis during pregnancy, infants must be closely examined at birth and tested at periodic intervals until tests are negative. However, infants may be infected and have a negative syphilis test at birth, particularly if they were infected late during pregnancy. Therefore, infants should be treated at birth if born to mothers in whom the type of syphilis treatment was unknown, inadequate, or treatment was with a drug or drugs other than penicillin.

The spinal fluid of infants with congenital syphilis should be tested for the presence of syphilis. If the spinal fluid is positive, or the infant has symptoms of congenital syphilis at birth, then aqueous crystalline penicillin G, 25,000 units per kilogram of body weight, should be given twice daily intramuscularly or intravenously, for a minimum of 10 days. Alternatively, procaine penicillin G, 50,000 units per kilogram of body weight daily, should be given intramuscularly for a minimum of 10 days. In infants who have normal spinal fluid and no symptoms of syphilis, benzathine penicillin G, 50,000 units per kilogram of body weight, can be given once intramuscularly. Children beyond the infant age who are diagnosed as having congenital syphilis should receive the same penicillin dosages as described for infants. For older children, the total penicillin dosage should not exceed the penicillin dosage recommended for adults with syphilis of greater than one year's duration.

Sexual partners of syphilis victims should be treated as if they have primary or secondary syphilis. They should also be tested for syphilis. Infected individuals who undergo successful treatment can be reinfected with syphilis; there is no "immunity" after having the disease. Prospects for development of a vaccine to prevent syphilis are not good.

There are usually few adverse effects associated with the use of penicillin for syphilis treatment. The most common adverse effect from penicillin is an allergic reaction. This can range from a mild rash to hives, swelling, and difficulty in breathing. Death may occur if the reaction is severe. Severe allergic reactions to penicillin occur in less than one percent of those who receive it.

In addition to the possible adverse effects from penicillin itself, up to 90 percent of those with secondary syphilis, 50 percent of individuals with primary syphilis, and 25 percent of those with early latent syphilis experience another type of adverse reaction. This reaction is characterized by fever, chills, muscle aches, headache, and a worsening of the skin and mucous membrane lesions. The reaction occurs within two to 12 hours of the initial treatment, with fever usually disappearing within a day. This is not an allergic reaction to the penicillin. It is thought to be caused by the rapid killing of *Treponema pallidum* and the resulting release of toxic substances that cause "flu-like" symptoms. If the reaction occurs, bed rest and aspirin or acetaminophen is generally all that is needed.

PREVENTION OF SYPHILIS

Since humans do not have any natural resistance to infection by *Treponema pallidum,* methods to help protect against syphilis must be used. The greater the number of sexual partners a person has, the greater the risk of acquiring syphilis. Therefore, the risk of syphilis can be reduced by minimizing the number of sexual partners.

Another effective method of preventing syphilis is for the male to use a condom during sexual intercourse. This is the only contraceptive device which has been shown to be unequivocally effective in preventing syphilis. However, in order to be effective it must be undamaged, correctly used, and worn throughout the interval of sexual contact. If properly and regularly used, the condom can be an important weapon in the fight against syphilis and other sexually transmitted diseases.

Douching or washing with soap and water following sexual contact is not an effective method for preventing syphilis development. Preliminary information suggests that certain vaginal contraceptive spermicides may be able to kill *Treponema pallidum;* however, further studies must be conducted to test their effectiveness in actually preventing syphilis transmission before their use can be recommended.

CONCLUSION

Although the discovery of penicillin produced the possibility of ultimate elimination of syphilis, the disease remains a significant health care concern in this country. Further awareness of ways to prevent syphilis is required. The signs and symptoms of all the stages of syphilis, including congenital syphilis, should be known. A physician should be consulted if signs and symptoms of syphilis occur. If a person is diagnosed as having syphilis, strict compliance with treatment is essential. The person must also return for follow-up testing to assure that the treatment was successful. With greater public awareness of syphilis, its prevention, treatment, and control will be substantially enhanced.

13

Nongonococcal Urethritis

INTRODUCTION

Nongonococcal urethritis (NGU) is defined as a sexually acquired infection of the male urethra (see Figure 3, Introductory Chapter) which is not gonococcal and is usually caused by infection with *Chlamydia trachomatis*, *Ureaplasma urealyticum*, or rarely, *Trichomonas vaginalis*, *Corynebacterium genitalium*, or *Candida albicans*. Approximately 50 to 60 percent of cases are due to *C. trachomatis*. *U. urealyticum* may account for 25 to 30 percent of cases, although the precise pathological role of this organism has not been defined. In approximately 25 percent of cases of nongonococcal urethritis, no specific cause of infecting agent can be identified. This nonspecific urethritis is assumed to be sexually transmitted and should be treated accordingly.

After treatment for a gonococcal infection (gonorrhea), some men develop a syndrome known as postgonococcal urethritis. This is actually nongonococcal urethritis that coexisted with gonorrhea before treatment. If urethritis continues after treatment of gonorrhea, this usually means the drug chosen to kill *Neisseria gonorrhoeae* (generally a penicillin) was not effective against the other organisms. Postgonococcal urethritis generally suggests infection by *C. tracho-*

matis. Approximately 20 percent of males and nearly 35 percent of females with gonorrhea also have chlamydial *(C. trachomatis)* infections of the genital tract.

Women may experience nongonococcal urethritis, but in women it is not a primary infection. Rather, it is generally a complication of a primary infection occurring elsewhere. For example, chlamydial and nonchlamydial infections may not only cause urethritis in women, but also produce cervicitis (inflammation of the cervix), endometritis (inflammation of the uterus), acute salpingitis (inflammation of the fallopian tubes), and perihepatitis (inflammation around the liver). Nongonococcal urethritis in women is usually a secondary complication of cervicitis. A counterpart of nongonococcal urethritis (NGU) in females is trichomoniasis. Trichomoniasis is addressed in Chapter 15. The complications of gonococcal and nongonococcal infections of the female reproductive tract are addressed in Chapter 14 (Pelvic Inflammatory Disease).

PREVALENCE OF NONGONOCOCCAL URETHRITIS

Nongonococcal urethritis (NGU) is two to three times more common than gonorrhea in the general population. Approximately 4.0 to 5.0 million cases of NGU occur each year. NGU is about 10 times more prevalent than gonorrhea among college students. The age at which the incidence of chlamydia-related NGU is highest from the late teens to early twenties.

The prevalence of chlamydial urethritis in young men seen in a general medical practice is three to five percent. Over 10 percent of routine physical exams of young male soldiers reveal a chlamydial infection of the urethra. Approximately 20 percent of men seen for the treatment of sexually transmitted disease have a chlamydial infection of the urethra. Males who are indigent, nonwhite, unmarried, and between 18 and 24 years of age have the highest incidence of NGU.

DIAGNOSIS OF NONGONOCOCCAL URETHRITIS

NGU has been largely neglected as a disease until recently, even though it is substantially more prevalent than gonorrhea and infects hundreds of thousands of Americans annually. This neglect is attributable to many causes, including preoccupation with the diagnosis of more dramatic diseases such as gonorrhea, syphilis, genital herpes, and AIDS; a low diagnostic index of suspicion by physicians; absence of serious and painful symptoms; and lack of availability of accurate and easily applied diagnostic tests. Complications of NGU can be serious; early and accurate diagnosis is necessary if health risks are to be minimized.

Diagnosis of NGU is difficult because organisms which cause NGU may produce subtle symptoms, no symptoms, or symptoms that could be caused by numerous other organisms, and pinpointing the infecting organism is therefore difficult. One may have a mixed (multiple) infection, and identification of one organism may not reveal the entire infectious picture. Laboratories have traditionally had a difficult time identifying chlamydia, and the diagnosis of male urethritis seldom includes cultures for *C. trachomatis* or *U. urealyticum.*

The latest generation of chlamydia testing involves use of monoclonal antibodies to detect small numbers of organisms in urethral fluid. Advantages of this test include speed (15 minutes), accuracy (greater than 90 percent), relatively low cost, and convenience. Utilizing the monoclonal antibody test, one may be diagnosed and treatment begun before leaving the physician's office. Sexually active women may wish to request this test in conjunction with their annual Pap smear.

Early and accurate diagnosis of NGU is often difficult due to subtle or nonspecific symptoms, or the lack of symptoms. In men, chlamydial urethritis generally produces less severe symptoms than gonococcal urethritis, and women infected with chlamydia frequently develop no obvious symptoms until complications of pelvic inflammatory disease develop. Use of monoclonal antibody diagnostic testing will allow low cost, convenient, and early detection of the chlamydial organism. This will contribute substantially to prevention of the spread of this infection and the serious consequences of untreated infection. Hopefully monoclonal antibody testing for *Ureaplasma urealyticum,* and other organisms causing NGU, will become available in the near future.

SIGNS AND SYMPTOMS OF NONGONOCOCCAL URETHRITIS

Symptoms of male NGU may be minimal, nonspecific, or absent. Symptoms usually develop five to 20 days after infection. Clinical symptoms, when present, usually consist of a scant or moderate urethral discharge which may be yellowish, white, or clear; painful burning on urination; and urethral itching. The inner lining of the urethra may be red and tender. White blood cells may be present in the urethral discharge and the urine. Approximately one-third of males with NGU have no clinically overt symptoms of urethritis. The sexually active male carrier of *C. trachomatis* is likely to infect the female sexual partner. This "seeding" of the female may then lead to involvement of the female cervix, uterus, fallopian tubes, urethra, and peritoneum, and may produce symptoms and serious complications of pelvic inflammatory disease (see Chapter 14).

COMPLICATIONS OF NONGONOCOCCAL URETHRITIS

The complications of NGU in the male are numerous and can be quite serious. Furthermore, the complications can be very serious in the female sexual partner if the infection is transmitted to her. Finally, chlamydial complications in newborns whose mother was infected by a male sexual partner may occur.

Complications of NGU in the Male

Epididymitis (inflammation of the epididymis) is a relatively frequent complication of NGU. *C. trachomatis*, along with *N. gonorrhoeae*, is the most frequent cause of epididymitis. Epididymitis is usually unilateral (occurring on only one side) and is associated with fever, scrotal pain, swelling, and tenderness in the area. Bed rest and scrotal elevation may hasten relief of symptoms. Epididymitis associated with NGU is readily treated, but prompt diagnosis and treatment is essential because delays in diagnosis and proper treatment may lead to epididymal scarring and occlusion (blockage) of the epididymis. Scarring of the epididymis bilaterally (on both sides) could lead to sterility as sperm could not travel from testes to other parts of the male reproductive tract.

Proctitis (inflammation of the mucous membranes of the rectum) is a complication of NGU that is acute, most commonly due to *C. trachomatis*, and generally restricted to homosexual men and heterosexual women practicing receptive anal intercourse. Symptoms include rectal pain, bleeding, mucous discharge, and painful spasms of rectal muscle.

Urethral stricture due to scarring associated with untreated or recurrent episodes of NGU may occur. This may impair urination and produce a situation where the male is at greater risk for developing urinary tract infections.

Complications of Sexually Transmitted Urethritis in the Female

As mentioned previously, nongonococcal urethritis is not a primary disease condition in women. Rather, it is viewed as a secondary complication of a primary infection, usually involving the vagina or cervix of the uterus. Complications of nongonococcal infections in the female, especially those due to *C. trachomatis*, are numerous and may be extremely serious. These complications are presented in detail in the chapter on pelvic inflammatory disease (Chapter 14).

Complications of NGU in the Newborn Infant

Women who become infected with *C. trachomatis* risk transmitting the infection to newborns passing through the birth canal. Approximately 50 percent of the offspring of mothers with chlamydial infections of the cervix may be infected. Because males who infect women may not have symptoms, it is necessary that pregnant women be screened to see if they have a chlamydial infection. The simple monoclonal antibody test which is now available makes this screening test as practical as a Pap smear. The cost of this convenient test is inconsequential when one considers the risk to offspring of mothers who have untreated chlamydial infections.

Inclusion conjunctivitis (chlamydial conjunctivitis) involves the membrane lining the eyelids and eyeball. This infection may develop from five to 14 days after birth. The eyedrops most routinely used to prevent eye infection in newborns (1 percent silver nitrate) may not prevent chlamydial conjunctivitis. Approximately 30 to 40 percent of infants born to women infected with *C. trachomatis* may be infected. Symptoms are variable and nonspecific, generally develop rapidly, and may produce a profuse discharge consisting of mucus and pus. The infection is readily treated with erythromycin. Failure to treat chlamydial conjunctivitis may lead to pneumonia.

A distinctive infant pneumonia due to *C. trachomatis* has been identified. The pneumonia develops in 10 to 20 percent of offspring of mothers infected with chlamydia. Symptoms of the pneumonia begin four to 12 weeks after birth and consist of a rapid barking cough, chest congestion, rapid breathing, and abnormal chest sounds. The infant will not have a fever. X-rays provide further evidence of pneumonia. The pneumonia lasts several weeks. Chlamydial pneumonia has not been reported in children over six months old. About half the infants with pneumonia also have chlamydial conjunctivitis. Treatment of the pneumonia should begin as soon as possible.

TREATMENT OF NONGONOCOCCAL URETHRITIS

The antimicrobial agents found to have the greatest activity against *C. trachomatis* and *U. urealyticum* are tetracycline (Achromycin V®, Sumycin®, Tetracyn®), doxycycline (Vibramycin®), erythromycin (E-Mycin®, ERYC®, Ilosone®, Ethril®, Wyamycin E®), the sulfonamides (sulfa drugs), and rifampin (Rifadin®, Rimactane®). Table 30 includes the drugs recommended to treat the various types of infections presented in this chapter. It should be noted that several drugs commonly effective in treating gonococcal infections are of limited or little value in treating chlamydial infections. The penicillins (including penicillin G, ampicillin, and amoxicillin) are of intermediate value, as is clindamycin (Cleocin®). The cephalosporins (cefoxitin, cefotaxime, moxalactam), aminoglycosides (gentamicin, tobramycin), spectinomycin (Trobicin®), and trimethoprim (Proloprim®, Trimpex®) are of limited value in treating chlamydial infections.

Rifampin, although effective, is seldom used to treat *C. trachomatis* infections because resistance to it emerges rapidly. Erythromycin appears to be somewhat less effective than tetracycline in treating nongonococcal urethritis due to *C. trachomatis* and *U. urealyticum*, and 14 days of therapy may be required. If an adult with NGU contaminates an eye with the infecting microorganism and symptoms develop, the eye infection should be treated the way urethritis is treated.

Treatment is not enough. Follow-up to treatment is essential to determine success of therapy. Ideally, those treated would be seen one week after beginning treatment to determine compliance to the drug regimen, occurrence of drug-induced side effects (if any), and whether evidence of the infection is disappearing. If symptoms have not improved or been eliminated after one week, a second week of therapy should occur. Failure of a two-week course of therapy requires a decision of whether to continue the drug or change to another drug. If symptoms are improved but still remain after two weeks of treatment, most clinicians will continue with the same drug. When symptoms disappear and the drug is discontinued, appropriate microbiological tests should be performed to determine whether the organism causing the infection has been eliminated.

A major part of follow-up care is the attempt to identify and treat all sexual partners of patients with NGU. Sexual contacts should be treated, whether they have symptoms or not, with the regimen for urethritis included in Table 30. Recurrence of NGU may be due to failure to treat the sexual partner(s). Persistent or recurrent signs of NGU after adequate treatment of patient and sexual partner(s) warrant further evaluation for less common causes of the symptoms.

PREVENTION OF NONGONOCOCCAL URETHRITIS

Steps to prevention of NGU and its complications are very straightforward and include:

1. Avoiding multiple sexual partners. This increases the probability of acquiring an infection.

TABLE 30
TREATMENT OF NONGONOCOCCAL URETHRITIS AND ASSOCIATED COMPLICATIONS

	Affected Area	Drug	Dose	Alternative Treatment
MALE	Urethritis[1]	Tetracycline[2]	500 mg orally 4 times daily for 7 days	Sulfisoxazole 500 mg orally 4 times daily for 10 days
		Doxycycline	100 mg orally 2 times daily for 7 days	
		Erythromycin[3]	500 mg orally 4 times daily for 7 days	
	Epididymitis[1]	Tetracycline[2]	500 mg orally 4 times daily for 10 days	
		Erythromycin[3]	500 mg orally 4 times daily for 10 days	
	Proctitis[1]	(same treatment as for urethritis)		
FEMALE	Cervicitis (acquired from male with NGU)	(For details of treating gonococcal and nongonococcal cervicitis on both an outpatient and inpatient basis see Chapter 14 on Pelvic Inflammatory Disease		

NEWBORN			
Newborn Conjunctivitis[4]	Erythromycin[5]	12.5 mg/kg of body weight orally or intravenously (i.v.) 4 times daily for 14 days	Sulfisoxazole, 100 mg/kg of body weight per day orally or intravenously (i.v.) in divided doses (for children older than 4 weeks)
Newborn Pneumonia[4]	Erythromycin	10 mg/kg of body weight orally or intravenously (i.v.) 4 times daily for 14 days	

[1] Due to *C. trachomatis* or *U. urealyticum*.
[2] Also a first line drug to treat *N. gonorrhoeae*.
[3] A 14-day course of therapy may be required.
[4] When *C. trachomatis* is the causative organism.
[5] Application of erythromycin or sulfonamide ointment directly to the eye does not appear to be very effective. There is no need to supplement oral or injectable therapy with eye ointment.

2. Identifying and treating sexual partners of victims of NGU. Others may have been infected, but have no symptoms. Treatment is essential to the prevention of complications. People who identify sexual partners may have their identity held confidential if they wish.

3. Seeking medical attention as soon as symptoms develop. Delays in diagnosing NGU may create unnecessary suffering from the urethritis and numerous complications. Physicians will regard the infection confidentially. In most states physicians do not need permission of a parent to treat a sexually transmitted infection in anyone over the age of 12. This law, which assures confidentiality of treatment, is generally known as the minor consent law.

   For obvious reasons, many young people living at home would not want to seek medical attention from the family physician if they suspected they had a sexually transmitted disease. There are other excellent ways to acquire care. Nearly every county or city in the U.S. has a clinic devoted to the prevention and treatment of sexually transmitted disease. The clinic in a particular area may be located by looking up "Health Department" or "Venereal Disease Clinic" in the telephone directory. Individuals may also seek outpatient care at a local hospital emergency room or outpatient clinic. For information on the treatment facilities in a particular area one may call the county medical society or national VD Hot Line (1-800-227-8922).

4. Following the treatment prescribed. Do not skip doses. Get the entire prescription filled. Tell the doctor or a clinic worker if you miss a dose or the drug makes you feel ill. Successful treatment are essential to preventing further infections.

CONCLUSION

Nongonococcal urethritis is often overlooked as a sexually transmitted disease. In most instances, treatment is relatively simple and effective. Prompt diagnosis and treatment are essential if serious complications in the male and female reproductive tract are to be avoided.

14

Pelvic Inflammatory
Disease (PID)

INTRODUCTION

Pelvic inflammatory disease (PID) is almost exclusively a disease of sexually active women. PID typically refers to cases of infectious and secondary inflammatory complications involving the upper genital tract (cervix, endometrium, and fallopian tubes) and is usually caused by bacteria, many of which are sexually transmitted. These bacteria migrate from the vagina or cervix of the uterus higher into the female reproductive system. Pelvic inflammatory disease is generally preventable if certain precautions are observed and risk factors avoided. If PID does develop, early diagnosis and aggressive treatment is necessary to prevent serious complications of this increasingly common sexually transmitted disease. The focus of this chapter is to assist you in recognizing risk factors which increase the chance of developing PID, reveal precautions which may be exercised to prevent development of PID, increase awareness of the symptoms of PID, reveal the serious complications of untreated or ineffectively treated PID, and present the most effective approaches to treatment of PID.

PREVALENCE OF PELVIC INFLAMMATORY DISEASE

Pelvic inflammatory disease has reached epidemic proportions in the United States. In the mid-1970s it was estimated that over 850,000 cases occurred each year. It is now estimated that there are over 2 million visits to physicians in this country each year because of PID. Approximately 10 cases of PID per 1000 women of childbearing age occur annually. Sexually active teenagers and women in their early twenties experience approximately 20 cases per 1000 women. Between 1975 and 1981, an estimated average of 267,200 women were hospitalized annually for treatment or management of complications of PID. The number of PID-associated hospitalizations now exceeds 300,000 annually. The cost of this disease in terms of physical suffering and mental anguish is untold. The economic impact of PID, in direct and indirect cost, is estimated to exceed $4 billion annually. The incidence and severity of PID will fall only when women understand more fully the steps which must be taken to prevent the disease—or to treat the disease if it occurs.

CAUSES OF PELVIC INFLAMMATORY DISEASE

Pelvic inflammatory disease may be caused by many bacteria, some of which are normally present in the vagina. The overwhelming majority of PID cases are due, however, to two organisms which are not normal inhabitants of the female or male genital tract. These two

---

TABLE 31
RISK FACTORS FOR DEVELOPMENT OF PELVIC INFLAMMATORY DISEASE

- Multiple sexual partners

- Use of an intrauterine device (IUD)

- Age (It is theorized that younger women may have lower immunity and less resistance to infection by bacteria that are sexually transmitted.)

- History of gonorrhea or another sexually transmitted infection (such as *Chlamydia trachomatis*)

- Delays in seeking appropriate medical attention when evidence of infection (increased vaginal discharge), frequent and painful urination, lower abdominal pain, and/or abnormal menstrual bleeding is present in the lower genital tract

- Invasive intrauterine diagnostic or therapeutic procedures which may carry organisms into the upper genital tract

---

organisms may be sexually transmitted; they are *Neisseria gonor-rhoeae* and *Chlamydia trachomatis.* First episodes of PID are particularly likely to be due to one of these two organisms, especially among young, sexually active women with multiple sexual partners. Factors which increase risk of developing PID are included in Table 31.

In the United States the gonococcus, *Neisseria gonorrhoeae,* has been isolated in a high percentage (45 to 70 percent) of women with acute (rapidly developing) PID. *Chlamydia trachomatis* has been isolated in approximately 20 to 50 percent of women with acute PID. In one study, 79 percent of PID victims who had positive cervical cultures for *N. gonorrhoeae* also had positive cervical cultures for *C. trachomatis.* Since infections leading to PID may be due to more than one bacterium, treatment should reflect this possibility.

How infectious organisms of the lower genital tract ascend from the vagina and endocervix (inner lining of the cervix of the uterus) to produce endometrial, tubal, and ovarian infection is not well understood. Invasive diagnostic or therapeutic procedures requiring insertion of instruments into the uterus could explain a small percentage of cases. One study suggests that bacteria may attach themselves to spermatozoa and ride "piggyback" through the cervical mucus to their eventual destination. Regardless of how infecting organisms reach the upper female genital tract, a woman must appreciate that failure to promptly and adequately treat sexually transmitted diseases, particularly those due to *N. gonorrhoeae* and *C. trachomatis,* greatly increases the risk of PID and its host of complications.

SIGNS AND SYMPTOMS OF PELVIC INFLAMMATORY DISEASE

It is very important that you be aware of the signs and symptoms of PID so you can seek appropriate medical attention, receive diagnosis, and begin treatment as soon as possible. The symptoms of PID may vary from person to person, depending on which organism is infecting the woman and which part of the pelvic region is most affected. Table 32 lists typical symptoms of PID according to the area affected.

A pelvic examination by a physician can usually detect cervicitis. Abnormal tenderness is typically associated with stretching and movement of the cervix during the examination. The white blood cell (WBC) count is elevated in approximately 60 percent of women with salpingitis. Evidence of a lower genital tract infection, as indicated by the fact that white blood cells outnumber all other cells in the vaginal fluid, may be useful in diagnosis. Over one-third of women with PID and acute salpingitis will have a fever of 38°C (100.4°F) or greater. Fever may subside if PID is not promptly treated and may not serve as a useful diagnostic measure. Specimens of the endocervix should be cultured for *N. gonorrhoeae* and *C. trachomatis*. A positive culture is not diagnostic of PID, but is highly suggestive if other symptoms are present.

PID associated with IUD use is often gradual in its onset, seldom associated with fever, and may be preceded by a foul smelling vaginal discharge. PID due to *N. gonorrhoeae* is typically more rapid in its onset than chlamydial PID, and symptoms of gonococcal PID are often associated with the menstrual period. Metrorrhagia (irregular bleeding during the menstrual cycle) precedes or coincides with the onset of pain in 30 to 40 percent of women with PID. PID and salpingitis associated with chlamydial infections tend to produce

TABLE 32
TYPICAL SYMPTOMS OF PID ACCORDING TO AREA AFFECTED

Area	Effect	Symptoms
Cervix	Cervicitis (inflammation of the cervix of the uterus)	—mucopurulent vaginal discharge —frequent and painful urination if urethra involved —abnormal menstrual bleeding —lower abdominal pain —possible rectal discharge, bleeding, and itching
Endometrium	Endometritis (inflammation of the inner lining of the uterus)	—midline abdominal pain (dull or aching) —abnormal vaginal bleeding
Fallopian Tube(s)	Salpingitis (inflammation of one or both fallopian tubes)	—pelvic pain (moderate to severe) —fever (in about one-third of cases)
Peritoneum	Peritonitis (inflammation of the lining of the abdominal cavity)	—nausea and vomiting —tender abdomen —generalized abdominal pain —fever (in some cases)

milder symptoms of longer duration, and with less fever, than gonor-rhea-associated PID and salpingitis. Laparoscopic (visual) examina-tions of fallopian tubes of PID victims suggest that chlamydia-associated salpingitis is a more severe inflammatory reaction than that induced by the gonococcus.

Although not financially feasible, laparoscopic examination is the best way to diagnose salpingitis due to pelvic inflammatory dis-ease. By physically viewing the fallopian tubes through a laparoscope inserted into the abdominal cavity, salpingitis can be diagnosed with a high degree of accuracy. Laparoscopic criteria for diagnosing sal-pingitis include local inflammation of the fallopian tube as evidenced by redness and swelling and secretion of a pus-containing fluid from the finger-like projections (fimbrae) of the fallopian tube or from the surface of the fallopian tube.

Only about 20 percent of women with salpingitis associated with PID exhibit the classic signs and symptoms discussed above. Diag-nosis is further complicated by the fact that PID may mimic the symptoms of appendicitis, endometriosis, or ectopic pregnancy. Early diagnosis and treatment are essential to minimizing tubal scar-ring, however. Most physicians tend to overdiagnose and overtreat when PID and salpingitis are suspected. This is medically appropriate due to the serious consequences associated with the progression of the disease and the low risk of treatment. Presence of lower abdomi-nal pain of several weeks' duration, cervical tenderness on pelvic examination, and evidence of lower genital tract infection, coupled with one or more "typical symptoms" (for example, fever, abnormal vaginal discharge, abnormal menstrual bleeding, abdominal tender-ness, positive cervical culture for *N. gonorrhoeae* or *C. trachomatis,* and a swelling of one or both fallopian tubes) is highly suggestive of salpingitis and PID. Medical information which may aid in confirming a diagnosis includes a history of sexual exposure to a male with urethritis; gynecological history of endometriosis, salpingitis and/or ectopic pregnancy; and presence of an IUD. Comprehensive evalua-tion of facts related to sexual history, medical history, and current clinical condition should lead to an accurate diagnosis in most cases. Improper diagnosis will likely result in inappropriate treatment, or no treatment, and the progression of PID until serious medical complica-tions develop.

COMPLICATIONS OF PELVIC INFLAMMATORY DISEASE

The most serious consequence of salpingitis associated with pelvic inflammatory disease is bilateral (both sides) tubal occlusion (blockage of fallopian tubes due to tubal scarring) and sterility. A single episode of tubal infection results in tubal closure and subsequent infertility in 11 to 17 percent of women. The rate of infertility seems to be related to age and number of episodes of salpingitis. One study revealed a sterility rate due to tubal occlusion of 14 percent for women 15 to 24 years of age. For women 25 to 34 years of age, the sterility rate secondary to tubal occlusion was 26 percent. Women in the older age group were more likely to have experienced more than one episode of salpingitis. In another study women who had experienced only one episode of salpingitis had a sterility rate of 11 percent; two episodes of salpingitis produced a sterility rate of 23 percent. Three or more episodes of salpingitis may produce a sterility rate of 55 to 75 percent.

Another complication of pelvic inflammatory disease, which is associated with tubal scarring without occlusion, is ectopic pregnancy (tubal pregnancy). Approximately four to five percent of women who develop salpingitis as a component of pelvic inflammatory disease and who subsequently become pregnant will experience an ectopic pregnancy. This represents an ectopic pregnancy rate which is six to 10 times greater than in women who have not experienced pelvic infections.

Long-term complications of pelvic inflammatory disease after treatment and recovery may include chronic abdominal pain, menstrual disturbances, and painful intercourse. The recurrence rate of salpingitis after treatment may be as high as 15 to 25 percent. Having had PID confers no immunity on a woman. Reinfection is probable unless the life-style is modified. Psychological trauma, time off work, and cost of medication and follow-up care also extract a toll.

TREATMENT OF PELVIC INFLAMMATORY DISEASE

Goals of Treatment

The two primary goals of treatment are to resolve symptoms and preserve functional ability of the fallopian tubes. This is best accomplished by early diagnosis and initiation of aggressive antibiotic therapy. Both early diagnosis and effective therapy are necessary to prevent tubal damage and the subsequent risk of ectopic pregnancy. Treatment failure rates run as high as 15 to 25 percent; this is simply not good enough. Conscientious efforts are required to treat victims of PID more effectively and aggressively. This requires hospitalization in some instances.

Criteria for Hospitalization

Dr. William Droegemueller of the University of North Carolina, while recognizing that hospitalization of women with PID is ideal, is practical enough to recognize that it is not always logically pragmatic, or financially feasible. He has developed some excellent criteria for deciding when hospitalization is required. Dr. Droegemueller recommends hospitalization when one or more of the following criteria are met:

1. Nulliparity. Nulliparity means having no previous pregnancy. Tubal scarring and occlusion can lead to infertility very prematurely. If hospitalized and treated aggressively with injectable antibiotics, the chance for effective treatment and no significant tubal scarring or blockage is greater than if treated as an outpatient.
2. Abscess or Tubo-ovarian Involvement. Such a medical condition is quite serious and requires aggressive antibiotic therapy that is best administered by injection. In the rare but serious event of a rupture of the abscess, it is appropriate that the condition be managed in a hospital and intravenous antibiotics administered.
3. Pregnancy. A uterine infection is often not localized to the uterus in a woman who is in or beyond the fourth month of pregnancy. The infection may become widespread and serious. Injectable antibiotic therapy in the hospital setting is generally required.
4. Uncertain Diagnosis. Because symptoms of PID are often confused with symptoms of appendicitis, endometriosis, and ectopic pregnancy, it is best to determine the specific diagnosis in a hospital, then begin aggressive treatment of the diagnosed condition.
5. Gastrointestinal Symptoms. The mainstay of treatment of PID on an outpatient basis is oral antibiotic therapy. If a woman has a gastrointestinal disorder which includes nausea and vomiting, she may be unable to tolerate medication orally. Rather than delay treatment of PID, it may be more appropriate to hospitalize the woman and treat her with injectable antibiotics.
6. Peritonitis in the Upper Abdomen. Peritonitis in the upper abdomen, associated with tenderness of the liver, develops in about five percent of women with PID. This inflammation may be caused by *N. gonorrhoeae* or *C. trachomatis,* should be viewed as a serious condition, and should be treated with injectable antibiotics.

7. Presence of an IUD. Pelvic infection in women utilizing an IUD is usually more severe than pelvic infections not associated with an IUD. Women often attribute early symptoms of pelvic infection to the presence of an IUD, therefore, pelvic infections in IUD users are often advanced. IUD-associated PID is best treated in the hospital with injectable antibiotics.

Some physicians recommend that the IUD be removed immediately if a pelvic infection is present. The International Planned Parenthood Federation recommends removal of the IUD if improvement does not occur within 48 hours after the start of antibiotic therapy.

8. Vaginal Diagnostic Procedures. Pelvic infections that occur after various vaginal or uterine diagnostic procedures are usually caused by one or more of many different bacteria that are normally present in the vaginal area. Because of the wide variety of possible infecting bacteria, it is best to hospitalize such women and utilize injectable antibiotics in treatment.

9. Lack of Response. Women should be examined within 48 hours after outpatient therapy is started. If the therapeutic response is poor, or the woman is not complying strictly with the prescribed oral antibiotic therapy, she should be hospitalized and switched to injectable antibiotic therapy.

Treating Outpatients with PID

The treatment of choice is not established. No single antibiotic is effective against the entire spectrum of potential infecting bacteria. The Centers for Disease Control have developed guidelines for initial outpatient therapy, and these are included in Table 33. All outpatient treatment should be reevaluated in 48 to 72 hours. Women not responding appropriately should be hospitalized.

Treating Hospitalized Patients with PID

Several different regimens may prove effective if the woman is hospitalized. A treatment that has proven effective against a wide spectrum of bacteria (for example, N. gonorrhoeae, penicillinase-producing N. gonorrhoeae (PPNG), and C. trachomatis) consists of doxycycline (Vibramycin®), 100 mg administered twice daily by the intravenous route plus cefoxitin (Mefoxin®), 2.0 grams four times daily by the intravenous route. This regimen should be continued for

TABLE 33
GUIDELINES FOR INITIAL TREATMENT OF OUTPATIENTS WITH PELVIC INFLAMMATORY DISEASE

First Dose: Cefoxitin (Mefoxin®), 2.0 grams injected intramuscularly

or

Procaine penicillin G, 4.8 million units injected intramuscularly (2.4 million units into each of two different injection sites). This injection should be accompanied by a 1.0 gram oral dose of probenecid (Benemid®), which will allow blood levels of penicillin to be sustained at a higher level for a longer period of time.

or

Ceftriaxone (Rocephin®), 250 mg injected intramuscularly

or

Amoxicillin (Amoxil®, Larotid®, Polymox®, Trimox®, Utimox®, Wymox®), 3.0 grams by mouth. This dose should be accompanied by a 1.0 gram oral dose of probenecid.

or

Ampicillin (Amcil®, Polycillin®, Principen®, Omnipen®, Totacillin®), 3.5 grams by mouth. This dose should be accompanied by a 1.0 gram oral dose of probenecid.

Followed By: Doxycycline* (Vibramycin®) 100 mg by mouth, twice daily for 10 to 14 days.

---

*Tetracycline (500 mg four times daily) could be used in place of doxycycline, but its antibacterial spectrum is not as broad, and it requires more frequent dosing.

at least four days and at least 48 hours after the woman begins to improve. Doxycycline (Vibramycin®) should then be continued after discharge, to complete 10 to 14 days of therapy, at an oral dose of 100 mg twice daily.

A hospital regimen that is not particularly useful in treating PID due to *C. trachomatis* or *N. gonorrhoeae*, but may be useful in treating pelvic infections due to certain other organisms, includes clindamycin (Cleocin®), 600 mg four times a day, intravenously, plus gentamicin (Garamycin®), 2.0 mg/kg of body weight given intravenously, followed by 1.5 mg/kg of body weight three times per day intravenously. These doses, which are only recommended in women with normal renal function, should be continued for at least four days and at least 48 hours after the woman begins to improve. Clindamycin (Cleocin®) should be continued after discharge at a dose of 450 mg orally, four times a day to complete a 10- to 14-day course of therapy.

A hospital regimen that is generally effective against *C. trachomatis,* but not optimal against *N. gonorrhoeae,* is doxycycline (Vibramycin®), 100 mg twice daily, intravenously, plus metronidazole (Flagyl®), 1.0 gram twice daily, intravenously. This combination should be continued for at least four days and at least 48 hours after improvement begins. After discharge from the hospital, both drugs should be continued in the oral dosage form at the same doses as given intravenously. The oral therapy should be continued to complete a 10- to 14-day course of therapy.

Treating Sexual Partners of PID Victims

Ideally, the male sexual partner(s) of women with PID should be treated. Frequently the male sexual partner has no symptoms, but is a carrier of *C. trachomatis* or *N. gonorrhoeae.* Men should be encouraged to visit a physician or local health department for examination. They should be treated if they have been a sexual partner of a PID victim during the previous six to 12 weeks. Men should receive one of the following treatments:

1. Doxycycline (Vibramycin®), 100 mg capsule by mouth twice daily for seven days
2. Tetracycline (Achromycin V®, Sumycin®, Tetracyn®), 500 mg capsule by mouth four times daily for seven days
3. Erythromycin (E-Mycin®, ERYC®, Ilosone®, Ethril®, Wyamycin E®), 500 mg tablet by mouth four times daily for seven days

PREVENTION OF PELVIC INFLAMMATORY DISEASE

Many behavioral and clinical measures may be taken to prevent the development of PID, including:

1. Avoid engaging in intercourse with multiple sexual partners. Such activity greatly increases the probability of

acquiring a sexually transmitted infection, which may
progress to pelvic inflammatory disease.

2. Avoid using an IUD. IUD users have a two- to fourfold
   higher incidence of pelvic infections than nonusers.
   Women should consider either oral contraceptives or
   barrier methods of contraception such as condom, diaphragm, foams, creams, jellies, or contraceptive
   sponge, as the risk of PID in users of such devices
   appears to be one-third to one-half as great as in women
   who do not use such contraceptives. Sexually active
   teens and women in their early twenties who have not
   borne children are not ideal candidates for use of an IUD.

3. Treat lower genital tract infections promptly and effectively since they usually precede and may lead to upper
   genital tract infections and PID.

4. Administer antibiotics prophylactically (before symptoms of infection) following a vaginal or uterine diagnostic or surgical procedure. Physical manipulation of
   the female reproductive tract may introduce bacteria of
   the vaginal area into the upper genital tract.

5. Treat sexual partners of PID victims. Male sexual partners may be carriers of infecting organisms, but the male
   may have no symptoms of gonorrhea, chlamydial infection, or other sexually transmittable infections. They
   should be treated according to the guidelines presented
   previously in this chapter.

6. Control gonococcal and chlamydial infections. Gonococcal and chlamydial infections lead to the majority of
   cases of PID if not properly treated. Prompt and effective
   diagnosis and treatment when symptoms of genital tract
   infection occur in the female are critical to controlling
   PID.

CONCLUSION

Pelvic inflammatory disease (PID) is an infectious and inflammatory condition of the upper genital tract of women. PID is both
preventable and treatable. This chapter reviews common causes,
factors which increase the risk of developing PID, symptoms, complications, and treatment. Steps which may be employed to prevent
PID from occurring or recurring should be recognized, as the disease
can have very serious medical consequences.

15

Trichomonas
Vaginalis

INTRODUCTION

Trichomonas vaginalis is a common parasite which feeds off living cells and is found in both men and women. It can cause vaginal infections in a large number of women, particularly when hygienic practices are poor. *Trichomonas vaginalis* can also infect the genitourinary tract of men. The organism is usually transmitted during sexual intercourse. However, infections can also occur through the use of contaminated towels, contaminated douche apparatus, unsterilized pelvic examination equipment, and so forth. Most individuals who are infected with *Trichomonas vaginalis* experience minimal to moderate discomfort. It is imperative that sexual partners be treated in order to effectively eradicate the organism and prevent reinfection of one sexual partner by another.

Prior to the availability of effective drugs, *Trichomonas vaginalis* infected many millions of women and men. Even now, approximately 3.0 million new infections are diagnosed each year in the U.S. Twenty to 30 percent of all cases of infectious vaginitis is due to trichomoniasis, the infection caused by *Trichomonas vaginalis*. Since the problem is so widespread and the financial burdens high (physician visits, medication costs, and lost work time), a thorough understanding of this disease and its treatment is necessary.

THE MEANING OF VAGINITIS

Vaginitis is defined as an inflammation and/or infection of the vagina. Vaginal secretions and the cells lining the vagina may be affected. The vagina is a canal with many folds which leads from the external genitalia to the uterus of the woman (see Figure 1, Introductory chapter). It serves as a passageway for the fetus from the uterus to the outside world during the birthing process.

When a woman experiences vaginitis, the external genitalia (vulva) may or may not be involved. A woman who complains of vaginitis will experience some or all of the following symptoms: vaginal discharge with a foul odor, vaginal itching, painful urination, or painful intercourse. A vaginal discharge per se does not automatically mean that an infection is present.

VAGINAL RESISTANCE TO THE DEVELOPMENT OF INFECTIONS

The normal vagina is usually resistant to infection by various organisms, particularly during the time from puberty to menopause. During this time, estrogens produced in the body maintain the vaginal epithelial cell thickness. The vaginal pH (acidity) is normally between 3.8 and 4.2; a pH in the range of 3.5 to 5.0 is compatible with vaginal health. This acidity inhibits the growth of most disease causing organisms. Acidity is maintained by the production of acids from the breakdown of glycogen (a carbohydrate) by bacteria (Döderlein's bacilli), which are normally present in the vagina. Additionally, the thickened vaginal epithelium acts as a protective barrier to bacterial invasion, thus contributing to a healthy vagina. Anything that influences the vaginal pH, estrogen production, or the concentration of Döderlein's bacilli will weaken the normal resistance to infection.

FACTORS WHICH CONTRIBUTE TO THE DEVELOPMENT OF VAGINITIS

Many factors have been implicated in contributing to the development of vaginitis, including poor vaginal hygiene, vigorous intercourse, sexually transmitted disease, foreign bodies, pregnancy, tight fitting undergarments, altered ability to fight infections due to drugs or diseases, and suppression of normal vaginal/bowel organisms with antibiotics. The major causes of infectious vaginitis are

Candida albicans (a fungus) and *Trichomonas vaginalis* (a one-cel-led, protozoal parasite).

Many women purchase douches which are promoted as feminine hygiene preparations. They are used for cleaning of the vaginal area; deodorizing; relieving itching, burning, or redness; removing secretions or discharge; and for psychological reasons. Many of the ingredients can cause vaginal or perineal (area between vaginal opening and anus) irritation leading to vaginitis-like symptoms. Feminine deodorant sprays, if not used properly, can also cause vulvovaginal irritation. Vaginal itching and burning may be symptoms of infectious vaginitis and should not be treated with available nonprescription douches or feminine hygiene products (see Chapter 22). Medical attention should be sought prior to the purchase of one of these products.

TRICHOMONAS VAGINALIS INFECTIONS

CAUSE AND LOCATION OF INFECTION

Trichomonas vaginalis belongs to a group of microscopic organisms called trichomonads. These parasitic, one-celled protozoa have flagella (antenna-like projections) with which they move about (see Figure 35). An infection with this organism does not lead to immunity or resistance to future infections.

The organism grows best in an environment which lacks oxygen. The optimal pH for growth is 5.5 to 6.0. *Trichomonas vaginalis* cannot live in the acid pH found in the normal postpubertal, premenopausal female. The organism has been found alive on inanimate surfaces for 60 to 90 minutes, in urine for three hours, in seminal fluid for six hours, and in swimming pool and toilet bowl water after 24 hours.

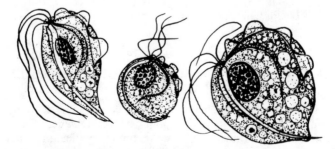

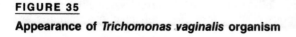

FIGURE 35

Appearance of *Trichomonas vaginalis* organism

Trichomonas vaginalis is not considered a normal inhabitant of the vagina of women or of the lower urinary tract of the male. The organism is more likely to be found in people with other sexually transmitted diseases. It also has a high prevalence in prostitutes and female prison inmates. Approximately 10 percent of women may be carriers without experiencing any symptoms. Since the vast majority of males who are infected have no symptoms, it is not known how many males harbor the organism.

The organism inhabits many genitourinary structures of both the male and female. In addition to the vagina, the organism can be found in the urethra, bladder, rectum, and Skene's glands of the female. Skene's glands surround the urethra of the female, and are the counterpart to the male prostate gland. In the male, trichomonas is found in the vas deferens, seminal vesicles, prostate gland, and urethra (see Figure 3, Introductory chapter). Any local or topical treatment is likely to fail since the organism inhabits so many lower urinary tract structures.

SIGNS AND SYMPTOMS OF TRICHOMONAS VAGINALIS INFECTION IN WOMEN

Women who develop trichomonal infections of the vagina often experience a wide variety of symptoms. The infection is considered a chronic condition with periodic relapses in some women. Some have harbored the organism for more than 20 years. Infections may be noted immediately after menstruation or during pregnancy. As many as 50 percent of infected patients (male and female combined) may not develop symptoms, however. Females are more likely to develop symptoms than males. Vulvar tissue swelling and complaints of intense itching may be noted. Women with trichomoniasis will usually have a malodorous vaginal discharge which may be watery, bubbly, frothy, and greenish, gray, or yellowish in color. The discharge can be heavy enough to cause the woman to complain that she is constantly wet. The irritation from the discharge may cause painful urination or intercourse.

SIGNS AND SYMPTOMS OF TRICHOMONAS VAGINALIS INFECTIONS IN MEN

Most men who are infected with *Trichomonas vaginalis* do not have any symptoms. One physician estimates that only approximately 12 percent of males will experience symptoms such as urethral burning and irritation following urination and/or intercourse. *Trichomonas vaginalis* has been implicated by clinicians in numerous other conditions afflicting the male. These include urethral strictures; urethral, epididymal, and prostatic infections; penile ulcers; and male infertility.

It is very important to note that, despite a lack of symptoms, most men who have sexual intercourse with a woman having trichomoniasis will subsequently harbor the organism. Therefore, the male serves as a source of reinfection for the female if he is not adequately treated.

Any man who develops a discharge from the urethra of the penis should seek prompt medical attention. Gonorrhea in the male is often associated with a urethral discharge (see Chapter 9). Other sexually transmitted diseases (STDs) may also produce a urethral discharge. Chlamydial infections and other causes of nongonococcal urethritis may be associated with a discharge (see Chapter 13). *Trichomonas vaginalis* may produce a thin, whitish urethral discharge in approximately 10 percent of men infected with the organism. The discharge may be copious and pus-like on rare occasions.

TREATMENT OF TRICHOMONAS VAGINALIS INFECTIONS

LOCAL (TOPICAL) APPLICATION OF ANTI-INFECTIVE MEDICATION

Since trichomonads inhibit many areas of the male and female genitourinary tract, the local application of vaginal antimicrobial creams or gels, or use of medicated douches, will not generally prove effective. The use of such products may temporarily relieve symptoms of trichomoniasis, but will not eliminate the organism. *Trichomonas vaginalis* infection *must* be treated with oral medication obtainable only with a prescription from a physician.

TREATING THE SEXUAL PARTNER(S) OF AN INDIVIDUAL WITH A TRICHOMONAS VAGINALIS INFECTION

Men and women having trichomoniasis must be properly treated to eradicate the organism from the genitourinary tract. Interestingly, it has been established that approximately 30 to 80 percent of male sexual contacts of infected women will harbor the organism. If the male or female sexual partner is not treated, he or she will serve as a source of reinfection for the sexual partner during intercourse. Whenever a sexually transmitted disease is the cause of vaginitis, all male sexual contacts should be found and treated. Conversely, if trichomoniasis is first diagnosed in the male, the female sexual partner(s) must also be treated, even if no symptoms are readily apparent.

THE DRUG OF CHOICE FOR TREATING TRICHOMONAS INFECTIONS

Metronidazole (Flagyl®, Protostat®, Metryl®) remains the drug of choice for the treatment of *Trichomonas vaginalis*. It kills trichomonads and several other organisms, including amebas and some bacteria. This prescription drug is available for intravenous use and in 250 mg and 500 mg tablets.

CONVENTIONAL THERAPY VERSUS SINGLE-DOSE THERAPY

Traditionally, the accepted treatment for men and women has been to administer 250 mg of metronidazole orally three times a day for seven days. However, despite the success with this regimen, single-dose therapy has been found to be nearly as effective and is now recommended as initial therapy. Single-dose therapy involves administration of a specified amount of the drug only once. Two grams (2,000 milligrams) of metronidazole (eight 250-mg tablets or four 500-mg tablets) are administered to both the male or female and the sexual partner(s) in single doses. Two 500-mg or four 250-mg tablets taken twice daily may also be given. Usual cure rates of approximately 95 percent with single-dose therapy approach cure rates with the multiple-dose, multiple-day regimen. Single-dose therapy offers the advantages of reduced cost and enhanced patient willingness to take all the tablets due to convenience. It is a well-known fact that as the number of tablets taken per day increases, and the length of therapy increases, the likelihood of missing doses will also increase. This may result in ineffective treatment. The seven-day treatment, although possibly more effective than single-dose therapy, has been associated with alteration of the vaginal flora and subsequent development of *Candida albicans* (fungal) vaginitis in some women.

Single-dose metronidazole therapy offers the advantage of convenience, good compliance, and reduced cost, but may be associated with disadvantages. Nausea and vomiting can occur, but the incidence is probably only slightly greater than that seen with the seven-day course of therapy. It has been suggested that the single-dose regimen may be associated with an increased rate of reinfection, particularly if the sexual partner is untreated.

Single metronidazole doses of less than 2.0 grams have also been used in the treatment of trichomonas vaginitis. Smaller doses may be associated with lower cost and less toxicity. Single doses of 1.5 or 1.0 grams have been studied, but cure rates do not appear to be as high as with the 2.0 gram single-dose or seven-day multiple-dose regimen. In one study, single doses of 1.0 gram were associated with cure rates of only 55 percent (42 of 77 patients).

METRONIDAZOLE AND CANCER

Metronidazole has been shown experimentally to be carcinogenic (cancer-causing) in rodents and mutagenic (causing cell mutations) in Salmonella bacteria and fungi. Despite the appearance of lung tumors in mice and breast tumors in female rats treated with metronidazole, there is no evidence to implicate metronidazole as a cancer-causing agent in humans. In 1979, a group of investigators from the Mayo Clinic studied 771 women who had received metronidazole for vaginal trichomoniasis. They concluded that these women did not have an appreciably increased risk of developing any form of cancer when assessed approximately 10 years following treatment.

SAFETY OF METRONIDAZOLE IN PREGNANCY

Teratogenicity refers to the ability of a drug or other substance to cause abnormal fetal development. Teratogenicity due to metronidazole has not been seen in animals. There are no adequate human trials to determine the teratogenicity of metronidazole in man. The use of metronidazole during the first trimester, and possibly the second and third trimesters of pregnancy, should be avoided, however. The use of the single-dose regimen is not recommended in pregnancy since the large single dose may result in high concentrations of the drug in the fetus.

An alternative management includes vaginal acidification with appropriate products, such as water and vinegar douches or Aci-Jel®, a prescription vaginal acidifier. Before such treatment is attempted, it is important that the woman contact a physician for approval and learn proper administration techniques. Micronized aluminum powder instilled into the vagina has also been advocated as an effective means of treating trichomoniasis in women. This treatment is only available from a physician, and is not yet accepted by all clinicians as a useful means of eradicating certain vaginal infections. If the patient still has symptoms after treatment, an alternative medication may be prescribed.

While clotrimazole vaginal tablets (Gyne-Lotrimin®, Mycelex-G®) are normally used to treat fungal vaginitis, their use in trichomoniasis during pregnancy may be beneficial. One 100-mg tablet inserted into the vagina at bedtime for seven days has resulted in cure rates of approximately 50 percent. The ability of this regimen to eradicate trichomonads from other genitourinary structures is questionable; further research is required to determine the proper role of clotrimazole in the management of trichomoniasis. The vaginal tablets are available only by prescription from a physician.

SAFETY OF METRONIDAZOLE IN NURSING MOTHERS

Metronidazole is excreted in breast milk. The concentration found in the nursing mother's blood is similar to that found in her milk. Since the drug is carcinogenic in animals and mutagenic in bacteria and fungi, its use should be avoided in nursing mothers, if possible. If a nursing mother requires the drug, she should consult with her physician regarding the appropriateness of breast-feeding. The Centers for Disease Control recommend that a breast-feeding woman with trichomonal vaginitis be treated with the 2.0 gram single-dose regimen. She should also be discouraged from breast-feeding for at least 24 hours following the single dose of metronidazole.

SIDE EFFECTS OF METRONIDAZOLE

A metallic taste may be noted by patients taking metronidazole. This reaction is more likely to occur following a large single dose. Metabolites (breakdown products) of the drug may darken the urine (dark yellow to brown). The discolored urine is no reason for concern. A reaction may be associated with the use of this drug following alcohol consumption. The user may experience stomach cramps, nausea, vomiting, headache, or flushing. These symptoms occur because metronidazole interferes with the metabolism of alcohol. Alcohol consumption should be discouraged during the multiple-dose regimen and for a week following therapy. Alcohol could be consumed 24 to 48 hours following a large single dose of metronidazole. Metronidazole may alter the taste perception of alcoholic beverages. Strict abstinence from alcohol is especially important during pregnancy. Acetaldehyde, a chemical which accumulates when metronidazole inhibits the metabolism of alcohol, may cause birth defects in the developing fetus.

HOW TO TAKE METRONIDAZOLE

If you are receiving metronidazole, try to take the medication with food to avoid stomach upset. It is very important that you take the full course of therapy. If a seven-day supply is given, it is important not to miss a single dose, and the tablets should be taken at evenly spaced times during the day (for example, 9 A.M., 1 P.M., 5 P.M., and 9 P.M.). A missed dose should be taken as soon as possible, but not taken if it is almost time for the next dose. Doses should not be doubled.

If no improvement is noted after a few days, your physician should be consulted. Alcoholic beverages should be avoided while taking metronidazole, especially during pregnancy.

Males and females who are to take two grams of metronidazole as a single dose should take them at the same time. Male partners who are not treated should be encouraged to use a condom during intercourse for the week following use of the single-dose regimen in the woman. The woman should abstain from intercourse during single-dose or multiple-dose metronidazole therapy.

CONCLUSION

Trichomonas vaginalis remains one of the most frequent causes of sexually transmitted disease. The organism is not considered a normal inhabitant of the human body, and its presence leads to infection in both men and women. Since the organism inhabits many structures within the male and female genitourinary tracts, local or topical therapy can only offer symptomatic improvement. Without successful treatment, the possibility of repeated infections is high. The best treatment available is metronidazole which, when taken orally, kills the organisms throughout the genitourinary system. Effective eradication of the trichomonads requires the concurrent treatment of sexual partners. Metronidazole remains an effective and relatively safe agent. Questions regarding its mutagenic, carcinogenic, and teratogenic potential await further study.

16

Other Sexually Transmitted Diseases

INTRODUCTION

When thinking of sexually transmitted diseases, AIDS, syphilis, gonorrhea, and herpes generally come to mind. However, there are many other infections that may be transmitted through sexual contact. These include scabies, hepatitis B, pediculosus pubis ("crabs"), epididymo-orchitis, and ophthalmia neonatorum.

SCABIES

Scabies is a condition caused by infestation of the skin with a small parasitic mite known as *Sarcoptes scabiei*. Scabies may occur in localized outbreaks within families, schools, institutions, or communities. A wide variety of dermatologic lesions, which may be confused with other skin diseases, may be produced. The mite is extremely small; it is nearly impossible to see with the naked eye. It has a rounded body and four pairs of legs (see Figure 36). The female burrows into the outer layer of human skin and deposits eggs for several weeks before she dies. The eggs hatch within two to three days; these mites then travel to the surface of the skin where sexual reproduction occurs, and a new life cycle begins. The mite lives its

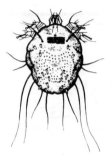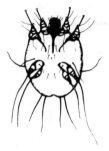

0.2 mm

FIGURE 36

Appearance of Sarcoptes scabiei, the mite that causes scabies

entire life on the human and can survive for only short periods of time when not in human contact.

TYPICAL SYMPTOMS OF A SCABIES INFESTATION

Symptoms of a scabies infection do not usually appear until four to six weeks after the initial infestation. This is the time required for the mite population to increase, and for the body's defense mechanisms to react to the parasites. Usual symptoms are rash and itching. Skin lesions may appear as scales, crusts, or nodules. The most commonly affected areas of the body include the area between the fingers, the hands, wrists, elbows, armpits, feet, ankles, buttocks, female breasts, and male genitals (see Figure 37). The scalp and the face are usually not involved. The most characteristic lesions are the burrows produced by the mite. They may be slightly elevated, with a small blister or pimple on one end. The itching is thought to be due to the body's response to either the mites, their metabolic waste products, or both. The itching is often very intense; many people aggravate the condition by vigorous scratching, which may result in bleeding, ulceration of the skin, or bacterial infections. The itching is most severe at night and may awaken the individual. This is thought to be due to increased activity of the mites caused by the warmer skin temperatures that occur during sleep.

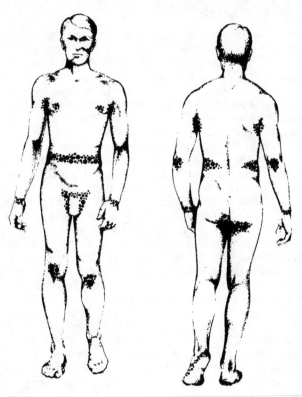

FIGURE 37
Areas of the body most likely to be infested by the scabies mite

SPREAD OF SCABIES

The usual method of spread is by close personal contact, including sexual contact. Members of a household, school children, and residents of nursing homes are frequent victims. Although direct personal contact is the most frequent form of transmission, mites may also be spread by contaminated clothing and bedding as they may live for a short period of time away from human skin. Sharing a bed with an infested person, with or without sexual contact, may result in transmission of the mite.

TREATMENT OF SCABIES

All persons in whom mites, mite eggs, or fecal matter of the mite are identified from burrows by examination under a microscope should be treated. In addition, family members, close personal contacts, and sexual partners should be treated, even if they have no obvious symptoms of scabies. This should be done because it may take up to six weeks to develop symptoms after the mite is transmitted. There are four drugs which may be used to treat scabies infestation—lindane (gamma benzene hexachloride, Kwell®), crotamiton (Eurax®), sulfur, 5–10 percent ointment, and permethrin (Nix®).

Lindane (Kwell®) is the preferred and most frequently used agent to treat scabies. You should first take a hot soapy bath using a rough washcloth. In order to minimize toxicity, lindane should not be applied immediately following a bath or shower. The skin should be thoroughly dry to prevent excessive absorption of the drug through the skin. After the skin is dry, a thin layer of lindane cream or lotion (one percent) should be applied over the entire skin surface (normal and affected skin) from the neck down. Special care should be taken to apply the drug thoroughly between fingers and toes, and on the soles of the feet. Lindane should not be used above the neck unless scabies is diagnosed on the face or scalp. The drug should remain on the skin overnight, or for at least eight to 12 hours. You should then bathe again to remove the medication. Lindane should be reapplied to the hands after each handwashing.

If applied carefully and thoroughly, one application of lindane is usually sufficient to treat scabies infestation. Another application may be employed in one week, if necessary. One ounce of lindane lotion, thinly applied, will cover an adult. People generally tend to apply the drug more frequently, and over longer periods of time than recommended. This may lead to irritation of the skin and should be avoided. Lindane is not recommended for pregnant or lactating women.

Crotamiton (Eurax®) is slightly less effective, but it is a good alternative to lindane. It not only acts by killing the mites, but also reduces itching as well. Crotamiton (as a 10 percent lotion or cream) should be applied in the same manner as lindane. However, a second application should be made in 24 hours. You should then take a bath 24 hours after the second application.

Sulfur ointments may also be useful in the treatment of scabies. Generally, a five percent concentration is used in children and 10 percent in adults. Sulfur ointments should be applied to the entire skin surface, from the neck down, every night for three consecutive nights. You may bathe before reapplying and should bathe 24 hours after the last application. The primary disadvantage of sulfur is that it has an unpleasant odor, is messy, and stains clothing easily.

For infestation of the scalp, permethrin (Nix®) is available as a one percent cream rinse. It is retained on hair shafts, and the therapeutic effect persists for up to two weeks, regardless of normal shampooing. It should be applied to freshly washed hair after drying, left on the hair and scalp for 10 minutes, then rinsed off. Less than one percent of users require retreatment.

DANGERS OF LINDANE

Lindane is a moderately toxic substance; animal studies have shown that in large doses it may cause central nervous system toxicity, including muscle spasms and convulsions. In addition, there is conflicting evidence regarding the possibility that lindane may cause cancer. However, when *used as directed*, there is minimal risk of toxicity in humans.

HEPATITIS B

Most persons associate viral hepatitis, particularly hepatitis B ("serum hepatitis"), with the use of contaminated needles and blood transfusions. However, there are many other ways by which viral hepatitis may be transmitted, including sexual contact.

Hepatitis is an inflammation of the liver. It may be caused by a number of different viruses, the most common being hepatitis A virus, hepatitis B virus, and non-A non-B viruses. Hepatitis A virus is excreted in the stool and, as a sexually transmitted infection, is seen mainly in homosexual men who engage in oral-anal contact. Non-A non-B hepatitis may also be transmitted by sexual contact, particularly in homosexuals. The hepatitis B virus has been shown to be present in the bloodstream, saliva, menstrual blood, semen, and the vaginal discharge of infected patients. It is not surprising that hepatitis B may occur as a sexually transmitted disease. Like hepatitis A and non-A non-B hepatitis, hepatitis B is most common in homosexual men. The incidence is highest in people with multiple sexual partners, and in those who engage in anal intercourse. In addition, there is a "carrier state" which consists of people who have never had symptoms of hepatitis, yet chronically have a substance in their blood and body secretions known as hepatitis B surface antigen (HBsAg). These carriers are capable of passing HBsAg, and therefore hepatitis B, to their sexual contacts.

Among homosexuals, those who engage in anal-genital intercourse seem to be at a much greater risk of contracting hepatitis B. This is somewhat surprising since HBsAg may also be present in saliva, semen, and vaginal discharge. However, one study revealed that approximately five percent of homosexual men had a positive test for HBsAg, and about 50 percent had developed antibodies to HBsAg. These rates are substantially higher than those seen in the general population. The higher incidence associated with anal intercourse may be due to the trauma to the rectum that frequently occurs, allowing the virus easier entry into the body than through the vaginal wall or digestive tract.

SYMPTOMS OF HEPATITIS B

Viral hepatitis of the three types mentioned produce a similar array of symptoms. Symptoms usually occur four to six weeks after infection with hepatitis A, six to eight weeks after non-A non-B, and about 12 weeks after infection with hepatitis B virus. In approximately 90 percent of cases, symptoms are mild and include fever, fatigue, headache, mild abdominal discomfort, loss of appetite, and jaundice. Jaundice is a yellow discoloration which may be present in the skin, whites of the eyes, or mucous membranes of the mouth. If jaundice is present, the stool may become clay-colored and the urine dark. In most cases, these symptoms, associated with inflammation of the liver, will disappear within six to 12 weeks. In less than two percent, a severe inflammation of the liver known as fulminant hepatitis may develop. In this case, there is rapid destruction of the liver, which leads quickly to bleeding, coma, and frequently death. In the remaining five to 10 percent who have viral hepatitis, there is a chronic course. Some may have persistent, mild abnormalities of the liver for many years. Others may have a chronic, continuous deterioration of the liver, known as chronic active hepatitis. Patients may initially complain of mild flu-like symptoms (such as loss of appetite or fatigue), but eventually this condition worsens and leads to cirrhosis of the liver.

TREATMENT OF VIRAL HEPATITIS

In 90 percent of cases, viral hepatitis will be mild, and recovery will occur without specific treatment. Generally, you should have bed rest during the initial phases of the disease, and a high protein–low fat diet may be recommended. In all those with hepatitis, alcohol and drugs which may damage or irritate the liver should be avoided until recovery is complete. In cases of chronic or fulminant hepatitis, steroid drugs, such as prednisone, may be used, although the benefits of their use are controversial.

There are now methods of *preventing* hepatitis B infections. It has been suggested that use of condoms and avoidance of anal contact may significantly decrease the risk of developing a hepatitis B infection. Passive immunization with hepatitis B immune globulin (HBIG) has been shown to be effective in preventing hepatitis B infection in sexual contacts of persons with hepatitis B. This immune globulin must be given within 14 days of sexual contact with an infected person in order to be effective. A hepatitis B vaccine has recently been developed. This vaccine has been shown to be 90 percent effective for five years with minimal side effects. In one study, the use of three doses of the hepatitis B vaccine resulted in 96 percent of recipients developing antibodies to hepatitis B surface antigen, and a 92 percent reduction in clinical hepatitis. Both HBIG and the hepatitis B vaccine are expensive, with the cost for the three doses of hepatitis B vaccine at approximately one hundred dollars. The hepatitis B vaccine will not eliminate the chronic carrier state.

PEDICULOSIS PUBIS

Pediculosis pubis ("crabs") is an infestation of the genital region by lice. There are many species of lice, but only three frequently infest humans. These are *Pediculus humanus capitis* (head lice),

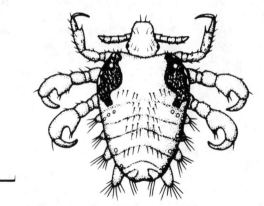

0.4 mm

FIGURE 38

Appearance of Phthirus pubis, the louse that causes pediculosis pubis

Pediculus humanus corporis (body lice), and *Phthirus pubis* (pubic lice, "crabs"). About one to two mm in length, the pubic louse is a flat, oblong, wingless insect (see Figure 38). Lice are parasites which feed on human blood.

SPREAD OF "CRABS"

Pubic lice are spread primarily through close contact with an infested person, particularly during sexual intercourse. Normally, pubic hair and the hair of the upper legs and abdomen are involved in transmission. However, facial hair including eyebrows, eyelashes, mustaches, and beards may also be affected. That lice are caused by a lack of good hygiene and that lice can "jump" from one person to another are both myths. Although sexual contact is the most common way of getting "crabs," the parasites occasionally may be transmitted through clothing, bedding, and even toilet seats. However, this is not usually the case as lice that fall off onto clothing or bedding are usually close to death. Pubic lice live only on humans and cannot be acquired from animals or vegetation.

Once a person is infested, the female louse begins to lay eggs, also referred to as nits. The female lays between three and ten eggs every night. These nits (eggs) are attached to hair shafts or fibers of clothing by a cementlike substance. The nits are usually attached close to the skin as warm temperatures are necessary for the eggs to hatch. Normally, a young louse, known as a nymph, emerges from the egg within one to two weeks. These nymphs attempt to feed themselves by piercing the skin and sucking blood from the human host. Within approximately 15 days, the nymph matures to an adult louse, shedding its skin (molting) several times in the process. The adult does not generally travel to other parts of the body, but remains attached to hair shafts by its claws. Here the adult lives for an average of about one month before dying and falling off the body.

SYMPTOMS OF PUBIC LICE

The most common symptom produced by pubic lice is itching. When a louse bites, its saliva enters the wound and causes irritation which results in itching. The saliva may also cause symptoms such as a mild fever, swollen lymph glands, and muscle aches. Vigorous scratching of the infested area may result in abrasion of the skin and secondary bacterial infections. Infestation with pubic lice may cause the development of bluish-gray patches on the skin of the abdomen, genital region, and thighs. These patches do not itch, and they fade gradually.

TREATMENT OF PUBIC LICE

Three agents are effective in the treatment of pubic lice infestation—lindane (Kwell®), malathion (Prioderm®), and pyrethrins (A-200 Pyrinate®, Rid®, and others). It is a myth that washing with brown soap or applying kerosene to the skin are the best ways to treat lice. All sexual and close personal contacts of the infested person should be treated. Furthermore, all bedding, towels, and clothing should be washed in hot water and machine dried (hot cycle), or dry cleaned.

Lindane (Kwell®) shampoo, lotion, or cream is available by physician's prescription in a one percent concentration. Normally, one ounce of the shampoo is applied to the affected and adjacent areas and worked into the hair and skin. When the affected area is thoroughly covered, small amounts of water should be added to produce a lather. It is recommended that the shampoo be in contact with the skin for four to five minutes before rinsing thoroughly and drying the area. When the hair is dry, a fine-tooth comb should be used to remove nits from the hair shafts. If the eyebrows or eyelashes are involved, an alternate form of therapy, such as petroleum jelly (Vaseline®), should be utilized instead of lindane. Vaseline applied twice daily for 10 days should suffocate the lice and their nits.

If lather from the shampoo should accidentally enter the eyes, they should be flushed with water. Generally, only one application of shampoo is necessary. However, treatment with lindane may be repeated one time only, in one week, if necessary. Itching may persist for a period of time after the lice are killed; this should not be interpreted as a sign that the treatment was unsuccessful.

The one percent lindane lotion or cream should be applied in a thin layer to the infested and adjacent hairy areas, and thoroughly washed off after eight hours. Treatment may be repeated in seven days, if necessary.

Malathion (Prioderm®), possibly the most effective agent to treat pubic lice, has recently been released in the United States, and is available only by prescription as a lotion in a 0.5 percent concentration. The drug should be applied to dry hair of the affected area (excluding eyebrows and eyelashes) and gently worked in until the area is thoroughly wetted. The area should then be left uncovered and allowed to dry naturally for at least eight hours. A blow-dryer should *not* be used since heat will decrease the effectiveness of malathion. After this period of time, the area should be washed thoroughly with soap and water and dried with a towel. When the hair is dry, a fine-tooth comb should be used to remove the dead lice and nits. One application is usually sufficient but may be repeated in seven to nine days.

Side effects of malathion are rare when the drug is used as

directed, the most common being mild irritation and dryness of the skin. It should not be used on persons with involvement of the eyelashes and eyebrows, as the drug may be rapidly absorbed through the eye if accidental contact occurs.

Pyrethrins (A-200 Pyrinate®, Rid®, and others) are available for use without a prescription. They are moderately effective against lice, but not against scabies. A solution, gel, or shampoo containing pyrethrins should be applied to the affected and adjacent areas and worked into the hair and skin. Care should be taken to avoid the eyes and mucous membranes, but if contact does occur, the eyes or affected areas should be flushed with water. After ten minutes of contact, the hair and skin should be washed thoroughly with soap and water and dried. After the hair is dry, a fine-tooth comb should be used to remove any remaining nits. Although one application is usually effective, treatment should be repeated in one week.

When used as recommended, pyrethrins have few side effects. Local irritation of the skin may occur in some cases. Furthermore, some patients will develop an allergy to pyrethrins.

ACUTE EPIDIDYMITIS AND EPIDIDYMO-ORCHITIS

Acute epididymitis and epididymo-orchitis refer to inflammation of the epididymis and of the epididymis and testicles, respectively. The epididymides are long, coiled tubules located adjacent to each testicle (see Figure 3, Introductory chapter). Acute inflammation of the epididymides or testicles may occur as a complication of several conditions, the most frequent being bacterial infection.

In men under 35 years of age, acute epididymitis or epididymo-orchitis usually occurs after infection of the urethra or bladder. The bacteria implicated in this population are primarily *Neisseria gonorrhoeae* (Chapter 9) and *Chlamydia trachomatis* (Chapter 13). These bacteria are transmitted via sexual intercourse. After having infected the male urethra, the bacteria travel through the vas deferens to the epididymis and testicle, where acute inflammation develops.

In men over the age of 35, epididymitis or epididymo-orchitis occurs primarily in those who have undergone recent urologic surgery or instrumentation or who have a structural defect in the urinary tract. The bacteria implicated most frequently in older men are *Escherichia coli* and *Pseudomonas aeruginosa*. These organisms are generally not transmitted by sexual contact.

SYMPTOMS OF ACUTE EPIDIDYMITIS AND EPIDIDYMO-ORCHITIS

Prior to the development of epididymitis, there may be symptoms of an inflamed urethra, including a urethral discharge, which is usually colorless or mucus-like in appearance, and painful urination. The typical patient is a sexually active male in his 20s or 30s. The onset of epididymitis and epididymo-orchitis is characterized by the rapid development of pain and enlargement of the contents of one or both sides of the scrotum. In most cases, only one testicle is involved, and the epididymis is hard and tender. Fever may also exist.

TREATMENT OF ACUTE EPIDIDYMITIS AND EPIDIDYMO-ORCHITIS

The infection in men under 35 is most often due to *Neisseria gonorrhoeae* or *Chlamydia trachomatis*. Therefore, antibiotic therapy designed to eradicate these bacteria should be started. The federally approved treatment schedule, particularly if the infection is thought to be due to *N. gonorrhoeae* or *C. trachomatis*, is as follows:

Amoxicillin (Amoxil®, Larotid®, Polymox®, Trimox®, Utimox®, Wymox®), 3.0 grams *or* ampicillin (Amcill®, Pfizerpen-A®, Polycillin®, Principen®, SK-Ampicillin®, Totacillin®, Omnipen®) 3.5 grams taken by mouth with 1.0 gram of probenecid (Benemid®) by mouth.

Injectable antibiotics may be used instead of the initial dose of oral penicillin (amoxicillin or ampicillin) mentioned above. For example, 4.8 million units of aqueous procaine penicillin G given intramuscularly (as 2.4 million units into each of two injection sites) plus 1.0 gram of oral probenecid (Benemid®) may be used. Two grams of spectinomycin (Trobicin®) or 250 mg of ceftriaxone (Rocephin®) administered intramuscularly may also be used.

The single large dose of an oral or injectable antibiotic should be followed by another antibiotic such as:

1. Tetracycline HC1, 500 mg by mouth four times daily for 10 days
2. Doxycycline, 100 mg by mouth twice daily for 10 days
3. Erythromycin base or stearate, 500 mg by mouth four times each day for seven days if tetracycline or doxycycline is not well tolerated or should not be used

Other treatments are available, but most individuals respond to the drugs previously presented if they are conscientious about taking the medication.

In people in whom the infection is thought to be sexually transmitted, all sexual partners should be examined and treated with an antibiotic regimen. In pregnant females, erythromycin is preferred over either tetracycline or doxycycline.

If the man is over 35 and *Escherichia coli* or *Pseudomonas aeruginosa* is suspected, oral ampicillin, amoxicillin, sulfa drugs, or sulfamethoxazole-trimethoprim would be appropriate initial therapy. If the infection does not respond to these antibiotics, hospitalization and treatment with injectable gentamicin, tobramycin, or another antibiotic may be necessary.

In addition to appropriate antibiotic therapy, treatment should include scrotal elevation and immobilization by a scrotal supporter or elastic tape, and bed rest for several days. Application of an ice pack during the first 24 hours also may be beneficial. Oral analgesics and/or nonsteroidal anti-inflammatory agents should be administered to provide pain relief.

In the vast majority of patients, therapy will bring about a dramatic improvement in symptoms within several days. However, if improvement is not noted in three days, the diagnosis and treatment should be reevaluated. Hospitalization may be necessary.

LONG-TERM COMPLICATIONS OF EPIDIDYMITIS AND EPIDIDYMO-ORCHITIS

In most cases, prompt treatment will result in resolution of the symptoms with no complications. However, if treatment is delayed or inadequate, chronic inflammation of the epididymides may occur, leading to fibrosis and sterility. In cases of chronic infection and inflammation, surgical removal of the epididymides may become necessary.

OPHTHALMIA NEONATORUM

Ophthalmia neonatorum is an infection of the eyes, occurring in children who have been born within the previous month. In most cases, ophthalmia neonatorum is manifested as an inflammation of the conjunctiva, the thin membrane that lines the inside of the eyelids and covers the eyeball.

CAUSE OF OPHTHALMIA NEONATORUM

This condition is usually caused by either a bacterial infection or chemical irritation. A bacterial infection may be transmitted during birth as the child passes through the birth canal of an infected mother. However, children born by cesarian section may also develop ophthalmia neonatorum if the bacteria migrate into the uterus after rupture of the membranes. The vast majority of bacterial infections are due to *Neisseria gonorrhoeae* and *Chlamydia trachomatis.* However, other bacteria, including *Staphylococcus aureus, Streptococcus pneumoniae,* and *Streptococcus pyogenes* have been implicated in some cases. Ophthalmia neonatorum may be caused by chemical irritation due to the instillation of 1% silver nitrate solution in the eyes at birth, a standard procedure in many hospitals to prevent the development of gonococcal ophthalmia neonatorum.

SYMPTOMS OF OPHTHALMIA NEONATORUM

Ophthalmia neonatorum due to *N. gonorrhoeae* is the most destructive form of the disease. The symptoms of this condition, which generally appear one to four days after birth, are: a profuse thick discharge, redness, and swelling of the conjunctiva and eyelids of both eyes. It is estimated that approximately 30 percent of children born to infected mothers will develop gonococcal ophthalmia neonatorum if unprotected. If untreated, this condition may lead to perforation of the cornea and blindness.

With the widespread use of silver nitrate to protect against the development of gonococcal ophthalmia neonatorum, *Chlamydia trachomatis* has become the most common infecting organism. Symptoms of this type of infection, also known as "inclusion blennorrhea," generally occur one to two weeks after birth and include discharge, inflammation and redness of the conjunctiva, and swelling of the lid of one or both eyes. Some children may simultaneously develop a pneumonia due to *Chlamydia trachomatis* as well. Approximately 20 to 40 percent of children born to mothers infected with this organism will develop ophthalmia neonatorum if unprotected. If the acute infection is untreated, a chronic, smoldering inflammation may develop, which occasionally leads to scarring of the cornea or damage to the conjunctiva.

In contrast to the bacterial causes of ophthalmia neonatorum, chemical irritation secondary to the use of silver nitrate has a rapid onset (often within six hours), lasts 24 hours or less, and resolves without serious complications. Because of the self-limiting nature of this irritation, the condition is probably underreported, and the actual incidence is unknown.

STEPS TO PREVENT BACTERIAL OPHTHALMIA NEONATORUM

If a pregnant woman or her sexual partner are found to be infected with either *N. gonorrhoeae* or *C. trachomatis* prior to birth of the child, they should both receive appropriate antibiotic therapy (either penicillin or erythromycin in most cases). However, many parents are infected, but do not realize it because they have no symptoms.

Therefore, preventive therapy (prophylaxis) is recommended for all newborn children. Prior to 1980, one percent silver nitrate was the standard approach to preventing gonococcal ophthalmia neonatorum. However, silver nitrate is not effective in preventing chlamydial infections and may be irritating to the eye. In 1985, the Centers for Disease Control recommended that either one percent silver nitrate solution, one percent tetracycline ophthalmic ointment, or 0.5 percent erythromycin ophthalmic ointment be applied to the eyes of all newborns. The erythromycin and tetracycline ophthalmic ointments have the advantage of providing protection against both *Neisseria gonorrhoeae* and *Chlamydia trachomatis,* and they do not cause chemical irritation. Tetracycline has not been as extensively evaluated as erythromycin, but appears to be effective. Whatever approach to prevention is employed, the medication should be applied no later than one hour after birth.

TREATMENT OF OPHTHALMIA NEONATORUM

Newborns who develop gonococcal ophthalmia neonatorum should be hospitalized and isolated for at least 24 hours as *N. gonorrhoeae* may be transmitted to others. Treatment with intravenous penicillin should be started and continued for a total of seven days. Also, the eyes should be irrigated with a saline or other buffered solution every hour in order to wash away the discharge. Ophthalmic antibiotic ointments are unnecessary. Both parents or sexual partners should simultaneously be treated for gonorrhea (see Chapter 9). Infants born to mothers who subsequently are found to have a positive cervical culture for *N. gonorrhoeae* may develop ophthalmia neonatorum, even if preventive treatment (silver nitrate, tetracycline ointment, or erythromycin ointment) has been used. Therefore, these children should receive a single intravenous or intramuscular injection of penicillin.

If chlamydial ophthalmia neonatorum develops, the recommended treatment is erythromycin either intravenously or orally for a total of 14 days. As in gonococcal infections, topical ophthalmic ointments are unnecessary. At the same time, parents should be treated with either a tetracycline or erythromycin (see Chapter 13).

In the event of chemical irritation caused by the use of one percent silver nitrate, no treatment is necessary. The condition usually resolves rapidly and is not associated with severe or permanent complications.

CONCLUSION

Numerous diseases of a bacterial, viral, and parasitic origin may be transmitted through intimate sexual contact. All these diseases are not addressed in this book, but the most prevalent have been presented. You should utilize other sources for information on the less frequently occurring sexually transmitted diseases such as chancroid, lymphogranuloma venereum, and anogenital warts.

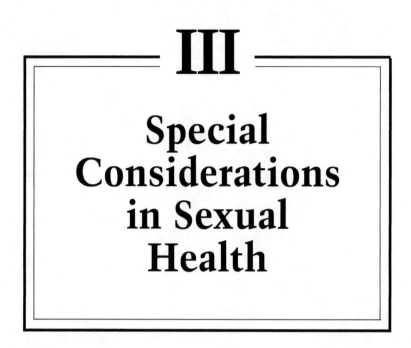

III

Special Considerations in Sexual Health

17

Premenstrual Syndrome (PMS): A Therapeutic Enigma

INTRODUCTION

Most people are not aware of the tremendous chemical (especially hormonal) changes that take place in a woman's body during each menstrual cycle. What occurs in women is entirely different from what men experience; hormone concentrations in males remain relatively constant from puberty to middle age. In women, hormone levels fluctuate throughout a period of approximately one month, causing what we know as the menstrual cycle. The periodic bleeding that occurs only marks the end of a series of internal events that begin anew after the menstrual period. The days just prior to or during the periodic bleeding are often associated with a complex array of aches, pains, mood changes, and other common maladies otherwise known as the premenstrual syndrome (PMS). Other names for PMS are premenstrual tension and congestive dysmenorrhea. Slang terms used to explain the syndrome have been "her time of the month" and "the curse."

An exact definition of PMS remains elusive because this medical disorder does not affect each woman the same way or with the same severity. The fact that PMS can cause a variety of symptoms complicates treatment.

293

Premenstrual syndrome (PMS) is perhaps best defined as a complex, recurring medical disorder caused by hormonal changes that affect various systems of the body (particularly the nervous system) resulting in physical and/or psychological symptoms that may produce temporary disruption of the personal and professional lives of a substantial number of women throughout their reproductive years.

It is very difficult to pinpoint exactly how widespread PMS is. Nonetheless, a very large percentage of women are affected. Most researchers report that somewhere between 30 and 50 percent of all menstruating women experience PMS to some degree.

The popular press has made PMS a "trendy" and "in" disorder. Since PMS is a poorly understood although widely experienced medical condition, it is excellent fuel for exaggerated, sensational, and speculative journalism. PMS is often blamed for behavior and/or medical symptoms that are unrelated to hormonal shifts.

Although a popular health subject today, PMS is not a new disorder. Primitive tribes have banished their women just before and during their menstrual periods for thousands of years. For example, ancient Hawaiians provided special huts on the edge of villages for intolerable females undergoing "the siege." Women have been suffering through PMS since prehistoric times, but few women have fully understood or openly acknowledged what was happening to them. Until recently medical science has been poorly responsive to the severity of this syndrome and the need for therapeutic intervention.

ECONOMIC CONSIDERATIONS

Aside from the physical and/or mental discomfort experienced by women with PMS, the economic implications of PMS are quite significant. As women become an increasingly larger segment of the work force, the effect of PMS on work efficiency and absenteeism is becoming a major economic concern. As early as 1969, it was estimated that economic loss from absenteeism due to PMS was $5 billion annually and this figure is considerably higher today. The 10 to 15 million American women who experience PMS should take effective steps to cope with the disorder and treat its symptoms.

SYMPTOMS OF PMS

One noted medical authority has referred to PMS as "the storm before the calm," because numerous physical and psychological manifestations of PMS may begin as early as seven to 10 days before menses (the menstrual period). Table 34 lists the various physical and psychological symptoms most frequently reported.

TABLE 34
MOST FREQUENTLY ENCOUNTERED PHYSICAL AND
PSYCHOLOGICAL SYMPTOMS OF PMS*

Physical Symptoms	Psychological Symptoms
Bloated Feeling	Irritability
Breast Tenderness	Anger
Weight Gain	Aggression
Dull Ache in Lower Abdomen and/or Lower Back	Anxiety
	Tension
Change in Bowel Habits	Fatigue
Nausea and Vomiting	Lethargy
Swelling of Hands, Feet, Ankles, and Abdomen	Depression
	Insomnia
Hot Flushes	Increased Appetite/Thirst
Skin Disorder	Loss of Concentration
Headache	Poor Coordination
Pelvic Pain	Change (usually a decrease) in Libido (sex drive)
Runny Nose	Craving for Sweets
	Crying

*Frequency of occurrence and severity of symptoms is highly variable from woman to woman. A woman can be in one or more of four subgroups: about 80 to 90% of women who experience PMS are in the PMS-A subgroup and experience anxiety, irritability, and/or nervous tension; 60 to 65% are in the PMS-B subgroup and experience abdominal bloating, edema, weight gain, and/or breast tenderness; approximately 40% are in the PMS-C subgroup and experience increased appetite, craving for sweets, fatigue, and/or headache; only approximately 3% are in the PMS-D subgroup and experience severe depression and withdrawal.

Over 150 symptoms have been associated with PMS. The symptoms that occur in one woman with this disorder may overlap or be completely different than those experienced by another woman with PMS. The severity of the symptoms of PMS also vary. Many experience only minor discomfort, while others may be severely impaired or even incapacitated (see Figure 39). Others report no symptoms. Still others may report positive changes immediately prior to the period, such as mood elevation, increased sexual desire, extra energy, and a general feeling of well-being. Perhaps the only common denominator of PMS sufferers is that symptoms occurring in the days prior to menses almost always subside within 24 hours after the onset of bleeding.

The majority of women who experience PMS suffer only mild to moderate symptoms (see Figure 39). However, it is estimated that 20

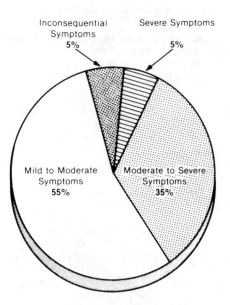

FIGURE 39

Approximate severity of PMS symptoms among U.S. women

to 40 percent of women experiencing PMS are temporarily incapacitated, either psychologically or physically, to a degree that is disruptive of occupational performance or social function.

Breast tenderness, lower abdominal bloating, fatigue, mood swings, and depression may occur as early as seven to 10 days prior to menses. Symptoms may intensify as the menstrual period approaches, resulting in loss of concentration, forgetfulness, and decreased dexterity and agility. As the menstrual cycle progresses, anxiety, restlessness, irritability, and hostility may occur. Some women report their self-confidence is decreased during this time. With the onset of menses, psychological symptoms of PMS generally subside, while relief of physical symptoms is slightly more delayed.

If symptoms associated with PMS occur at times other than the seven to 10 days prior to menses, it is probable that the symptoms are not due to PMS. Symptoms that continue beyond the early part of menses or into the first week or two of the menstrual cycle could be due to a major gynecological or even a psychiatric illness. Prompt medical attention should be sought if symptoms of PMS persist continuously or for long periods of time (one to two weeks) after menses.

CAUSES OF PMS

Historically, physicians, family members, and friends of PMS sufferers have not recognized PMS as an organic condition, and have not been particularly empathetic or supportive when symptoms arise. Evidence has shown, however, that the theory that PMS is psychogenic, "all in your head," is false. PMS is a bona fide medical disorder. Although hormonal changes occur that may affect a woman's mental attitude and perception (as well as produce physical changes), PMS is not a psychiatric illness.

Theories about the exact cause of PMS are numerous and varied. Factors that have been evaluated as possible causes of PMS include excess estrogen, deficiency of progesterone, vitamin deficiency, hypoglycemia (low blood sugar), allergy to hormones, fluid retention, fluctuating prostaglandin levels, and excess prolactin. Alterations in brain chemicals and their effects on internal organs have also been implicated in causing PMS. The hormonal changes that take place in a woman's body just before menses appear to be at the root of the problem, although exact cause and effect relationships between changes in hormone levels and physical and psychological symptoms of PMS are poorly defined.

Clinical studies have suggested that some of the symptoms of PMS may be the result of sudden changes in the levels of the body's own morphine-like (pain-relieving) substances called endorphins. Distributed throughout the body, endorphins are capable of producing a surge in many of the hormones associated with PMS symptoms. Elevated endorphin levels have been measured in women experiencing PMS symptoms. There is no available evidence, however, that reduction of endorphin activity alleviates PMS symptoms.

A deficiency of vitamin B_6 has been implicated as a possible cause of PMS because of the role vitamin B_6 plays in the production of chemicals (dopamine and serotonin) in the brain that affect the hypothalamus and pituitary gland. Dopamine also inhibits prolactin, another substance implicated in development of PMS symptoms.

Fluid retention has been cited as an underlying cause of PMS. According to this theory, certain symptoms of PMS—such as breast soreness and headache—are believed to be the result of swelling at different sites in the body due to fluid retention. It is hardly likely that fluid retention is a cause of PMS; it is just a symptom of the condition.

The fact of the matter is that the cause or causes of PMS are poorly defined. Until specific causes of PMS are identified, precision in treatment will be difficult.

COMPLICATIONS OF PMS

Possible consequences (complications) of PMS are stressful marital and other interpersonal relationships, a tendency toward social isolation, decreased work efficiency and productivity, and increased absenteeism. Worldwide attention focused on PMS when it was used in England as a defense for crimes of arson, assault, and manslaughter by three different women. Each woman claimed she only committed crimes during the days just prior to menses. Their defense lawyers pointed out that future episodes of antisocial behavior were avoided when the women took high doses of progesterone, a hormone used to treat severe PMS. In a similar case in the U.S., a woman was found innocent of murder; the principal defense was stress of PMS.

TREATMENT OF PMS

At the present time there is no "cure" for PMS. Frequency and severity of symptoms vary. You should consider treatment on an individual basis, as what might work for another woman may not work for you.

You can assist your physician in diagnosing PMS if you maintain a menstrual chart. By recording weight gain and the onset, duration, and severity of physical and psychological symptoms throughout the menstrual cycle you can better understand your PMS, as well as assist in the diagnosis.

The best approach to treatment consists of awareness of symptoms, avoiding environmental stress, observing dietary precautions, engaging in daily exercise, and treating specific symptoms with drug therapy when necessary and appropriate.

AWARENESS

If you suffer from PMS, you should become familiar with its symptoms. Additionally, your sexual partner, family, and friends (if appropriate) should be made aware of PMS and its symptoms so they can assist you in coping. Although formal psychiatric consultation is probably not of great value in treating PMS and is seldom warranted, discussing the problem openly with your physician may prove helpful in relieving some of the symptoms or coming to terms with the condition.

ENVIRONMENT

Developing an environment in which sexual partners can discuss PMS openly increases understanding. Both partners may then anticipate the time symptoms may occur, thereby reducing the level of tension. What the woman needs is understanding, not condescension. Mates should attempt to provide a stress-free environment for the woman approaching menstruation. Bear in mind that stress and anger are often the result of physical (*not* mental) internal events that are cyclical in nature.

DIET

If you experience PMS, you should cut down your salt intake for the two weeks prior to menstruation. Salt reduction might reduce some of the symptoms associated with fluid retention and weight gain. During the week prior to menses you should also reduce the amount of sweets you eat and increase the amount of protein to help maintain steady blood sugar levels. Minimize daily caffeine intake as well, as this may reduce abdominal cramping, tension, and nervousness. You may wish to limit your daily intake of coffee, tea, colas, and any nonprescription medication containing caffeine at this time.

Some women may experience symptoms of hypoglycemia (low blood sugar) during the premenstrual period. Evidence suggests that hypoglycemia may be due to an increase in the body's ability to use glucose (sugar); this may account for the craving of sweets that some women experience.

EXERCISE

Victorian attitudes and lack of information has led many women to believe that the time before menses is not a time for strenuous activity. In reality, daily exercise will help reduce excess body fluid. For some women, daily exercise reduces abdominal cramping; others find it helpful in working off anxiety, stress, and depression. Daily exercise is strongly encouraged.

DRUG THERAPY

To date, a varied selection of medicines from harsh laxatives to male hormones has been used to treat PMS. The treatment picture is distorted by the high rate of success of placebos (inert or inactive substances). In some studies, placebos have offered relief of PMS symptoms to as many as 50 percent of the subjects tested. In addition, the great number of possible causes of PMS has given rise to a host of theoretically justifiable treatments.

The use of *psychoactive (mind affecting) drugs* is a holdover from the days when PMS was considered a psychiatric condition. Tranquilizers such as Valium® and Librium® may be used to treat anxiety and tension in PMS sufferers. Studies have shown that they are poorly effective in managing the symptoms of PMS, however, and probably worsen depression and lethargy. Other drugs, such as amphetamines, barbiturates, and antidepressants have also been examined for effectiveness in treating the mental symptoms of PMS. Once again, studies have provided no conclusive evidence that any of these drugs is of significant value in relieving the psychological symptoms of PMS. In the case of amphetamines, abuse potential and strict federal controls have played a part in reducing their use. Lithium, more commonly used for severe mood swing disorders (manic depression), looks no more promising than a placebo in relieving the mental symptoms of PMS.

Oral contraceptives appear to relieve some of the discomfort associated with PMS in about half of women taking the pill. If a woman doesn't wish to have children at the time and side effects from the contraceptive are acceptable, oral contraceptives may be used as a short-term drug therapy for PMS.

PMS symptoms often become worse as levels of progesterone decline in the days just prior to the onset of bleeding. This has led doctors to treat some women with PMS with extra *progesterone,* especially women whose symptoms interfere with normal life-style on a frequent basis. Progesterone is generally supplied in suppository form for vaginal or rectal insertion. Progesterone taken by mouth is not absorbed well enough to be effective. Because progesterone accumulates in the body, the drug appears to be most beneficial if therapy begins five days prior to when symptoms are anticipated. If therapy is begun as early as 10 to 14 days prior to the usual onset of symptoms, spot bleeding at midcycle may occur. On occasion, progesterone therapy shortens the length of the menstrual cycle. Other side effects from progesterone supplementation (such as cramps and backache) are rare.

The misconception that fluid retention is a *cause* of PMS has resulted in *diuretics* (agents used to remove excess body fluid by increasing output of urine) being overprescribed by doctors more than any other group of drugs used to treat this disorder. Although use of diuretics often proves helpful in reducing fluid retention and relieving certain symptoms, side effects from these drugs can be serious (complicating control of diabetes or removing too much potassium from the body). Additionally, some women who have taken diuretics for PMS have ended up abusing them (taking more than prescribed and using them for weight control). Therefore, diuretics should not be employed casually for treatment of PMS.

Some women who suffer from PMS experience craving for salty foods before menses, which may account for fluid retention and weight gain and possibly some of the mood changes that occur. Before commonly used prescription diuretics such as hydrochlorothiazide (HydroDIURIL®) and spironolactone (Aldactone®) are used, personal eating habits should be explored as a possible contributing factor to fluid retention.

Diuretics (also known as water pills) are contained in many nonprescription products as well. They are marketed for the management of symptoms associated with the menstrual cycle. Pamabron and caffeine, both very weak diuretics, are most commonly included. Caffeine intake has, of course, been associated with nervousness, tension, and irritability. For this reason, it may be appropriate to avoid drugs and beverages (including colas) containing caffeine prior to the onset of the menstrual period.

Ammonium chloride is another diuretic contained in certain nonprescription drugs. Generally, these nonprescription products contain about one-fourth the dose needed for diuresis (increased urination). If taken in larger doses, ammonium chloride may cause nausea and vomiting. In fact, the effective dose of ammonium chloride is so close to the toxic dose that if a woman takes large amounts over a period of several days, she may experience nausea, vomiting, headache, hyperventilation, drowsiness, and mental confusion. A woman with kidney or liver disease or impairment is more prone to experience these adverse effects.

Other "diuretics" in "menstrual products" are holdovers from the 19th century and are of very questionable effectiveness. Such agents include powdered buchu leaves, couch grass, uva ursi, corn silk extract, and powdered hydrangea. Even if these substances *were* proven useful for treatment of PMS symptoms, they are not present in high enough concentration to be effective.

While a diuretic may provide some symptomatic relief of PMS, nonprescription products often take a "shotgun" approach to diuresis; the safety and efficacy of such products is questionable. In addition, over-the-counter diuretics are relatively expensive. If you experience premenstrual edema (excess fluid), you would be much better off seeing a physician than rushing to a drug store. If a diuretic is needed, your doctor can prescribe a mild prescription diuretic such as hydrochlorothiazide (HydroDIURIL®).

Some investigators believe that a relative shortage of *vitamin B_6* (pyridoxine) exists in PMS sufferers and that this deficiency results in depression. Supplemental vitamin B_6 supposedly increases the production of chemicals in the brain that may effectively treat depression and alter estrogen metabolism which may, in turn, relieve fluid retention, breast swelling, bloating, and headache. To date there is little conclusive evidence to support this theory, and the use of vitamin B_6 in PMS remains controversial.

Some researchers believe that the hormone prolactin may be the culprit responsible for some of the symptoms of PMS, such as tenderness and swelling of the breasts. In fact, the prescription drugs *bromocriptine* (Parlodel®) and *danazol* (Danocrine®), which lower prolactin levels in a woman's bloodstream, have been found to be effective in controlling the breast swelling and tenderness. Unfortunately, however, these drugs are of limited value in treating other PMS symptoms. It is also important to note that use of these drugs in treating PMS is still investigational; they have not been approved by the FDA for this use. In addition, both drugs are expensive and may produce troublesome side effects.

High levels of the hormones known as *prostaglandins* may also be responsible for some PMS symptoms. Although there have been no studies conducted on the levels of prostaglandins present in the blood during the time symptoms of premenstrual syndrome appear, prostaglandins are known to affect the concentration of certain hormones and stimulate contractions of the uterine wall and the gastrointestinal tract. Too much prostaglandin can result in lower abdomen cramping. The use of prescription antiprostaglandin drugs, such as mefenamic acid (Ponstel®), naproxen (Naprosyn®), indomethacin (Indocin®), tolmetin (Tolectin®), and ibuprofen (Motrin®, Rufen®; now available without a prescription under the brand names Advil® and Nuprin®) have all been found effective in relieving premenstrual and menstrual cramping. Combinations of codeine with aspirin or acetaminophen, or aspirin or acetaminophen alone, may also be effective in relieving premenstrual cramps and headache. None of the drugs listed above have been approved by the FDA for use in treating PMS; however, doctors often prescribe these antiprostaglandins for PMS sufferers.

A host of nonprescription (over-the-counter) drugs (in addition to diuretics) are marketed to treat the symptoms of PMS. Nonprescription drug products commonly purchased to treat the symptoms of PMS are included in Table 35. Some of these products contain combinations of ingredients of questionable value. Those products that do contain potentially useful ingredients often do not contain enough of the drug to be effective in relieving symptoms.

The most effective ingredients in these over-the-counter products for treating symptoms of PMS are the pain relievers aspirin, acetaminophen, and ibuprofen. Both aspirin and acetaminophen are rated as safe in treating PMS when taken at recommended doses of 325 mg to 650 mg every four hours (assuming, of course, there are no contraindications to their use). You should not exceed a dose of 4,000 mg of aspirin or acetaminophen in any 24-hour period. The recommended dose of ibuprofen is 400 mg every six hours. The maximum dose of ibuprofen should not exceed 2,400 mg per 24 hours. You should not continue to consume any of these nonprescription drugs at the upper dosage limit for more than 10 days without consulting your physician.

Occasionally aspirin or ibuprofen use will be inappropriate; women with aspirin or ibuprofen allergy or any health situation that makes their use risky (asthma, ulcers or a history of ulcers, bleeding disorders, or drug therapy that will interact with aspirin or ibuprofen) may wish to consult with their pharmacist or physician. Acetaminophen is an acceptable alternative in most instances.

Selected menstrual products contain various amounts of *antihistamines,* such as pyrilamine maleate, supposedly to produce sedation (a side effect of antihistamines) and therefore relieve nervousness and irritability caused by PMS. The nonprescription drug products available generally contain only ⅛ to ½ the adult dose needed to achieve such results.

Some nonprescription preparations contain *sympathomimetic amines* (ephedrine, cinnamedrine) which, in theory, will relax the uterus, thus relieving the symptoms of cramping. There is virtually no evidence to support the use of these drugs in the treatment of PMS, however. In addition, sympathomimetic amines may produce adverse effects (such as nervousness, restlessness, and headache) that are symptoms associated with the premenstrual syndrome. Sympathomimetic amines may also complicate the management of such coexisting medical disorders as diabetes, heart disease, high blood pressure, and thyroid disease. Finally, sympathomimetic amines may interact adversely with a number of other widely prescribed drugs (reserpine, guanethidine, methyldopa, propranolol). For these reasons it is best to avoid products containing sympathomimetic amines in the treatment of PMS.

Various other drugs have been used to treat PMS. These include clonidine (Catapres®), vitamin A, calcium, atropine sulfate, magnesium, and ergotamine. These drugs are of unproven value in treating PMS, and their routine use is not recommended.

CONCLUSION

As the title of this chapter indicates, treatment of PMS is truly an enigma. Treatment is complicated by the fact that PMS is poorly defined. The exact causes are not clear, and occurrence of symptoms and severity of symptoms are highly variable from woman to woman. Women find the most effective treatment for PMS is treatment that is

TABLE 35
PARTIAL LISTING OF NONPRESCRIPTION (OVER-THE-COUNTER) DRUGS USED TO TREAT PMS

Product	Analgesic	Diuretic	Antihistamine	Caffeine	Other Ingredients
Acetaminophen (generic)	acetaminophen 325 mg	—	—	—	—
Acetaminophen Extra Strength (generic)	acetaminophen 500 mg	—	—	—	—
Advil	ibuprofen 200 mg	—	—	—	—
Anacin	aspirin 400 mg	—	—	32 mg	—
Anacin-3	acetaminophen 325 mg	—	—	—	—
Anacin-3 Maximum Strength	acetaminophen 500 mg	—	—	—	—
Aqua-Ban	—	ammonium chloride 325 mg	—	100 mg	—
Ascriptin	aspirin 325 mg	—	—	—	magnesium hydroxide 75 mg aluminum hydroxide 75 mg
Aspirin (generic)	aspirin 325 mg; 500 mg	—	—	—	—
Bufferin	aspirin 325 mg	—	—	—	calcium carbonate, magnesium oxide, magnesium carbonate
Bufferin Extra Strength	aspirin 500 mg	—	—	—	magnesium carbonate 150 mg aluminum glycinate 75 mg

304

Cardui	acetaminophen 325 mg	pamabron 25 mg	pyrilamine maleate 12.5 mg	—	—
Datril Extra Strength	acetaminophen 500 mg	—	—	—	—
Diurex	potassium salicylate	uva ursi; buchu	—	amt. not stated	salicylamide, juniper berries, methylene blue, magnesium trisilicate
Diurex-2	same as above	same as above	—	amt. not stated	same as above plus iron
Femcaps	acetaminophen 325 mg	—	—	32 mg	ephedrine sulfate 8 mg atropine sulfate .03 mg
Flowaway Water 100	—	uva ursi 78 mg buchu extract 24 mg	—	20 mg	potassium nitrate 171 mg
Midol	aspirin 454 mg	—	—	32 mg	cinnamedrine 14.9 mg
Nuprin	ibuprofen 200 mg	—	—	—	—
Pamprin	acetaminophen 325 mg	pamabron 25 mg	pyrilamine maleate 12.5 mg	—	—
Panadol	acetaminophen 500 mg	—	—	—	—
Percogesic	acetaminophen 325 mg	—	phenyltoloxamine 30 mg	—	—
Trendar	acetaminophen 325 mg	pamabron 25 mg	—	—	—
Tri-Aqua	—	—	—	100 mg	—
Tylenol	acetaminophen 325 mg	—	—	—	—
Tylenol Extra Strength	acetaminophen 500 mg	—	—	—	—
Vanquish	aspirin 227 mg acetaminophen 194 mg	—	—	33 mg	magnesium hydroxide 50 mg aluminum hydroxide 25 mg

individualized to their own personal needs and directed toward relief of symptoms, whether physical or psychological. If you suffer from PMS, many steps can be taken to relieve symptoms before trying drug therapy, including better understanding of this disorder, avoiding stressful situations, implementing dietary restrictions, and exercising. If you feel drug therapy is required, seek the advice and counsel of a pharmacist or physician who can assist in selecting proper drugs to help you manage your particular symptoms.

18

Toxic Shock
Syndrome (TSS)

INTRODUCTION

A great deal has been written and said about toxic shock syndrome
(TSS) over the last several years, but many people remain relatively
confused about this syndrome. TSS was first reported in 1978. The
first reports were not in mature women, but rather in seven female
children, ages eight to 17. After these initial reports, there were other
similar case reports from around the country. By May 1980, the
Centers for Disease Control (CDC) had reviewed reports of 55 new
cases. Of these 55 reports, 52 involved women, and the majority of
cases developed during the menstrual period. New cases continue to
be reported, although the incidence is declining.

Toxic shock syndrome, a rarely occurring but serious illness,
develops very suddenly. Most cases occur in women between the
ages of 10 and 30, and in the large majority of cases, symptoms start
between the second and fifth day of the menstrual period in women
using tampons.

Although much of the original fear and panic about TSS has
abated, there is still a great deal of public confusion about TSS
related to the cause, rate of occurrence, role of tampons in causing
the disease, symptoms, what you should do if symptoms occur,

treatment, and what you can do to prevent TSS. Well-informed people are at reduced risk. If symptoms do occur, it is imperative that you recognize the symptoms and seek medical attention promptly. Early treatment is crucial to complete recovery, and may be lifesaving.

DEFINITION AND CAUSE

Toxic shock syndrome (TSS) is a fever-producing illness that is often associated with rash, low blood pressure, and involvement of several of the organs of the body. It is viewed as a type of "blood poisoning." TSS is indirectly caused by the common bacteria known as *Staphylococcus aureus* in almost all cases. This bacteria is normally present on skin and mucous membranes, but generally causes no symptoms.

In women who develop TSS, *Staphylococcus aureus* may be present on the walls of the vagina. Once the bacteria start to grow in an area, they give off one or more waste products which are toxic (poisonous) if they reach various parts of the body. Certain tampon fibers that are highly absorbent (for example, polyester foam and polyacrylate rayon) apparently "soak" up large amounts of magnesium normally present in vaginal fluid and tissue. The removal of magnesium appears to allow *Staphylococcus aureus* to churn out larger quantities of deadly toxins.

The toxic waste product(s) cannot produce TSS unless they enter the bloodstream. They may enter the bloodstream through tiny lesions or wounds that exist where the bacteria are present. The toxin, once in the blood, travels throughout the body. The reaction to the toxin is rapid and can be relatively mild, extremely severe, and even life-threatening.

OCCURRENCE OF TOXIC SHOCK SYNDROME

Over 3,000 cases of toxic shock syndrome (TSS) had been reported to the Centers for Disease Control (CDC) up to 1986. Approximately 35 to 50 new cases are reported each month. Tampon-users appear to be at greatest risk for developing TSS. Approximately 80 to 90 percent of all cases reported have involved young, healthy menstruating females. Of the menstruation-associated cases, approximately 99 percent have occurred in tampon-users. Approximately 35 percent of cases involve menstruating females between 15 and 19 years of age. The majority of cases occur in women under 30. After 30, even though the incidence of tampon use remains high, the probability of developing TSS appears to decrease. This may be due to the development of a type of "immunity" that young women have not acquired.

Toxic shock syndrome does not occur exclusively in menstruating females who use tampons. Approximately 5 percent of all cases are reported in men, and by 1982 over 20 percent of cases occurred in men, children, and nonmenstruating women (see case report which follows). Although documentation is poor, other factors may increase the probability that TSS will occur. The role of a high frequency of intercourse, frequency of intercourse during menstruation, use of the diaphragm or contraceptive sponge for prolonged periods of time, history of herpes and other genital infections, and use of douches and deodorizing chemicals during menstruation are being evaluated to see if they increase the risk for developing TSS among women. There is no conclusive evidence that the items listed above are major risk factors for developing TSS, but isolated reports justify investigation into possible causative relationships.

As the tampon-using female has become more knowledgeable about precautionary measures which may be taken to prevent the development of TSS, the proportion of cases associated with menstruation has decreased very substantially. Nonmenstrual TSS accounted for 7 percent of cases reported in 1980, 18 percent in 1981, and 22 percent in 1982. Evidence of better hygiene among female tampon-users is demonstrated in the fact that the number of cases of TSS decreased each year from 1980 to 1982. The fact remains, however, that of menstruation-associated cases of TSS, approximately 99 out of 100 will involve use of tampons.

Most menstruating women prefer to use tampons for reasons of convenience and aesthetics. Approximately 70 percent of menstruat-

---

Case Report of Toxic Shock Syndrome in a Nonmenstruating Woman

N. R., a 55-year-old postmenopausal female who had not worn a tampon in 11 years began vomiting and felt weak after dinner. Symptoms worsened during the night; vomiting continued, and profuse diarrhea developed. An ambulance was called, and N. R. was hospitalized, diagnosed correctly before all the classic symptoms of TSS developed, and was treated promptly and appropriately with intravenous fluids and antibiotics.

This was a rapidly progressive and serious case. In spite of the promptness of the diagnosis and treatment, N. R. developed gangrene in eight fingers which had to be partially amputated. This case underscores the extreme importance of seeking medical attention at the first sign of diarrhea, vomiting, and high fever, especially if this symptom complex develops during a menstrual period.

ing U.S. women use tampons. The TSS scare produced a brief drop in tampon use, but tampon use is higher today than ever. Tampon use should not be discouraged, but safe and appropriate use must occur to minimize health risks. You must read and follow the precautionary labels and package insert—and talk with your physician or pharmacist if you have any questions—to minimize risks.

ROLE OF TAMPONS IN CAUSING TOXIC SHOCK SYNDROME

Tampons, in themselves, do not cause toxic shock syndrome. Tampon use is associated, however, with development of TSS, as is explicitly indicated in the statistics of the previous section (99 percent of menstruation-associated cases of TSS involve tampon use). Exactly how tampons increase risk for developing TSS in menstruating women is not known, but several theories have been proposed:

1. Many bacteria thrive in a warm, moist environment. It is possible that a blood-soaked tampon may produce a good medium upon which *Staphylococcus aureus* may grow and produce its toxins.
2. The more absorbent tampons soak up vaginal magnesium. Decreased magnesium may allow *Staphylococcus aureus* to produce larger quantities of the toxin, which may be absorbed.
3. Small nicks and areas of local trauma may be made in the wall of the vagina when tampons are inserted and removed. These nicks may allow bacterial toxins to enter the bloodstream more readily.
4. The tampon may be contaminated by bacteria from the woman's hands, or bacteria from the area between the anus and vaginal opening or from the external genitals. The tampon will carry bacteria into the vagina where they may grow and produce toxins at an accelerated rate, thus increasing the chance of their entering the bloodstream.
5. Some feel that TSS is caused by toxins contained in menstrual blood. By blocking the vaginal outlet, some investigators feel that the accumulated toxins have a greater chance of being absorbed into the bloodstream to produce TSS.
6. Absorbency of most tampons was increased in the early and mid 1970s by changing the composition from rayon or rayon-cotton fibers to more absorbent synthetic materials (carboxymethyl cellulose, rayon-cellulose, polyacry-

late fibers, and polyester foam). This change occurred just prior to the recognition of TSS as a distinct and major disease. A disproportionately high number of cases were reported in the late 1970s and early 1980s among users of some brands of tampons that were super-absorbent. The FDA does plan to proceed with a labeling requirement for absorbency that will be a better guide for the consumer than vague terms such as "regular" and "super." All tampons containing the "superabsorbent" polyester foam and polyacrylate rayon have been re-moved from the market.

SYMPTOMS OF TOXIC SHOCK SYNDROME

In the typical victim of toxic shock syndrome, the symptoms may include:

1. A high fever (102°F or higher) that develops suddenly (chills may also occur).
2. Heavy vomiting and diarrhea, which usually accompany the fever.
3. A sunburn-like rash may develop a few days after the onset of fever, vomiting, and diarrhea. This rash most often develops on the palms of the hands and soles of the feet, but may also develop on the face and trunk.
4. About two to three days after symptoms first appear, the TSS victim may feel faint or dizzy and may even faint when changing body position (sitting to standing). These are symptoms of low blood pressure. In severe cases, blood pressure may drop to dangerously low levels and result in shock which, if not treated properly, may be life-threatening.
5. Other common symptoms of TSS which occur early in the progression of the illness are sore throat, muscle aches, swelling and redness of the eyes, disorientation, and mental confusion.

Most of these symptoms subside over a period of 7 to 10 days if properly treated. After about two weeks, the rash becomes scaly and peels off. Some TSS sufferers also suffer temporary loss of hair about two to six weeks after symptoms first appear. Gangrene may be a complication of inadequate blood supply to the extremities due to severe drops in blood pressure. Return of energy levels to that before the development of TSS may take several weeks.

As is obvious in the above description of the disease, TSS can have an adverse effect on numerous parts of the body including the brain (fever, disorientation, mental confusion), skin (rash), gastrointestinal system (diarrhea, vomiting), muscles (aches), eyes (redness, swelling), cardiovascular system (low blood pressure, dizziness, fainting, shock), and the liver and kidney. All victims of TSS do not develop all of these symptoms, and in some individuals the symptoms are often so mild they go unrecognized. In its most severe form, however, TSS may prove fatal if not recognized and treated rapidly.

ACTION TO TAKE IF SYMPTOMS OF TOXIC SHOCK SYNDROME OCCUR

The victim can never predict how rapidly progressive or serious the symptoms of toxic shock syndrome may become. Early recognition of symptoms and prompt reporting of these symptoms to a physician is critical. Early diagnosis, hospitalization, and effective treatment greatly decrease the chance that severe complications or death may occur.

The association between TSS and tampon use in menstruating females is unequivocal. Because of this, women using tampons during the menstrual period who develop a high fever (102°F or greater), vomiting, diarrhea, or a sunburn-like rash should stop using tampons and seek medical attention immediately. If such symptoms occur at night or on weekends and your regular physician is not available, you should be taken to the emergency room of a hospital. Not every bout of fever, vomiting, or diarrhea in a menstruating female means TSS is present, but potential health risks warrant a conservative approach to diagnosis.

TREATMENT OF TOXIC SHOCK SYNDROME

The importance of prompt and appropriate treatment cannot be overemphasized. Patients usually require hospitalization and monitoring in an intensive care unit until their body functions are normalized and stable. The key elements of treatment are fluids and drugs to support blood pressure and antibiotics to kill the bacteria which produce the toxins.

Victims of TSS often lose a large amount of fluid because the illness causes the smallest blood vessels of the body (capillaries) to "leak" fluid out of the blood vessels into the surrounding tissues of the body. This loss of fluid inside blood vessels causes the blood pressure to drop. Hospitalized women must receive fluids directly into the vein (intravenously) to maintain blood pressure until the capillary leaks stop. Large volumes of intravenous fluid may be necessary to get the blood pressure up. Sometimes as many as 12 to 15 liters of intravenous fluid may be given in a 24-hour period. This may cause some swelling (edema) of body tissues, but most of the excess fluid will eventually be converted to urine and eliminated from the body.

In some instances, intravenous fluids alone will not be sufficient to raise blood pressure. In this instance, it may be necessary to administer a blood pressure elevating drug along with intravenous fluid. The drug which is most often employed to raise blood pressure in shock is dopamine.

Antibiotics injected intravenously or into the muscle (intramuscularly) are an important part of the treatment of TSS. Women should receive broad spectrum antibiotics that are effective against penicillin-resistant *Staphylococcus aureus* and effective against other organisms that may produce symptoms which may be mistaken for toxic shock syndrome (Rocky Mountain spotted fever, scarlet fever, meningococcemia, for example). Any local infection that might harbor *Staphylococcus aureus,* such as a boil or abscess, should be drained.

Surprisingly, the antibiotics selected do not appear to contribute greatly to the successful treatment of TSS during the seven to 10 day period when symptoms are most serious. The use of appropriate antistaphylococcal antibiotics during the seven to 10 day acute phase of TSS does appear, however, to dramatically reduce the risk of a repeat attack.

A third approach to treatment is more controversial than intravenous fluid replacement and antibiotic therapy. This approach involves the administration of large doses of steroids for three to four days early in the course of the illness. It is alleged that steroid administration may produce a shorter and milder case of TSS. The value of steroid therapy has not been clearly demonstrated and requires further study.

DEATH RATE OF TOXIC SHOCK SYNDROME

As stated previously, toxic shock syndrome may be fatal. The death rate is highest if symptoms are not recognized or are ignored. Prompt hospitalization and effective treatment are essential to an optimal health outcome. Prior to 1980, the death rate from TSS was approximately 10 percent. The death rate was 5 percent in 1980, 3 percent in 1981, 3 percent in 1982, and 5 percent in 1983.

RISK OF HAVING TOXIC SHOCK SYNDROME MORE THAN ONCE IF TAMPON USE CONTINUES

Toxic shock syndrome may occur again if certain precautions are not taken. The recurrence rate is a remarkably high 30 percent in women who are not properly treated with antibiotics during the acute phase of the illness and continue to use tampons during menstruation. The rate of recurrence of TSS can be reduced to near zero if broad spectrum antistaphylococcal antibiotics are administered during the seven to 10 day acute phase of the illness and tampons are not used for three to four months after the initial illness. If a woman has had, or believes she has had, toxic shock syndrome, she should discuss tampon use with her physician before using them. In most instances the physician will authorize renewal of tampon use after appropriate precautions have been taken.

HOW TO DECREASE CHANCES OF EVER GETTING TOXIC SHOCK SYNDROME IF YOU USE TAMPONS

One can entirely avoid the low risk of developing tampon-associated toxic shock syndrome by not using tampons. Most menstruating U.S. women prefer to use tampons, however, so numerous specific precautionary measures should be taken to reduce the risk of developing TSS. The FDA requires that certain warnings and precautions to be observed by users of tampons be placed on either the tampon package or in the informational leaflet inside the package.

Appreciation of the warnings and precautions listed below can be very helpful in preventing the development of toxic shock syndrome in tampon users.

1. Early warning signs of toxic shock syndrome are high fever (102°F or higher), nausea, vomiting, diarrhea, rash that looks like a sunburn, dizziness, and/or fainting. If these symptoms occur, remove the tampon immediately and contact a physician.
2. Women between the ages of 10 and 30 years should be aware of the fact that use of tampons may increase the risk of developing TSS in their age group. All women, and women in this age group in particular, should be encouraged to change tampons relatively frequently (every six to eight hours) and consider using a sanitary napkin or minipad at night. This should minimize the ability of *Staphylococcus aureus* to multiply.

3. Evidence suggests that the risk of TSS appears to be less when the least absorbent tampons are used. Consider using tampons with the lowest absorbency that are still effective.
4. If TSS has occurred in the past, tampon use should not be continued for at least three to four months after the illness *if* the patient received effective antistaphylococcal antibiotics during the acute phase of the illness. Re-institution of tampon use after a case of TSS should be discussed with a physician in every case as relapse rates may be very high (up to 30 percent) if antibiotics were not used properly and/or tampon use is reinstituted too soon after an episode of TSS.
5. Discuss tampon use with a physician if any warning signs of TSS have occurred in the past.
6. Women who have recently given birth should not use tampons for at least six to eight weeks after birth.

CONCLUSION

Toxic shock syndrome is a rare but serious disease that can be fatal. Menstruating women who use tampons are the group at by far the greatest risk. A thorough appreciation of TSS, its warning signs and symptoms, the importance of prompt and effective treatment, and measures which may be taken to prevent development of the disease can prevent untold amounts of physical suffering, mental anguish, and even death.

19

Drugs and Diseases That Affect Sexual Function

INTRODUCTION

Sexual competence is a significant aspect of your health. In the past two decades, sexual attitudes and values have undergone radical change, resulting in additional emphasis on adequate sexual function.

Feelings of inadequacy and loss of self-esteem are frequent complaints in men who, because of sexual impairment, feel like "only half a man." Women are experiencing more societal pressures concerning sexual competency. The ability to achieve orgasm has become an increasingly important benchmark of female sexual competence.

Much of the difficulty involved in sexual behavior, whether or not a bona fide sexual impairment exists, is due largely to ignorance, unrealistic expectations of one's own sexual performance, and the inability to convey needs and desires to one's sexual partner. This chapter is intended to facilitate understanding about human sexual response while presenting some of the causes of sexual dysfunction induced by drugs and diseases.

MALE AND FEMALE RESPONSE TO SEXUAL STIMULATION

To understand the various types of sexual dysfunction, it is important to understand sexual response. Sexual response in humans is divided into four basic phases (see Table 36).

TABLE 36
THE FOUR PHASES OF SEXUAL RESPONSE IN HUMANS

| Phase | Sexual Event | |
	Male	Female
Arousal	Penile Erection	Clitoral and Vaginal Swelling
Lubrication	Mucous Secretion	Mucous Secretion and Lubrication
Orgasm	Emission, Bladder Relaxation and Closure of Internal Urethral Sphincter Muscle	Pelvic, Vaginal and Anal Muscle Contraction
Resolution	Present	Absent

AROUSAL

Both sexes respond similarly during the arousal phase. The first sign of sexual arousal in men is erection. In women, the vagina, labia minor, and clitoris become swollen during this phase of sexual response.

Sexual arousal in the female involves the vagina, clitoris, and external area around the vaginal opening. The clitoris is the female counterpart of the male penis. It contains erectile tissue and a high concentration of nerve endings. Much like the penis, the clitoris becomes erect due to dilation of blood vessels and the subsequent compression and trapping of blood. Massaging the clitoris during lovemaking is a major source of sexual arousal for the female.

LUBRICATION

Secretions in the male urethra, seminal vesicles, and prostate gland combine with sperm to form semen. In the female, there are no mucus-producing glands in the vaginal wall. Small glands at the opening of the vagina and urethra contribute to vaginal lubrication.

ORGASM

In the orgasm phase of sexual response, men and women differ. Orgasm in the male consists of emission and ejaculation. Contractions of the prostate gland, seminal vesicles, and vas deferentia cause emission of semen into the urethra. During these contractions the internal, ringlike muscle between the urethra and the bladder closes. The closing of this muscle prevents mixing of urine and semen, and what is known as retrograde ejaculation.

Pressure exerted by the semen in the urethra triggers nerve impulses which cause contractions of genital muscles, which produce ejaculation. Ejaculated fluid is made up primarily of secretions from the prostate and seminal vesicles. The average volume of ejaculated fluid is three to five milliliters (two-thirds to one teaspoonful); this volume may contain 100 to 300 million, or more, sperm in fertile men.

In women, contraction of vaginal and anal muscles occurs during the orgasm phase. Orgasm in both the male and female is accompanied by a rapid increase in heart rate, breathing, and perspiration.

RESOLUTION

The phase of sexual response following orgasm, the resolution phase, is a period during which sexual intercourse is difficult, if not impossible, for the male to perform. The female does not appear to, at least physically, undergo the resolution phase of sexual response. This phase has also been referred to as the evaluation phase in which each partner may experience feelings of pleasure, contentment, guilt, embarrassment, or failure.

THE EFFECT OF THOUGHTS AND EMOTIONS ON SEXUAL RESPONSE

Although direct physical stimulation can initiate erection in the penis or clitoris (reflexogenic erection), what is thought and felt emotionally also plays a large role in sexual response. Mental activity secondary to sight, sound, smell, and imagination is sometimes enough to trigger the arousal or lubrication phase—and even orgasm. Emotions and thoughts may also reduce or totally inhibit sexual response, even during direct physical stimulation.

THE EFFECT OF HORMONES ON SEXUAL RESPONSE

Alterations in hormone levels may affect sexual function. The hormone testosterone maintains the process of sperm production and is responsible for development and maintenance of male characteristics such as height, weight, beard growth, body hair distribution, and muscle mass. Testosterone is also necessary for normal libido (sexual desire) in men.

Hormone alteration in females can affect sexual function significantly. Estrogen plays a primary role in female sexual response. Adequate vaginal lubrication is dependent on maintaining sufficient estrogen levels in the bloodstream. Female libido (sexual desire) is more dependent on the level of androgens ("male hormones") in the body than on estrogen ("female hormone"). This is supported by the fact that female libido is usually not significantly affected by removal of the ovaries. However, libido can be reduced greatly by removal of the adrenal glands, a primary source of androgens in females.

TYPES OF SEXUAL DYSFUNCTION

Sexual dysfunction involves difficulties in, or impairment of, the normal sexual response. Until recently, 95 percent of sexual dysfunction was believed to be of psychogenic (of the mind) origin. Research now suggests that organic (physical) conditions are responsible for up to 50 percent of cases of sexual dysfunction. Psychogenic sexual dysfunction is often a result of emotional and/or social stress such as marital problems, loss of job, bereavement, fatigue, or mental illness. Organic conditions which may produce sexual dysfunction include surgery, a physical handicap, and acquired sexual dysfunction due to prescribed drug therapy, substance abuse, physical exhaustion, acute or chronic illness, and aging. The onset of psychogenic sexual dysfunction may be abrupt and can be intermittent or constant. Organic sexual dysfunction is usually a slow, persistent, and progressive deterioration. Psychogenic and organic dysfunction may coexist.

The term "impotence" will not be used in this chapter because its meaning is frequently misunderstood; more specific terms will be used. Impotence is frequently used to describe either a male's inability to have an erection or to ejaculate semen, or both. Therefore, the terms erectile difficulty or ejaculation difficulty will be used because they are more descriptive.

CATEGORIES OF MALE SEXUAL DYSFUNCTION

Loss or decrease in libido (sexual desire) is a common sexual problem that goes largely unreported. Reduced libido in males may result from a decrease in testosterone, sedation, fatigue, or drug-induced depression.

Erectile difficulty is the most common form of sexual dysfunction in men, and is defined as a frequent or constant inability to obtain or maintain an erection prior to ejaculation that is sufficiently rigid for vaginal penetration and completion of the sex act. Impaired erectile function can result from reduced testosterone, increased prolactin hormone, which ultimately reduces the testosterone level, and damage or interference with the nervous system controlling this phase of sexual response.

If penile erection is possible during sleep (nocturnal erection), masturbation, or when having sex with another partner, the erectile difficulty is of psychogenic origin. A man with a previous history of erectile difficulty may continue to be unable to achieve or maintain an erection, even after the cause of the problem has been removed.

Ejaculation difficulty is a broad term used to describe several sexual abnormalities that may occur in males. The normal male biological response is to ejaculate within two minutes after vaginal penetration. Since few women are able to attain orgasm within two minutes, most men must learn to delay emission and ejaculation. Ejaculatory difficulties include:

1. Premature ejaculation—when the male ejaculates semen during a process of foreplay, understood by both partners to be leading toward sexual intercourse; when the male ejaculates semen just before or during the act of penetration; when the male ejaculates semen during the first penile thrusts following penetration
2. Retarded ejaculation—when ejaculation is very slow or the male is virtually unable to ejaculate. Retarded ejaculation is usually limited to an inability to ejaculate during sexual intercourse. In many cases, normal ejaculation is possible via masturbation.
3. Retrograde ejaculation—when semen is ejaculated into the bladder due to paralysis of the internal urethral sphincter muscle, a ringlike closure between the bladder and urethra.

Gynecomastia is the abnormal growth of one or both breasts in the male. The psychological response to gynecomastia is probably more of a deterrent to normal sexual activity than the condition itself.

Priapism is a condition in which there is a persistent abnormal penile erection, usually without sexual desire. This condition is often accompanied by pain and tenderness of the penis. Priapism is frequently the result of spinal cord injury or obstruction of the outflow of blood from the penis.

Oligospermia is a condition of reduced sperm count in the semen. The most common cause of oligospermia is use of certain drugs that may affect any one of several stages of sperm production.

Although sexual function may not be strictly dependent on fertility, many men equate sexual competence with the ability to induce pregnancy and produce offspring. A barren marriage, therefore, can have detrimental psychological effects that may affect libido in both partners.

Hormone alteration that may affect male sexual function involves primarily the hormones of the hypothalamus and pituitary gland. Any drug or medical disorder that affects production of hormones by these structures may alter sexual function.

Gonadotropin-releasing hormone (GnRH), a hormone secreted by the hypothalamus in the brain, stimulates the pituitary gland, also located in the brain, to release another hormone called luteinizing hormone (LH). The level of testosterone secreted from the testes into the blood stream is controlled by LH. A hormone called prolactin, originating in the pituitary gland, reduces the responsiveness of the testes to LH, thereby reducing the level of testosterone in the bloodstream.

An adequate level of androgens (especially testosterone) plays a significant role in male sexual activity. However, the presence of penile erection in infants and preadolescent males indicates that erection is not solely dependent upon normal adult testosterone levels.

CATEGORIES OF FEMALE SEXUAL DYSFUNCTION

Decreased libido (sexual desire) is a more frequent problem in females than in males. In women, a reduction in libido is frequently the result of pain, fear, depression, emotional disturbances, and/or hormonal imbalances.

One of the most common causes of organic sexual dysfunction in females is dyspareunia, a condition involving vaginal or pelvic pain occurring upon penile penetration and during sexual intercourse, often leading to interruption or termination of the sexual act. Most cases of pelvic pain upon penile penetration of the vagina are the result of organic disorders such as vaginal muscle spasm, pelvic congestion, pelvic inflammatory disease (PID), or some other infectious disease. Additionally, dyspareunia is frequently associated with the inability to achieve orgasm.

Orgasm dysfunction or anorgasmia (absence of orgasm) is a relatively common sexual problem in which a woman is unable to reach orgasm on a frequent or consistent basis in situations that appear to be sufficiently stimulating. Roughly 10 percent of women never experience orgasm. About 75 percent of those who experience orgasm do so regularly. Approximately 45 percent experience orgasm during sexual intercourse. Orgasm dysfunction is frequently due to lack of understanding by one or both sexual partners of what is involved in effective sexual stimulation of the woman. Organic causes of orgasm dysfunction include genital or urinary tract infections, hormone imbalance, nervous system disorders, and muscular disorders.

Vaginismus is a term used to describe the partly voluntary, partly spontaneous spasm of the muscles in and around the vagina that make penile penetration difficult or virtually impossible. Most cases of vaginismus are of psychogenic origin. Painful lesions at the vaginal entrance may cause this disorder. Even though sexual intercourse may not be possible, women with vaginismus often enjoy clitoral orgasm.

Menstrual irregularities include amenorrhea (the absence or discontinuation of menses) and anovulation (absence of ovulation). Although menstrual irregularities rarely have a direct effect on sexual function, their psychological effects may cause a decreased desire for sex or decreased enjoyment of sex.

Inadequate vaginal lubrication is a little discussed and often overlooked part of the female sexual response. Sufficient vaginal lubrication is important for pleasurable and successful sexual intercourse. Artificial lubrication with a spermicidal cream or jelly or with K-Y Jelly® may be required.

Painful breast enlargement may lead to female sexual dysfunction. Several drugs are known to cause painful breast enlargement.

Hormone alteration in females can affect sexual function significantly. Elevated prolactin can prevent ovulation and cause amenorrhea. Adequate vaginal lubrication depends heavily on maintaining sufficient estrogen levels in the bloodstream.

DISEASES WHICH CAN AFFECT SEXUAL FUNCTION

Disease or illness of many types may affect sexual function, either physically, psychologically, or socially. Over 100 causes of sexual dysfunction are related to illness or trauma. The effects of diseases on sexual function, especially long-term, chronic illnesses, are many and varied. The degree of sexual impairment is often directly related to the severity of the disease.

CARDIOVASCULAR DISORDERS THAT AFFECT SEXUAL FUNCTION

The fear of overexertion and death is prevalent among many heart attack survivors. The belief that sex is "out" after a heart attack is generally incorrect. For the majority of heart attack victims, there are no physical reasons why sexual activity cannot be ultimately resumed under appropriate conditions. Physical energy expended during sexual intercourse is equivalent to such activities as scrubbing a floor or climbing a few flights of stairs. The heart beats an average of 117 beats per minute during orgasm. Death due to a heart attack during sexual activity typically occurs during overly vigorous extra-marital sex or after a large meal and considerable alcohol consumption. Resumption of sexual activity after a heart attack should be discussed with your doctor.

When an individual with hypertension (high blood pressure) experiences an adverse sexual effect, it is frequently assumed that an antihypertensive drug is responsible. If the drug is discontinued and the patient fails to recover, the sexual impairment is often labeled as "psychogenic." The fact that hypertension itself may be responsible is often overlooked.

With more than 400,000 people added to the list of stroke survivors each year, poststroke sexual function is certainly important. In males, a stroke appears to inhibit both erectile and ejaculatory function, with ejaculation being somewhat more affected. Female stroke victims are affected significantly more than males. In one study, only one of 11 females questioned experienced orgasm after a stroke episode. Eight of the 11, however, did have poststroke sexual activity they rated as "good" or "enjoyable."

HORMONAL DISORDERS THAT AFFECT SEXUAL FUNCTION

Medical disorders affecting the delicate hormonal balance in the body play a significant role in sexual health. Diabetes is not a disease that initially has a direct effect on the body's sexual system. Nonetheless, diabetes is the largest single cause of organic erectile difficulty, with 50 to 60 percent of all diabetic males experiencing erection difficulty at some stage of their sexual lives. As in the general population, however, approximately half of all diabetes-associated sexual impairment appears to be psychogenic. The incidence of sexual dysfunction in diabetes increases with age at a rate two to five times greater than that in the general population. Little is known about the effects of diabetes on sexual function in females.

Addison's disease results in a decrease in luteinizing hormone (LH) release and/or a decrease in testicular function. Cushing's syndrome, also known as "moon face" syndrome, is caused by abnormal adrenal gland activity or by prolonged intake of steroid medication. Approximately 70 percent of men with Cushing's syndrome have reduced libido and loss of erectile function. The disease causes a reduction in luteinizing hormone and testosterone levels.

Hyperprolactinemia (unusually high amount of prolactin production) can result from a number of medical disorders. This condition ultimately suppresses testosterone secretion by diminishing the response of the testicles to luteinizing hormone. Up to 90 percent of men with significant hyperprolactinemia experience gynecomastia and/or a reduction in libido.

Hypo-ovarianism (defective hormone production by the ovaries) causes a decrease in female estrogen levels. A reduction in estrogen production can result in decreased or inadequate vaginal lubrication.

Hypothyroidism (reduction in thyroid gland function) usually causes a reduction in sexual function if not treated. Hyperthyroidism (overactive thyroid gland) causes a reduction in libido in over 70 percent of those affected if not properly treated. More than half of all males with untreated or poorly treated hyperthyroidism suffer from a reduction in erectile function. Diminished sperm concentration in semen, gynecomastia, and reduced testosterone are other adverse sexual effects which may be seen in hyperthyroidism.

MALIGNANT DISORDERS THAT AFFECT SEXUAL FUNCTION

Feminizing tumors produce feminizing effects as a result of secreting high amounts of estrogen. This type of tumor is generally accompanied by reduced libido, altered erectile function, gynecomastia, and reduced testicle size in men. Gynecomastia is present in almost all men with a feminizing tumor.

Testicular cancer is also a cause of sexual dysfunction. It reduces fertility and may disrupt intimate sexual relationships. Some forms of testicular cancer require radiation therapy, which may also cause sexual dysfunction. To reduce the risk of birth defects, contraceptive measures must be used for at least six months after chemotherapy or radiation therapy has been discontinued.

Breast cancer now affects, or will affect, one in eleven American females. It is estimated that over 100,000 women develop the disease annually. Loss of one or both breasts may have adverse psychological effects on both the affected female and her sexual partner. However, sexual function is not impaired by breast cancer per se. Concerns such as "will a man want me" and feelings of sexual inadequacy occur in most women who must have a mastectomy (breast removal).

INFECTIOUS DISORDERS OF THE GENITOURINARY TRACT THAT MAY AFFECT SEXUAL FUNCTION

Infections of the genitourinary tract can have profound effects on sexual function. In some men, infection of the urinary tract may cause complete closure of the ducts leading from the prostate gland.

Pelvic inflammatory disease (PID), an infection which may involve the fallopian tubes, is the cause of sexual impairment in some females. Deep pelvic pain during intercourse may be due to current or previous PID. Guilt over past PID or frustration concerning sterility may cause dyspareunia (vaginal and/or pelvic pain associated with intercourse). Dyspareunia may also occur in the presence of genital herpes lesions.

MUSCULAR AND JOINT DISORDERS THAT AFFECT SEXUAL FUNCTION

Muscular dystrophy is characterized by progressive weakness and degeneration of muscle tissue. As muscular dystrophy progresses, it becomes increasingly difficult for an affected individual to engage in sexual activity.

Arthritis causes pain and deformities in the joints. The pain and deformities may make sexual intercourse difficult in some positions.

NERVOUS SYSTEM DISORDERS THAT MAY AFFECT SEXUAL FUNCTION

Multiple sclerosis is a disease which causes progressive destruction of the brain and spinal cord. The victims of multiple sclerosis (MS) are usually 19 to 30 years old, with 60 percent of the cases occurring in females. A series of symptoms in MS, such as slurred speech, impaired vision, loss of balance, muscle weakness, numbness, and paralysis may have a profound impact on sexual activity. In some MS victims, orgasm may be difficult to achieve. Women may experience a reduction in vaginal lubrication as well.

Parkinson's disease is a condition characterized by slowness, loss of voluntary movement, muscle rigidity, and tremor. The partial or total absence of voluntary movement affects sexual activity in much the same way as does muscular dystrophy.

PHYSICAL DISABILITIES THAT AFFECT SEXUAL FUNCTION

Not surprisingly, a disabling condition often causes a change in the frequency, enjoyment, and nature of an individual's sexual activity. Spinal cord injury does not mean complete loss of sexual function in all cases, however. With the exception of ejaculation, it is possible for many spinal-cord-injured males to experience much of the normal sexual response. Sexual function in spinal-cord-injured females has not been adequately studied.

PSYCHOGENIC DISORDERS AND THEIR EFFECT ON SEXUAL FUNCTION

Practically all organic diseases that affect sexual function are accompanied by a degree of psychological sexual dysfunction. The reasons for psychological impairment of sexual function are numerous and varied.

THE EFFECTS OF AGING ON SEXUAL FUNCTION

Scant information is available concerning the effects of aging on sexual function. Older healthy males may continue to be sexually active well into their 60s and 70s. Many cases of sexual impairment in older men result from the presence of disease or alcoholism. Some erectile dysfunction is present in approximately 75 percent of men over 60. Although the frequency of erection may be reduced somewhat by age, the ability to have an erection in an otherwise healthy male over the age of 60 generally remains.

Women have the capacity to achieve orgasm throughout life. Menopause does not mark the end of sexual activity. If the female is regularly exposed to effective stimulation, there is no reason why an otherwise healthy, older female is not capable of sexual activity and pleasure. Vaginal lubrication and speed of lubrication in a woman may be diminished somewhat after menopause, but is often restored to normal with estrogen supplements.

DRUGS WHICH CAN AFFECT SEXUAL FUNCTION

Unfortunately, drugs can affect more than the disease they are intended to treat. Numerous medications can adversely affect sexual function. The combined adverse effects of drugs and disease on sexual activity can be a major obstacle to sexual fulfillment.

Although a drug may be the cause of an adverse sexual reaction, the frequency and severity of that reaction often depends on the dose of the medicine, length of therapy, simultaneous use of other drugs, underlying medical disorder, how the medicine is taken, and the general physical health of the individual.

The two groups of drugs with the highest potential to alter sexual response are antihypertensive (blood pressure lowering) and psychoactive (mind-altering) drugs. Both groups of drugs are used by millions of Americans.

ANTIHYPERTENSIVE DRUGS

Hypertension (high blood pressure) produces few symptoms, but its long-term effects on internal organs and the circulatory system can be very harmful, particularly if not treated effectively with drug therapy. If you are being treated for hypertension, you may experience a greater frequency of sexual dysfunction than persons with untreated hypertension. Do not abruptly discontinue antihypertensive drug therapy when they suspect the cause of your sexual dysfunction is your medicine. You should discuss discontinuing antihypertensive drug therapy with your physician if you suspect it is contributing to sexual dysfunction. Other drugs or combinations of drugs that do not adversely effect sexual function may be used to control blood pressure.

Medicine used to control hypertension is the most common cause of erectile failure and retrograde ejaculation in men. The incidence of sexual side effects caused by antihypertensive medication has been estimated to range from five to 20 percent. Table 37 lists several commonly prescribed antihypertensives with the possible

TABLE 37
ANTIHYPERTENSIVE DRUGS THAT *MAY* ALTER SEXUAL FUNCTION*

	Male					Female	
Drug	*RL*	*ERD*	*EJD*	*GY*	*PRI*	*RL*	*PBE*
Clonidine (Catapres®)	x	x	x	x	—	—	—
Guanadrel (Hylorel®)	x	x	x	—	—	—	—
Guanethidine (Ismelin®)	x	x	x	—	—	—	—
Hydralazine (Apresoline®)	x	x*	—	—	x	—	—
Methyldopa (Aldomet®)	x	x	x	x	—	—	x
Metoprolol (Lopressor®)	x	—	x	—	—	—	—
Nadolol (Corgard®)	x	—	x	—	—	—	—
Pargyline (Eutonyl®)	x	x	x	—	—	—	—
Prazosin (Minipress®)	x	x	—	—	x	—	—
Propranolol (Inderal®)	x	x	x	—	—	—	—
Reserpine (Serpasil®)	x	x	x	—	—	x	—

RL = Reduced Libido
ERD = Erectile Difficulty
EJD = Ejaculatory Difficulty
GY = Gynecomastia
PRI = Priapism
PBE = Painful Breast Enlargement

Drugs are listed by generic name, with the most common brand name in parentheses. The frequency of sexual dysfunction induced by individual antihypertensive drugs is not well defined.

*only in high doses

effect of these drugs on sexual function. The most severe cases of sexual dysfunction in hypertensive patients are generally seen in patients on large doses of antihypertensive drugs.

ANTIANXIETY/ANTIDEPRESSANT/ANTIPSYCHOTIC DRUGS

Impaired sexual activity may occur with the use of drugs prescribed to treat behavioral disturbances. Table 38 lists several commonly prescribed tranquilizers and antidepressants with their possible effects on sexual function.

TABLE 38
ANTIANXIETY/ANTIDEPRESSANT/ANTIPSYCHOTIC DRUGS THAT
MAY **ALTER SEXUAL FUNCTION***

	Male				Female
Drug	*RL*	*ERD*	*EJD*	*GY*	*MI*
Amitriptyline (Elavil®, Endep®)	x	x	x	x	—
Chlordiazepoxide (Librium®)	x	—	x*	—	—
Chlorpromazine (Thorazine®)	x	x	x	x	x
Chlorprothixene (Taractan®)	—	—	x	—	—
Diazepam (Valium®)	x	—	x*	—	—
Doxepin (Adapin®, Sinequan®)	x	x	x	x	—
Fluphenazine (Prolixin®, Permitil®)	—	x	x	—	—
Haloperidol (Haldol®)	—	x	x	—	—
Imipramine (Tofranil®)	x	x	x	x	—
Nortriptyline (Aventyl®, Pamelor®)	x	x	x	—	—
Oxazepam (Serax®)	x	—	—	—	—
Perphenazine/amitriptyline (Etrafon®, Triavil®)	x	—	—	x	—
Protriptyline (Vivactil®)	x	x	x	—	—
Thioridazine (Mellaril®)	x	x	x	x	x
Thiothixene (Navane®)	—	—	x	—	—
Trifluoperazine (Stelazine®)	—	—	x	x	—
Triflupromazine (Vesprin®)	—	x	x	—	—

RL   = Reduced Libido
ERD = Erectile Difficulty
EJD = Ejaculatory Difficulty
GY   = Gynecomastia
MI   = Menstrual Irregularities

Drugs are listed by generic name, with the most common brand name(s) in parentheses. The frequency of sexual dysfunction induced by these individual drugs is not well defined.

*only in high doses

APPETITE SUPPRESSANTS

Appetite suppressants such as diethylpropion (Tenuate®), fenfluramine (Pondimin®), and phentermine (Fastin®, Ionamin®) may be associated with reduced libido and erectile difficulty. Diethylpropion has also been reported to cause gynecomastia. Fenfluramine may cause a reduction in sexual interest in as many as 85 percent of women who take it. Only approximately 5 percent of men who take fenfluramine experience sexual dysfunction.

ANTIHISTAMINES

Antihistamines are commonly used to relieve symptoms of colds and allergy. Almost all antihistamines have the ability to produce some degree of drowsiness, which may reduce libido. Diphenhydramine (Benadryl®) and hydroxyzine (Atarax®, Vistaril®) produce the greatest degree of sedation and, therefore, have the greatest potential to alter libido. Some antihistamines, taken in doses large enough to cause dry mouth, may also cause erectile problems. Difficult erection may also be caused by antinausea medicines such as dimenhydrinate (Dramamine®) and antivertigo medicines such as meclizine (Antivert®), if the doses are large.

MUSCLE RELAXANTS

Difficult erection can result from taking muscle relaxants such as orphenadrine (Norflex®) and cyclobenzaprine (Flexeril®). Baclofen (Lioresal®), a drug used to treat muscle spasms, may cause erectile difficulty as a result of its sedating effect.

NARCOTICS

Erectile difficulties and ejaculation problems are common in heroin addicts and men involved in methadone maintenance programs. Long-term use of narcotics may also be associated with a reduction in semen volume, reduced testosterone levels, and impaired sperm motility.

Narcotics induce a greater degree of sexual dysfunction in female addicts than in male addicts. Up to 90 percent of female narcotic addicts experience menstrual abnormalities. Less than half of all pregnancies in this group are completed successfully. Commonly abused narcotics include codeine, hydromorphone (Dilaudid®), meperidine (Demerol®), methadone (Dolophine®), and oxycodone (Percodan®).

RECREATIONAL DRUGS

Shakespeare's comment in Macbeth that drink "provokes the desire but it takes away the performance" is only partially accurate. Small amounts of alcohol depress brain centers which govern fear and anxiety. Therefore, moderate intake may serve as a disinhibitor and thereby may increase libido. Excessive short-term alcohol ingestion may increase libido, but may reduce the ability to attain satisfactory erection.

Long-term alcohol abuse is destructive to the nervous system, contributing to loss of erectile ability in nearly all long-term, heavy drinkers. Even though prolonged, heavy alcohol use causes erection difficulties, most male alcoholics maintain a strong desire for sex. Few women complain of sexual inadequacy due to their own alcohol abuse.

Marijuana may enhance sexual response in some individuals. Touch and taste are most likely to be enhanced by occasional marijuana use. Heavy, long-term use, however, may reduce male testosterone levels, causing erectile difficulty and oligospermia in isolated cases. Gynecomastia has been reported in a study involving three male patients using marijuana for extended periods.

Effects of cocaine on sexual function are similar to those induced by amphetamines, but are more intense and of shorter duration. Low doses by the nasal route may enhance sexual response in males, but may cause delayed ejaculation. Heavy, prolonged use may bring on a greatly reduced or total loss of interest in sexual activity.

Amyl nitrite, an illicit recreational drug, is known to relieve sexual inhibitions. Its ability to dilate blood vessels and produce a sudden drop in blood pressure, often accompanied by dizziness, supposedly causes a delayed, yet more intense orgasm.

MISCELLANEOUS DRUGS THAT MAY CAUSE SEXUAL DYSFUNCTION

A host of other drugs may affect sexual function. Erectile difficulty has been reported in approximately 10 percent of men taking lithium carbonate, a drug used to treat manic-depressive behavior. No sexual dysfunction has been reported to date in women taking lithium carbonate.

Aminocaproic acid, a drug used to treat uncontrolled bleeding episodes, may inhibit ejaculation without noticeable effect on libido. Drugs used in the treatment of Parkinson's disease, such as benztropine (Cogentin®), levodopa, and trihexyphenidyl (Artane®), may cause erectile difficulty and reduced libido. Anticancer agents may cause amenorrhea and alter the production of sperm. Metronidazole (Flagyl®) is believed to cause a reduction in libido in some cases.

Disopyramide (Norpace®), a drug used to stabilize the rhythm of the heart, may produce erectile problems in doses of 300 mg to 400 mg per day. Clofibrate (Atromid-S®), a cholesterol-lowering drug, may cause erection and ejaculation difficulties in some males, but has not shown any adverse sexual effects in women. Vaginal irritation may be caused by use of spermicidal jellies, creams, foams, and medicated douches.

OVERCOMING SEXUAL DYSFUNCTION

If one experiences what is believed to be drug- or disease-induced sexual dysfunction, professional medical help is encouraged. Even if sexual dysfunction from a drug or chronic illness is alleviated, the fear of failure may prevent resumption of normal sexual activity. Identifying misconceptions, minimizing fear of failure, and encouraging improved communications with the sexual partner may reduce existing and avoid potential sexual problems.

MANAGEMENT OF DISEASE-INDUCED SEXUAL DYSFUNCTION

Management of disease-induced sexual dysfunction is often no more complicated than successfully treating the disease. Medical management and conscientious application of treatment by the patient with thyroid disorders, diabetes, certain types of cancer, Parkinson's disease, cardiovascular disease, Addison's disease, Cushing's disease, hormonal imbalances, infections, arthritis, and psychiatric disorders will often eliminate or minimize sexual dysfunction.

MANAGEMENT OF DRUG-INDUCED SEXUAL DYSFUNCTION

When sexual impairment is due to a drug, the sexual dysfunction can usually be reversed by either adjusting the dose of the medicine downward or discontinuing that medicine altogether. One of the most formidable obstacles to identifying and solving sexual dysfunction problems arising from use of medicine is lack of awareness and hesitance of patients and doctors to discuss sexual problems openly. Many people feel perfectly comfortable reporting that a drug is upsetting their stomach or causing drowsiness, yet may shy away from reporting an adverse reaction affecting sexuality. You should not underestimate the many ways that drug therapy can be manipulated to avoid or minimize sexual dysfunction.

MANAGEMENT OF PSYCHOGENIC SEXUAL DYSFUNCTIONS

Psychogenic sexual dysfunction can result from tension, marital discord, anxiety, performance anxiety, performance embarrassment, distraction, nonsexual thought during sexual intercourse, preoccupation with homosexual ideas, perception or reception of inadequate stimulation, and many other factors.

Couples who are suffering from psychogenic sexual dysfunction may benefit from sex therapy. Although the format of sex therapy varies, the basic principles involved remain constant. Current sex therapy stresses learning and encourages improved communication and engaging in activities intended to aid mutual comfort and pleasure in sexuality. The emphasis on pleasure instead of performance enhances confidence and often reduces the symptoms of the original sexual impairment.

20

Methods of
Pregnancy Detection

INTRODUCTION

Pregnancy, if given time, can usually be detected quite readily from simple outward physical signs. The absence of menses or growth of the lower abdomen are not associated with pregnancy only, however. A great number of medical disorders are also associated with the classic signs of pregnancy, such as amenorrhea (absence of menstrual bleeding) and lower abdominal swelling. Furthermore, the adverse effects of tobacco, alcohol, drugs, and environmental pollutants upon the developing fetus, particularly during the first three months of pregnancy, have been widely reported. Women must realize when they are pregnant so they can take all necessary precautions to protect the developing fetus. Early pregnancy detection is not only desirable, but essential for the health and welfare of women and the developing fetus.

The ability to determine pregnancy in its early stages has fascinated people for centuries. Since the time of Hippocrates (460–370 B.C.), both distinguished physicians and quacks have pursued a variety of methods to determine whether conception has occurred.

For centuries, attempts to detect pregnancy in the first few weeks following conception have been directed at examining the woman's urine. Urine examination has proven to be a reliable, modern means of early pregnancy detection, but procedures used in ancient and medieval times were somewhat less than scientific. Ancient Egyptians, as early as the fourteenth century B.C., claimed the ability to not only confirm pregnancy, but determine fetal sex as well. Their method involved daily moistening of a bag of wheat and a separate bag of barley with the woman's urine. If the grains in either bag germinated, the woman whose urine was used was declared pregnant. Should the wheat grains germinate first, a male child was predicted; germination of barley grains indicated a female.

One of the most bizarre episodes in the history of pregnancy detection took place in medieval England, where men known as "piss-prophets" were held in high public regard. "Piss-prophets," not content with merely predicting pregnancy, professed the ability to diagnose a host of illnesses upon examination of the urine. Of course, "piss-prophets" were ultimately exposed for their medical quackery.

For brief periods during the eighteenth and nineteenth centuries, attention was again focused on new methods of urine examination. In 1831, for example, one such test entailed letting a urine sample from a pregnant woman stand for 30 to 40 hours. Scientists then observed the formation of a white, opaque film at the top of the sample, which they believed was formed by casein, an ingredient of milk. The film these scientists observed has never been shown to be relevant to the existence of pregnancy.

A scientific method for pregnancy detection was finally devised in 1928 by Ascheim and Zondek. This test was based on the presence of a hormone found in the urine of pregnant women. The hormone, known as human chorionic gonadotropin (HCG), caused a remarkably stimulating effect on the reproductive organs of infant mice injected over a 48-hour period with the urine from a pregnant woman. Although the Ascheim-Zondek procedure, or A-Z test, took five days to complete, it was considered a major breakthrough in the early detection of pregnancy.

Having learned of the A-Z test (mouse-test), M. H. Friedman at the University of Chicago developed a further refinement of pregnancy testing. Friedman's procedure involved injection of urine into an unmated mature female rabbit and took only 48 hours to complete. The Friedman test was soon the most widely used pregnancy test in the United States and became popularly known as the "rabbit test." Further modifications in the "rabbit test" reduced the waiting period to about 24 hours.

In 1960, the introduction of immunological assays (tests that utilize antibodies directed against a specific substance) marked the beginning of the present stage of pregnancy testing. Over the past 25 years, significant improvements have been made. The measurement of human chorionic gonadotropin (HCG) remains the focus of attention in the development of these improved methods of pregnancy detection.

SIGNS AND SYMPTOMS OF PREGNANCY

SIGNS AND SYMPTOMS A PREGNANT WOMAN MAY NOTICE

Many of the familiar signs and symptoms of pregnancy are a result of the changes that occur in a woman's body to protect and nurture the developing fetus. These changes are numerous (see Table 39). The most noticeable include such classic signs as a missed period (amenorrhea), nausea and vomiting (morning sickness), breast tenderness, lower abdominal congestion, and weight gain.

The sign of pregnancy most often noticed first is amenorrhea (absence of menstrual bleeding). However, not all pregnant women experience a complete absence of menstrual bleeding. One in four pregnant women may have some staining or slight bleeding, even though they are pregnant. Nausea and vomiting due to pregnancy occurs with greatest intensity in the first trimester (first three months) of pregnancy. This symptom has earned the name "morning sickness" because it is usually worse at breakfast; it generally subsides in the afternoon and may recur in the evening. Increased breast size and deepening of color of the pigmented area around the nipple (areola) are other commonly occurring signs of pregnancy. Other signs and symptoms of pregnancy are listed in Table 39.

TABLE 39
USUAL SIGNS AND SYMPTOMS OF PREGNANCY

Amenorrhea ("missed period")
Breast Tenderness
Constipation
Dislike of Smoking
Elevated Body Temperature
Fatigue and Exhaustion
Frequent Urination
Increased Pleasure During Sexual Intercourse
Increased Salivation
Nausea and Vomiting ("morning sickness")
Nipple (areola) Color Change
Pelvic Congestion (weight gain)

SIGNS AND SYMPTOMS THE PHYSICIAN MAY DETECT TO CONFIRM PREGNANCY

Your doctor looks for several telltale physical signs and symptoms that occur six to seven weeks after your last menstrual period. Softening of the lower segment of the uterus is sometimes evident as early as week six of pregnancy (about 42 days after the last normal menstrual period). Approximately seven weeks into pregnancy a pale violet coloration of the entrance to the vagina and the neck of the uterus may be observed. This is caused by blood engorgement in the vaginal area that may darken to blue, then to an almost blue-black tint as pregnancy progresses.

If you "feel pregnant," chances are 80 percent that you are correct. Even if correct, examination by a physician is necessary because amenorrhea, nausea, vomiting, pelvic congestion, enlarged breasts, raised body temperature, urinary frequency, and other symptoms of pregnancy may be caused by medical conditions other than pregnancy.

CURRENT METHODS OF PREGNANCY DETECTION

While early methods to predict pregnancy were somewhat misdirected, it was recognized that the urine of a pregnant woman possessed increased biological activity. During pregnancy, the body produces the hormone human chorionic gonadotropin (HCG). Approximately nine days after fertilization (conception), or about five days before the first expected day of menstruation, the urine contains detectable amounts of HCG. Essentially, this is the message from the fertilized egg saying it is present.

The initial role of HCG in pregnancy is to support the corpus luteum, which continuously secretes estrogen and progesterone until the developing placenta becomes sufficiently mature. Since rising levels of HCG occur after conception, its presence in urine has provided an excellent laboratory marker for early diagnosis of pregnancy. If elevated levels of HCG cannot be detected early in a suspected pregnancy, pregnancy is unlikely.

Only those detection methods that can provide a diagnosis of pregnancy in the first 42 days of pregnancy can be considered "early" pregnancy tests. After that point, classic signs and symptoms, as well as other methods of pregnancy detection, such as ultrasound, may confirm the diagnosis.

THE IDEAL PREGNANCY DETECTION TEST

Since the development of the A-Z test, methods of pregnancy detection have undergone numerous modifications. During the past fifty years, pregnancy testing has evolved from a cumbersome, complicated laboratory procedure into a rapid, convenient technique suitable for use in the physician's office. However, an ideal pregnancy test is yet to be discovered. If one is developed, it should possess the properties outlined in Table 40.

A false-negative result (when a pregnant woman obtains negative test results) is the most commonly occurring error in pregnancy testing. These errors occur most often in very early pregnancy because the HCG concentration is lower than the point at which current tests can detect its presence. If you are pregnant, but believe you are not due to a false-negative test result, you may unwittingly expose the fetus to potentially harmful situations and substances that may cause birth defects.

If a pregnancy test confuses another substance for HCG, a false-positive test results. The implications of a false-positive result can be as serious as a false-negative result. If you are incorrectly informed that you are pregnant, you may undergo unnecessary abortion procedures or stop using contraceptives and subsequently become pregnant.

Many of today's pregnancy tests provide fast, reliable results that can be interpreted easily. Commercial test kits are widely available at affordable prices and allow your physician to perform a pregnancy test in his office. To ensure accurate test results, you should follow the precautions outlined in Table 41 in collecting the urine sample to be tested.

TABLE 40
PROPERTIES OF THE IDEAL PREGNANCY TEST

1. Very sensitive to the presence of HCG at levels that occur prior to a missed period

2. Readily recognize HCG (should not confuse HCG with structurally similar substances)

3. Provide fast results that can be easily interpreted

4. Easy to perform

5. Relatively inexpensive

6. Widely accessible

TABLE 41
PROCEDURES FOR COLLECTING THE URINE SAMPLE

---

1. Use first or early morning urine, which contains the highest concentration of HCG.

2. Test may be more accurate if drugs and alcohol are omitted at least 12 hours prior to collection of urine sample. Eat only bland food the night before.

3. Freezing urine for more than 24 hours before testing can reduce accuracy of the test significantly.

4. Clean and rinse container for the urine thoroughly to remove foreign matter and detergents that may distort test results.

EARLY PREGNANCY DETECTION METHODS USED IN THE
LABORATORY AND THE PHYSICIAN'S OFFICE

Pregnancy can be detected by several methods. Biological assays require the use of laboratory animals and exact adherence to test procedure guidelines. In most cases, bioassays take several days to obtain results. Additionally, they are expensive and often require elaborate laboratory facilities for their completion.

Biological assays for HCG have been replaced by the more accurate, convenient, economical, and expedient immunological assays. Immunological assays also detect pregnancy by measuring HCG levels. They differ from bioassays, however, because they do not require the injection of urine or blood samples into laboratory animals. For the past two decades, immunoassays have been the mainstay of pregnancy detection methods.

In the 1950s and 1960s, hemagglutination assay (HIA) tests were developed. In one such test, called the direct hemagglutination assay, urine is mixed with antibody (directed against HCG) that is attached to red blood cells from an animal source (usually rabbit or sheep). If a certain level of HCG is present in the urine, the antibody binds to the HCG and the red blood cells adhere to each other and form visible clumps, signifying pregnancy. If insufficient HCG is present in the urine, clumping (agglutination) does not occur.

Indirect hemagglutination and latex agglutination inhibition tests differ from the direct hemagglutination method. In these tests, if a certain level of HCG is present, it will neutralize the antibody so that when red blood cells or latex particles coated with HCG are added to the solution, no clumping occurs, signifying pregnancy. If insufficient

HCG is present, the antibody reacts to the HCG attached to the red blood cells or latex particles and clumping takes place.

Developed in the early 1970s, radioimmunoassay (RIA) methods provided a means of detecting HCG at extremely low concentrations. This provided the opportunity to diagnose pregnancy before the missed period, earlier than was previously possible with biological and standard immunological assay methods.

In the RIA methods, antibodies directed against HCG are placed in blood or urine samples. HCG that is attached to radioactive iodine is then added to the solution. If no HCG is present in the sample, the antibody will react with the radioactive HCG upon its addition to the solution. If HCG is present in the sample, there will be less antibody to react with the radioactive HCG. The solution is then measured for its level of radioactivity to obtain results. Immunological assays are preferred over radioimmunoassay for routine pregnancy testing because they are less time consuming and less expensive.

The radioreceptor assay (RRA) is a more rapid form of RIA. Although not as sensitive to the presence of HCG, the RRA takes only one hour to complete and has near 100 percent accuracy. The RRA does not utilize antibodies against HCG. Rather, it allows HCG from a sample and radioactive HCG to compete for binding sites on a corpus luteum from a cow. As with RIAs, if HCG is present in the sample, less radioactive HCG will bind to the cow corpus luteum, and the resulting solution will exhibit higher radioactivity. Because the RRA method requires elaborate laboratory facilities, its use is restricted largely to urban areas in developed countries.

The next generation of pregnancy testing, enzyme immunoassay (EIA), incorporates the same principles as radioimmunoassay methods, but without the use of radioactive HCG. In EIAs, HCG from the woman and HCG attached to a nonradioactive enzyme compete to react with antibody that is directed against a subunit of HCG. After undergoing a series of laboratory procedures, the amount of HCG present in the patient sample is determined by measuring the intensity of the color generated through a special piece of equipment called a spectrophotometer. If the color intensity is higher than predetermined control solutions, the results are positive for pregnancy. If the color of the control solution is more intense, the results are negative.

The development of monoclonal antibody assays (MAA) for use in pregnancy testing may have solved some technical problems with HCG. Results from an MAA can be obtained in only 35 to 60 minutes. Additionally, they require no special laboratory equipment or radioactive materials. MAAs can detect very low HCG levels, making them useful at or just before the missed period.

OTHER METHODS OF PREGNANCY DETECTION

Although it is not useful as early in pregnancy as HCG measurement techniques, ultrasound may be useful in determining the status of fetal development (see Table 42). Ultrasound can be used in the sixth to eighth week of pregnancy, in combination with HCG tests, to clarify possible complications of pregnancy. It may also help diagnose developing spontaneous abortion, ectopic pregnancy, or incomplete abortion—all of which are difficult to diagnose during the first trimester with HCG detection methods alone. The HCG concentration in these situations does not continue to progress normally. Ultrasound may also be useful in confirming development of more than one fetus.

TABLE 42
MAJOR FETAL EVENTS IN EARLY PREGNANCY

Detection Method	Gestational Event	Gestational Week*
HCG Test	fertilized egg	2–4
Ultrasound	fetal sac visible	6–7
"	fetal heart formed	5–7
"	fetus visible	7–9
"	fetal heart visible	9–10
"	fetal head visible	9–11
"	fetal skeleton visible	14
"	fetal movement	18–22
"	fetal heartbeat heard	20

*Weeks from last normal menstrual period

HOME KITS FOR PREGNANCY DETECTION

In-home diagnostic kits and devices, which may be purchased without a prescription, have been found beneficial for detection of certain types of cancer, hypertension, diabetes, urinary tract infection, ovulation, and some sexually transmitted diseases. In years to come, in-home diagnostic kits and devices may be available for early detection of heart abnormalities (cardiac arrhythmias), stroke, anemia, stomach ulcers, glaucoma, and many other medical conditions. The usefulness of these kits should be judged on accuracy, simplicity, economy, and the relative importance to health their results may provide.

An accurate, simple, and reliable in-home pregnancy test is beneficial for some women, especially those residing in medically underserved areas. Their use requires a high level of literacy, however.

In-home pregnancy test kits are provided by several manufacturers (see Table 43). The first commercially available in-home kits were tube immunoassays. Results from these tests could be rendered inaccurate by vibration of the solution (from shaky furniture, fans, refrigerators, or even the ring of a telephone), direct sunlight, heat, or touching the test tube with the dropper tip. A multistep procedure in these kits provides ample opportunity for error. If a dark, doughnut-shaped ring (with a hole in the center) formed at the bottom of the test tube, the pregnancy test was considered positive.

More recent tests utilize a combination of monoclonal antibody and enzyme immunoassay methods to obtain results. This method is utilized in the e.p.t. Plus® kit. A positive result is seen when the original red solution turns to pink or gray. At least one kit (Advance®) uses a plastic stick coated with test chemicals that may change from white to blue if pregnancy exists. The format used in the Advance®, First Response®, and e.p.t. Plus® kits is not affected by minor vibration.

When used strictly according to a long list of directions, early in-home pregnancy tests are claimed to be 97 to 99 percent accurate if used 10 or more days after a missed period. In reality, they are approximately 80 percent accurate when used 10 or more days after a missed period. If results are positive, you should see your physician as soon as possible. If used nine days or less after a missed period, the average accuracy rate is only approximately 65 percent. Whether

---

TABLE 43
PREGNANCY TESTS FOR IN-HOME USE

Name	Manufacturer	How Supplied
Acu-Test	Beecham	1 or 2 tests/kit
Advance	Advance Care	1 test
Answer	Carter	1 test/kit
Daisy 2	Advance Care	2 tests/kit
e.p.t.	Warner-Lambert	1 or 2 tests/kit
e.p.t. Plus	Warner-Lambert	1 test/kit
Fact	Advance Care	1 test/kit
First Response	Tambrands	1 test/kit
Predictor	Whitehall	1 test/kit

or not you use a home pregnancy test kit, your physician should perform another pregnancy test to confirm the pregnancy.

In about the same amount of time it takes to purchase an in-home pregnancy kit and perform the test, you could drop off a urine sample at the physician's office and forego the cost of the kit. Furthermore, the cost of the very reliable physician's test and that of a kit are about the same. Home pregnancy detection kits currently cost the consumer between $12 and $25, depending on the type of kit.

If an in-home pregnancy test result is negative, and amenorrhea continues, the manufacturer offers no assurance that you are *not* pregnant. Additionally, instructions for in-home pregnancy test kits recommend using yet another test one week later. If results in the second test are still negative, the only assurance product pamphlets offer is that there is little chance you are pregnant. However, if you have yet to begin your period after the second test, you are instructed to see your physician. The missed period may be due to other health conditions that may or may not be related to pregnancy, such as an ovarian cyst, ectopic pregnancy (pregnancy outside the uterus), colds, flu, sudden or prolonged physical exertion, weight loss, drugs, or emotional upset.

Table 44 (next page) outlines the recommended action to take according to the product literature accompanying in-home pregnancy tests available in the United States. In most cases, a woman eventually checks with her physician anyway, making the practicality of using in-home pregnancy kits somewhat obscure.

If purchasing the first in-home pregnancy kit is impractical, the purchase of a second kit is less logical. Should amenorrhea continue, some manufacturers suggest a second kit be purchased one week later. Supposedly, the second kit is suggested because some women do not produce detectable concentrations of HCG in the urine early in pregnancy. Although the answer is obvious, this raises the question of why manufacturers recommend that in-home pregnancy kits be used so early. One study found that three commonly used brands were only 65.5 percent accurate when used nine days or less after a missed period. If product labels did not recommend testing quite as early as they do (most recommend using their test as soon as three days after the first day of the missed period), more accurate results could be obtained initially for more women using these kits and, possibly, negate the perceived need to purchase a second kit.

If you obtain a first-test, negative result with an in-home pregnancy detection test, you may find that avoiding the purchase of a second kit is a wise move. Since you are advised by product literature to seek medical advice should amenorrhea continue, the money for the second kit may best be used in obtaining a more accurate pregnancy determination from your physician.

TABLE 44
PROBABLE COURSE OF ACTION AFTER USING A HOME PREGNANCY KIT COMPARED TO HAVING TEST PERFORMED BY A PHYSICIAN

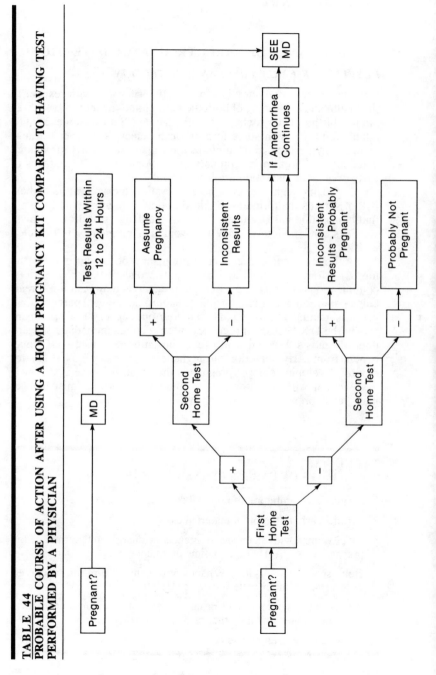

IMPORTANCE OF EARLY PREGNANCY DETECTION

BENEFITS OF EARLY PREGNANCY DETECTION

The earlier pregnancy is detected, the safer it is with respect to the health and well-being of both the mother and the fetus. Over three million births occur each year in the United States. Some 200,000 infants are born with some form of birth defect. A number of these defects may be avoided or minimized through use of early pregnancy detection and appropriate prenatal care. Some of the advantages of early pregnancy detection are listed in Table 45.

In the first eight weeks of pregnancy, the embryo is at its highest risk of serious malformations. All too often women may be unaware that conception has occurred. Many of the dangers of drugs, x-rays, vaccines, and pollutants may be avoided if pregnancy is detected early.

Although ectopic pregnancy (pregnancy occurring outside the uterus) is rare in the United States, it is one of the most serious complications of pregnancy. Ectopic pregnancy may be a life-threatening condition and is responsible for approximately 10 percent of all maternal deaths. Occurring in two to four out of every 1,000 pregnancies in the U.S., ectopic pregnancy often requires immediate surgery upon diagnosis. Women who use an intrauterine device (IUD) may benefit from early detection of pregnancy, as this group is at greater risk for developing ectopic pregnancy than non–IUD users.

Women with a history of spontaneous abortion (miscarriage) may begin prenatal care promptly with a very early diagnosis of

---

TABLE 45
ADVANTAGES OF EARLY PREGNANCY DETECTION

---

1. Permits early initiation of prenatal care.

2. Permits early initiation of maternal care.

3. Gives woman with an unwanted pregnancy the option to terminate the pregnancy at an early date—a time of minimal risk.

4. Helps screen patients for pregnancy prior to use of oral contraceptives or insertion of an intrauterine device (IUD).

5. Allows early detection and prompt treatment of ectopic pregnancy, threatened abortion, and other pregnancy-related disorders.

6. Reduces anxiety and tension.

pregnancy. A test that is sensitive to elevated HCG before the missed period would be helpful for women who suffer habitual spontaneous abortions. When pregnancy is detected this early, women with a history of spontaneous abortion may be placed on a hormone supplement to protect their pregnancy.

Presence of HCG, if you are not pregnant, should be carefully evaluated because it could be due to an HCG-secreting tumor. Cancer occurring in muscular tissue (myoma) may be mistaken for an enlarged, pregnant uterus. A test for HCG may help rule out pregnancy and hasten appropriate cancer therapy. Additionally, high levels of HCG are produced from tumors of the ovary and lung. Measurement of elevated HCG in the absence of pregnancy may alert the physician to these conditions.

False pregnancy (pseudocyesis) has occurred in a few women overanxious to become pregnant. These women experience some of the signs and symptoms of pregnancy without conception. Through a powerful, obsessive desire to have a child, the woman may somehow exhibit a state of pregnancy. Missed menses, breast enlargement, nausea, and vomiting may occur in false pregnancy. Only after conducting a test for HCG have some women experiencing false pregnancy become convinced they are not pregnant.

LIMITATIONS OF CURRENT EARLY PREGNANCY DETECTION METHODS

Measurements of HCG obtained before the eighth week of pregnancy can be used to predict the delivery date. However, values obtained after the eighth week fluctuate too widely to make an accurate determination of when the baby is due.

Early pregnancy tests capable of detecting pregnancy only after a missed period may not indicate that an ectopic pregnancy exists because HCG levels during an ectopic pregnancy are usually abnormally low. So low, in fact, that a false-negative result could occur.

The marked structural similarity between HCG and other hormones, such as luteinizing hormone (LH), could cause a false-positive result. Additionally, HCG may also be found in ovary, testes, pituitary gland, lungs, liver, kidney, spleen, and stomach. As pregnancy tests become increasingly sensitive to lower levels of HCG, results may become unreliable if they detect HCG from these organs.

Early pregnancy tests can be altered if you are taking certain psychoactive (mind altering) drugs such as chlorpromazine (Thorazine®), fertility enhancement agents such as clomiphene (Clomid®), or narcotic pain relievers such as methadone (Dolophine®). Elevated levels of protein (proteinuria) and red blood cells (hematuria) in the urine may also distort HCG measurements.

Geographical differences may also affect the accuracy of pregnancy tests. For example, women from the New Jersey pine barrens possess such a high iron content in their urine that if an agent that binds iron and removes it from the solution is not used first, the results can be inaccurate.

Teenage women 14 to 19 years old comprise a large portion of all women seeking pregnancy tests at family planning clinics. Menstrual irregularity frequently occurs in this age group. This inhibits HCG testing, which requires that a woman have a period at somewhat regular intervals for consistently accurate results.

CONCLUSION

A number of methods are currently available for the early diagnosis of pregnancy. Most offer results in a very short time.

In-home pregnancy detection kits are not as reliable as tests performed by a physician or laboratory. Potential users of pregnancy tests performed in the home may be well advised to take a urine sample to their physician for a more accurate test, thus sparing the expense of the in-home kit.

The advantages to early pregnancy detection are significant. Both the pregnant woman and the developing fetus can benefit. If you have a long-term medical condition, such as diabetes or a history of difficult pregnancy, you are particularly encouraged to seek early detection of a suspected pregnancy.

21

Pregnancy Termination (Abortion)

INTRODUCTION AND DEFINITIONS

Within the context of this chapter abortion is defined as "the voluntary and deliberate removal of fetal tissue from the uterus which results in the termination of pregnancy." This definition should not be confused with the terms spontaneous abortion or miscarriage, which describe an involuntary, passive event often viewed as the process by which the body naturally disposes of a malformed or improperly developing fetus. Approximately 15 percent of all pregnancies result in spontaneous abortion (miscarriage), and most of these occur during the second or third month of pregnancy.

Voluntary termination of pregnancy via an abortion should not be viewed as a primary means of family planning or population control. The abortion issue raises profound ethical, moral, religious, philosophical, legal, and political questions. The emotion-laden controversy surrounding abortion is based on questions such as:

1. Does a developing fetus have the status of a human being and, if so, when during pregnancy does the fetus reach that status?
2. Is abortion murder?

3. Does a pregnant woman have the right to terminate a pregnancy?
4. Does a woman have the right to control her reproductive potential?

Abortion has been voluntarily employed throughout recorded history. Legal decisions around the world have liberalized the accessibility of abortions. More than 20 million legal abortions have been performed in the U.S. since 1967. It is estimated that 50 to 70 million abortions occur annually throughout the world. Approximately 1.6 million legal abortions were performed in the U.S. in 1982. Legal abortion, when properly performed by skilled health practitioners, is one of the safest surgical procedures. Tonsillectomy results in death approximately 12 times more frequently than death of a female as a complication of a medical abortion.

Determination of the age of the developing fetus (gestational age) and when fetal viability begins (the time after which a fetus might possibly survive alone) are of major concern to individuals considering abortion. Gestational age is calculated by adding the completed weeks since the first day of the last menstrual period. Gestational age should not be calculated by adding the weeks from the time of presumed ovulation or conception. In the landmark decision legalizing abortion in 1973 (Roe vs. Wade), the U.S. Supreme Court suggested that fetal viability generally occurs between the 24th and 28th week of gestation. Due to sophisticated medical technology, an aborted fetus in the 24th to 28th week of gestation may survive. Women who desire an abortion should seek the abortion as early in pregnancy as possible, and preferably before 12 weeks of gestation, in order to minimize ethical questions, emotional risks, and health complications.

If you are pregnant, you have three basic options regarding the outcome of pregnancy. You can have the baby and keep it, have the baby and give it up for adoption, or have an abortion. If you decide to have an abortion, five major factors will determine the health outcome:

1. Your general physical and mental health
2. The method of abortion
3. The training and skill of the person performing the abortion
4. Length of the pregnancy leading up to the abortion
5. Quality and accessibility of medical facilities to treat possible complications of abortion

About the only common ground between pro-life and pro-choice groups is that abortion, as a voluntary means of pregnancy termination when the health of the mother is not in question, is an undesirable and crude solution to problems that would better be solved by other means, such as public education and more effective family planning (contraception). The author does not take a pro-life or pro-choice position on whether or not to undergo an abortion. The decision is an individual matter influenced by a host of medical and nonmedical factors. The goal of this chapter is to present the abortion issue in perspective and to provide health information so that decisions about abortion can be made with full consideration given to matters concerning health.

LEGAL STATUS OF ABORTION IN THE U.S.

Abortion is legal in the United States, but the legal system has imposed limits upon the legality of abortion at various times during a pregnancy. In the Roe vs. Wade decision of January 22, 1973, abortion was legalized during the first two trimesters (first six months) of pregnancy. In a seven-to-two decision the U.S. Supreme Court stated, in essence, that neither states nor the federal government could interfere with decisions regarding abortion during the first trimester (first 12 weeks of pregnancy). The Court considered such decisions regarding abortion a private matter between a woman and her doctor. Previous restrictions were declared unconstitutional.

The Court further stated that during the second trimester (the second 12 weeks of pregnancy) a state may impose regulations designed to protect a woman's health (for example, that second trimester abortions be performed only in properly licensed hospitals). The decision of whether to have an abortion, and how and when to have it, remains with the pregnant female.

The same Court decision allows individual states to place restrictions, or even outlaw abortions, after the 24th week of gestation (the beginning of the third trimester) when fetal viability begins. Few conditions exist where third trimester abortion is morally or medically justifiable. Extenuating conditions exist under which third trimester abortion may be legally performed, but there is a lack of unanimity among pregnant women and physicians about the appropriateness of these measures due to the potential viability of the fetus. The legal circumstances under which a third trimester abortion may be considered are as follows:

1. To preserve the life and health of the pregnant woman.
2. When the fetus is afflicted with a condition that is incompatible with survival for more than a few weeks.
3. When the fetus is afflicted with a condition that will leave the child totally or virtually absent of cognitive function.

TABLE 46
RECENT HISTORICAL EVENTS RELEVANT TO ABORTION

1915— Margaret Sanger was arrested for protesting care of indigent New York women dying of septic (infected) self-induced abortions.

1962— Sherri Finkbine sought a legal abortion in the U.S. because of birth defects induced by thalidomide.

1970— Hawaii and New York passed legislation placing the decision of whether or not to have an abortion in the domain of the pregnant woman and her doctor.

1971— Medicaid funding for abortion care was instituted in New York.

1973— The historic U.S. Supreme Court Decision (Roe vs. Wade) regarding the legalization of abortion was rendered.

1976— The U.S. Supreme Court ruled that husbands or parents could not affect their wives' or children's decision to abort a pregnancy.

1976— Congress passed the Hyde Amendment which restricts the use of Medicaid funds for abortion to those situations where the pregnancy endangers the life of the woman.

1977— The U.S. Supreme Court ruled that states may deny use of Medicaid funds for abortions that are not related to medical emergencies.

1979— The U.S. Supreme Court reaffirmed in Belloti vs. Baird that a minor, unmarried female does not need parental consent to obtain an abortion.

1980— The U.S. Supreme Court upheld the Hyde Amendment.

1981— The Human Life Bill (Helms-Hyde Bill) proposed enforcing the obligations of states under the 14th Amendment of the U.S. Constitution not to deprive persons of life without due process of law, and stated that human life exists from conception. Serious constitutional questions, including erasure of First Amendment right guaranteed in the Bill of Rights without the process of a constitutional amendment, were raised.

1985— The Reagan administration asked the U.S. Supreme Court to overrule its previous finding that a woman's decision to end a pregnancy is supported by a fundamental right of privacy.

1986— The U.S. Supreme Court overturned a Pennsylvania law designed to discourage women from seeking abortion, thus reaffirming Roe vs. Wade.

4. When highly reliable diagnostic procedures are available to determine that the fetus meets either condition in item 2 or 3.

No court decision has yet imbued a developing fetus (regardless of gestational age) with the status of a person, but the potential viability of the fetus in the third trimester has led to state legislation and ethical constraints which make third trimester abortions difficult to obtain.

A summary of relatively recent historic events surrounding abortion and the legality of abortion are included in Table 46. Pro-life and pro-choice groups are becoming highly polarized and incidents of violent protest and picketing of clinics where abortions are performed have increased sharply. Efforts to pass a constitutional amendment prohibiting abortion are underway, although public opinion suggests that such a prospect is unlikely. On July 15, 1985, the Reagan administration asked the U.S. Supreme Court to overrule its finding that a woman's decision to end pregnancy is supported by a fundamental right of privacy.

HISTORY OF VOLUNTARY PREGNANCY TERMINATION

Abortion is one of the oldest and, until recently, one of the most hazardous methods of preventing unwanted births. The earliest evidence of use of an abortifacient dates back to a Chinese medical text written between 2737 and 2696 B.C. It consisted of a mixture of various elements, probably including mercury, and was swallowed. Abortion was common in ancient Greece and Rome. The Greeks used various instruments and medicated tampons. The ancient Romans used curettage (scraping of the interior of the uterus), douches (often very caustic), and various oral agents (usually strong laxatives). Medical complications, such as infection and hemorrhage, were quite common.

Religious criticism of abortion is noted in the Old Testament, but became stronger in the Christian era. Under principles of common law, inducing abortion before "quickening" (the first perceptible movement of the fetus) was not an offense. While not condoned in the Middle Ages, abortion was rarely considered cause for legal action; abortion was generally regarded as a desperate, but understandable, alternative to pregnancy out of wedlock.

During the 19th century, abortion became more common and publicized. Dangers of the procedure received more attention. Many Western nations began to enact restrictive legislation. By 1868, most states in the U.S. had laws restricting abortion. These laws were prompted more by physicians trying to protect the public health than by religious opponents. The restrictive approach to abortion in the 19th and early 20th centuries has swung to a more permissive approach over the past few decades. Since 1950, more than 30 countries have amended legislation to permit abortion for social or sociomedical reasons.

The People's Republic of China, in a struggle for national survival, has invoked a policy of "one couple, one child." The effort to restrict population growth is the key to modernization, and births are a matter of state planning. The one-child policy was launched in 1979 and tightened in 1982 to contain China's population at 1.2 billion by the year 2000. In 1983 alone, 14.4 million abortions were performed in China, and approximately 53 million abortions (the population of France) occurred between 1979 and 1984. Many of the "abortions" were during the last trimester, or at term, and would be considered infanticide (murder of the child) by most.

The statistical gains in China are dramatic, but the one-child policy is extracting a heavy toll in broken lives and is tearing at the fabric of family-oriented Chinese society. The program is not restricted to abortion; mandatory contraception and an aggressive sterilization program are also components of the population control policy.

The 1973 U.S. Supreme Court decision decriminalized abortion significantly and clarified each individual's right of privacy. Approximately 3 percent of U.S. women of reproductive age (15 to 44 years) obtained an abortion in 1982 (1.6 million) and an estimated 26 percent of all pregnancies were terminated by abortion that year.

CURRENT ATTITUDES TOWARD ABORTION IN THE U.S.

The controversy surrounding abortion has increased since 1973. Bomb or arson attacks on abortion clinics by pro-life advocates increased from three in 1982 to 24 in 1984. Groups or individuals responsible for attacks on abortion facilities usually express a religious basis for their violent action. A perpetrator of four arson attacks in 1984 claimed he performed the attacks "for the glory of God." He received a 20-year sentence and a $298,000 fine. An accomplice in the bombing of a clinic on a Christmas day stated that the bombing was intended to be a "gift to Jesus on His birthday." Such violence is abhorred by the public at large, and is incongruous with a pro-life position. Bombings and arson directed against property are also potentially harmful to human life.

Despite the attention received by pro-life advocates, the public is still supportive of abortion. About one in four Americans support abortion under any circumstance; anywhere from 7 to 22 percent are strictly opposed to abortion under any circumstance. The remainder approve of abortion under certain conditions, such as rape, incest, or when a woman's life is in jeopardy. The Roman Catholic Church has the clearest position on abortion. Two papal encyclicals of the 20th century, Casti Connubii (1930) of Pius XI and Humanae Vitae (1968) of Paul VI, have condemned abortion under any circumstance. Many Catholics do not support the position of the Catholic church, however. A recent Gallup poll on abortion showed that 64 percent of U.S. Catholics oppose a ban on all abortions. This compares closely with the opposition to an abortion ban by the general American public (69 percent), all Protestant denominations (70 percent), and "evangelical" Protestants (58 percent) as determined by another poll.

Today's abortion debate is occurring in an environment that is very emotional and volatile. Since 1973 the abortion issue has taken on the tone of such historical moral issues as abolition and temperance. The present-day controversy, with its deep moral, religious, ethical, philosophical, and social questions unresolved, involves two primary organized groups, and both groups are dominated by women. The groups are highly polarized and represent pro-choice and pro-life viewpoints.

The pro-choice group is committed to:

1. Freedom of choice and the sovereignty of the individual conscience of the pregnant female in cases of moral doubt
2. The rights of individuals, who must bear the burden of their moral choices, to have the right to make those choices
3. Fostering enfranchisement of women to control their own destinies
4. Freeing procreational choices from the control of the state and giving the benefit of uncertainty in matters of conscience to the pregnant female
5. Removing childbearing from the realm of biological chance, accidental impregnation, or sexual inevitability

In short, the pro-choice position is heavily directed toward the maximization of individual choice and the privatization of moral judgment. The pro-choice position is compatible with the 1973 U.S. Supreme Court decision legalizing abortion and reflects the opinion of the majority of American society. Crass expediency and convenience do not represent the mainstream thinking of pro-choice advocates.

The pro-life group is committed to:

1. Respect for the right to life of individuals (including a developing fetus) even if there are questions about when life actually begins

2. Protecting the weak and powerless from the more powerful so they will have opportunities to develop to their full potential
3. The appropriateness of translating moral convictions and values into law (as in the civil rights movement)
4. Denial of a violent solution (abortion) to accidental or unwanted pregnancy, and acceptance of accidents as a part of life
5. Providing support (by the community, health care facilities, and state) to mediate hardship associated with an unwanted or unintended pregnancy
6. Supporting the conviction that moral values and ideas toward a developing person should be upheld, even at the cost of personal difficulty for the eventual mother

The pro-life movement is guided by a value system that is deeply moral. Religious overtones are very strong. Pro-life advocates espouse the rights of a developing fetus and believe the willingness to live with and accept externally imposed hardship should be accepted as a part of life.

The debate about abortion will continue. Abortion is not likely to ever fit into some overall coherent scheme of values. Arguments by both pro-choice and pro-life groups command respect. Society can only hope that the debate will become more controlled and not degenerate to the level of sustained violence or terrorism.

ABORTION SERVICES AVAILABLE IN THE U.S.

There are wide gaps in the geographic availability of abortion services. There are about 3,000 abortion providers in the U.S. Seventy-eight percent of all U.S. counties, containing 28 percent of women aged 15 to 44, had no identified provider of abortion services in 1982. Only 15 percent of all abortion providers are located in nonmetropolitan counties, and these facilities only conduct about 2.5 percent of all abortions. Abortion services are concentrated in urban areas and are most available on the east and west coasts. Approximately 18 percent of abortions are performed in hospitals and 82 percent in nonhospital clinics—clinics specializing in abortion services (56 percent), other clinics (21 percent), and physician's offices (5 percent).

Since legalization of abortion in 1973, women have obtained abortions earlier in pregnancy. By 1980, 91 percent of women who terminated their pregnancy did so within the first 12 weeks (first trimester) of gestation. Many providers of abortion services restrict abortions to women whose pregnancies have lasted no more than eight, 10, or 12 weeks. Only one-third of providers offer abortion services after 12 weeks of pregnancy. Private physicians are most likely to limit abortions to early gestations; only 11 percent will perform abortions after 12 weeks gestation. Hospitals are most likely to offer late abortions (past 16 weeks), but 10 percent restrict abortions to eight weeks, and 23 percent restrict abortions to 10 weeks gestation, or less.

Public funding for abortion services is decreasing. The so-called Hyde Amendment to the annual appropriation of the U.S. Department of Health and Human Services (DHHS) have limited Medicaid financing of abortion services to those instances in which the life of the pregnant woman is in jeopardy if the pregnancy is carried to term. In 1982, the federal government spent less than $1.0 million to provide medically necessary abortion services to approximately 500 indigent women. Eighteen states and the District of Columbia reported spending $67 million to provide 210,000 abortions for poor women in 1982. Seven states reported no publicly funded abortions in 1982.

The federal government has shifted its focus from abortion services to the provision of family planning and contraceptive services to patients eligible for Medicaid. The federal government pays 90 percent of the cost of family planning services under Medicaid and less than one percent of the cost of providing abortions to Medicaid-eligible women. In fiscal year 1982, the federal government spent $328 million to support contraceptive services, largely through Title X of the Public Health Service Act.

MEASURES WHICH SHOULD BE TAKEN BEFORE HAVING AN ABORTION

Four basic steps should be taken before an abortion is performed:

1. A woman should have a pregnancy test as soon as she suspects she may be pregnant. Pregnancy testing by an ethical laboratory is preferable to in-home pregnancy testing (see Chapter 20). By the time most women determine they are pregnant, they are four to six weeks into a pregnancy. Since the safest and simplest abortion procedures should be performed before 12 weeks gestation, the earlier a pregnancy is determined the more time a woman has to make a decision about whether to have an abortion.

2. A woman may wish to seek counseling about the appropriateness of an abortion and learn about the various abortion methods available. It is very important that a woman considering abortion be in touch with her own personal feelings and values. Reputable counselors will not try to influence a woman's ultimate decision, but may provide valuable information about options and abortion procedures. Uncertainty and ambivalence are likely to occur. After counseling, approximately five percent of women who had decided on abortion change their mind. If counseling is sought, a woman should reflect for a few days on considerations discussed during the counseling session before making the final decision on whether or not to have an abortion.

3. A thorough health history should be obtained from the women seeking an abortion by a physician or an associate of the physician. A health history should include relevant information from the following areas: (a) a statement about the nature of the problem or concern, (b) a statement about present or past health status, whether health problems are or were chronic or acute, and how they were treated, (c) a review of the developmental, sexual, menstrual, contraceptive, gynecological, and obstetrical history, (d) medical history of other family members, (e) a review of the psychological, social, cultural, and occupational history of the woman, and (f) the nutritional history and current nutritional status of the woman.

4. A thorough physical examination should be performed after a health history has been acquired and before an abortion is performed. A physical exam will assist in determining the cardiovascular, respiratory, neurological, gastrointestinal, gynecological, muscular, skeletal, breast, and hormonal health status of the woman. The exam will also assist in screening for infections, cancer, allergies, alcoholism, and a number of other factors that may increase risk during and after abortion. The physical exam may include a chest x-ray (especially if a woman wants general anesthesia during the abortion), analysis of blood (blood count), analysis of urine, pelvic examination, Pap smear, and test for the presence of gonorrhea or other sexually transmitted diseases (particularly if the woman is unmarried and has a history of multiple sexual partners).

If the woman is over 35, has borne one or more than one

child with a birth defect, has a personal or family history of birth defects, or engaged in intercourse with a potential father who has a personal or family history of birth defects, the physician may recommend analyzing a small sample of fluid from the sac surrounding the developing fetus. This process is known as amniocentesis and may allow detection of certain birth defects early in pregnancy.

METHODS USED TO PRODUCE AN ABORTION AND THEIR SAFETY

FIRST TRIMESTER ABORTION (FIRST 12 WEEKS OF GESTATION)

Postcoital "Contraception"

There are three accepted methods of postcoital (after intercourse) contraception. These are the "morning after pill" (diethylstilbestrol [DES], 25 mg two times daily for five consecutive days, beginning 24 to 72 hours after unprotected intercourse), the "morning after insertion of an IUD," and menstrual extraction (miniabortion). All appear to be very effective.

Diethylstilbestrol (DES) must be employed within a few hours to three days after unprotected intercourse. An IUD should be inserted within three days after unprotected intercourse. Menstrual extraction involves removal of the contents of the uterus within five to 14 days after a missed period. Menstrual extraction involves mechanical removal of the contents of the uterus by strong suction. Menstrual extraction can be performed in an office or clinic before pregnancy is confirmed, and the cost is not high. Cramping and/or bleeding may be experienced. The vaginal bleeding may last for a few days. Intercourse and douching should be avoided until bleeding has stopped. Strenuous exercise should be avoided for at least 48 hours after the procedure. Normal menstrual bleeding usually returns within four weeks.

There is debate about the appropriateness of calling these three techniques "contraceptive" measures. If fertilization has occurred, both postcoital DES and IUD insertion probably act as abortion inducers by preventing implantation of a fertilized egg. Menstrual extraction is definitely a form of early abortion. The semantics of identifying these procedures as "contraceptives" are very misleading, especially with menstrual extraction.

French scientists have developed an experimental pill—a steroid known as mifepristone, or RU 486—which appears to abort about 85 percent of pregnancies if taken in the first month of pregnancy. The drug seems to produce an abortion by blocking the action of progesterone, a hormone essential for a viable pregnancy. Availability in the U.S. is not expected for several years.

Abortion by Laminaria Digitala

Laminaria digitala is a form of sterilized seaweed which is made into a tampon-like object that can be inserted into the cervical canal. The device is left in the cervix of the uterus for six to 24 hours, during which it swells up to five to six times its regular size by absorbing moisture. This dilates (widens) the cervix. Once removed, a suction-scraping technique or injection of a drug which stimulates contractions of the uterus may be employed to remove the contents of the uterus.

Laminaria rods are popular in Japan and Northern Europe, but not in the U.S. The disadvantages of this method include possible infection, increased trauma to the cervix from unskilled use of the rods, and cramping.

Suction Curettage (Vacuum Abortion)

An abortion by suction is the most widely used method of terminating pregnancy up to 12 weeks after a missed menstrual period. This procedure seldom requires hospitalization (depending on the method of anesthesia employed). Most women receive local injections of anesthetic into the cervix and ligaments supporting the uterus. This may be preceded by a tranquilizer and/or pain medication. There is little or no pain associated with injection of the local anesthetic. The physician then typically dilates the opening of the cervix by inserting metal rods of increasing width. A hollow tube called a curette that is attached to a suction device is then inserted through the cervix and into the uterus, and the contents of the uterus are gently vacuumed out.

Women who receive local anesthesia may experience a slight tugging sensation. Toward the end of the procedure, which takes three to five minutes, the uterus contracts sharply. A strong cramping sensation may last for up to 20 minutes. Drugs may be given to keep the uterus contracted, thus minimizing bleeding. Some bleeding and occasional clots are to be expected and may begin again a few days later. Slow bleeding is indicated by dark blood. Bright red blood which soaks a pad in less than an hour is abnormal and should be reported to the physician immediately, as should severe lower abdominal cramping that begins a day or more after abortion, a temperature over 100.4°F, a green or foul smelling vaginal discharge, and/or burning on urination.

Most employed women return to work in a day or two, but rest and inactivity are strongly encouraged for at least 24 hours, and preferably 48 hours. Douching, tub bathing, and intercourse should be avoided for approximately two to four weeks, and tampons should be avoided for at least two weeks. Fertility returns rapidly; contraceptive measures should be employed when intercourse resumes. Menstruation should occur in four to six weeks. A follow-up exam should be scheduled two to four weeks after the abortion, even if there is no discomfort.

SECOND TRIMESTER ABORTION (13 TO 24 WEEKS OF GESTATION)
Dilation and Evacuation (D & E)

Dilation and evacuation (D & E) is the most frequently used method of second trimester abortion in the U.S. Approximately two-thirds of all second trimester abortions are by the D & E method, and some 90 percent of second trimester abortions at 13 to 15 weeks gestation are by D & E. This method may be employed beyond 15 weeks, and up to 24 weeks, of gestation, but D & E at these stages of pregnancy increases risk to the pregnant female. Popularity of D & E after 15 weeks of gestation is not high among physicians. Good alternatives to D & E are available if an abortion is required at 16 to 24 weeks of gestation.

Dilation and Evacuation (D & E) is a combination of suction curettage, done in first trimester abortions, and a surgical procedure in which a sharp curette is used to scrape the uterus to remove any remaining fetal tissue. The scraping with a curette is necessary at this stage of gestation due to the larger amount of fetal tissue.

D & E is usually performed under local anesthesia, but general anesthesia may be employed if that is the woman's preference. The cervix is first dilated with instruments, and uterine contents are then broken apart and vacuumed out. Scraping of the uterine wall and suction removal of the remaining debris completes the procedure. The procedure usually takes 20 to 30 minutes, and the recovery and precautions to be observed are similar to those presented in the section on first trimester suction curettage (vacuum abortion).

Amniocentesis Abortion (Instillation Abortion)

Amniocentesis (instillation) abortion is a procedure in which a hollow needle is inserted through the abdominal wall and uterine wall into the fluid-filled amniotic sac that surrounds the developing fetus. Approximately 180 to 240 ml (6 to 8 ounces) of amniotic fluid is removed and replaced by a similar volume of fluid containing a drug which will induce fetal death, uterine contractions, and expulsion of fetal tissue.

This procedure should be conducted in a hospital under sterile conditions as it involves more risk than abortion methods used earlier in pregnancy. The amniocentesis (instillation) abortion should not be attempted before 16 weeks of gestation because the amniotic sac will not contain enough fluid prior to that time for the procedure to be done effectively or safely. The optimal time for the performance of an abortion using this method is at 16 to 18 weeks of gestation, although it may be performed until the 24th week.

A two to three day hospital stay is generally required. General anesthesia cannot be used with this procedure; women must be alert so they can report unusual sensations to the physician. A local anesthetic may be injected into the abdominal area where the amniocentesis needle is to be inserted. Some physicians insert Laminaria rods into the cervical canal after the amniocentesis procedure, while others insert them before the procedure, so the cervix will be dilated, thus minimizing the risk of tearing the cervix when fetal tissue is expelled. Uterine contractions, similar to labor pains, usually begin spontaneously within six to 24 hours. If a concentrated solution of saline (salt solution) was injected into the amniotic sac, some doctors administer a drug (oxytocin) which induces uterine contractions and shortens the time interval between the amniocentesis procedure and expulsion of the fetus. This reduces the chance of infection and retention of the placenta (structure of uterine wall through which fetus is nourished). Pain medication may be administered to relieve the discomfort of uterine contractions. The length of time between the amniocentesis procedure and expulsion of the fetus is usually between 24 and 36 hours (perhaps as little as six to 12 hours if oxytocin is administered); well over 90 percent of women undergoing this procedure will abort in 72 hours. Since the fetus is relatively small at 16 to 18 weeks, the expulsion is not usually painful. Surgical widening of the vaginal opening (episiotomy) is not necessary. The placenta is usually expelled naturally within two to three hours after expulsion of fetal material. All expelled materials must be examined by medical personnel so completeness of expulsion may be determined. A woman should tell the nurse and/or physician if she does not want to see the expelled fetal material.

Women should remain in the hospital for at least 12 hours after expulsion. Most women will experience mild vaginal bleeding for seven to 10 days. Breast changes with swelling and discomfort may occur. A slight temperature elevation, approximately three days after abortion, may occur and last for one or two days; consult the physician if the fever is over 101°F for 24 hours or more. If bleeding is prolonged and/or heavy, consult the physician. Tampon use, tub bathing, douching, and sexual intercourse should be avoided until the follow-up gynecological examination (two to six weeks after the abortion).

Drugs contained in amniocentesis (instillation) abortion fluids are usually (1) a highly concentrated (usually 20 percent) solution of saline (sodium chloride or table salt) or (2) a fluid containing a urea-prostaglandin mixture or a prostaglandin alone. Urea-prostaglandin mixtures, prostaglandins alone, and concentrated saline induce uterine contractions. Saline appears more effective than prostaglandins in eliminating signs of fetal life in abortions late in the second trimester.

Retention of some products of conception (incomplete abortion), infection, excessive bleeding, injury to the cervix, and uterine perforation are the most likely complications of amniocentesis (instillation) abortion; complications may be severe, although they seldom are. In extremely rare instances, death may occur. Approximately 10 to 12 deaths per year occur as a result of legally acquired abortions in the U.S., and these deaths are usually due to infection. The act of childbirth is several times more likely to result in the death of the mother; the incidence of maternal death is approximately 8 to 12 deaths per 100,000 live births.

Both saline and urea-prostaglandin instillation are associated with low failure rates. In one large-scale, comprehensive study there were 1.71 failures per 100 urea-prostaglandin abortions and 1.93 failures per 100 saline abortions. Urea-prostaglandin abortions resulted in 1.03 significant complications per 100 procedures; saline abortion produced 2.88 significant complications per 100 procedures. Saline abortions appear to increase the risk of bleeding complications by almost five times. Saline abortions are more likely to lead to failure to expel the placenta than urea-prostaglandin abortions. The instillation of prostaglandins directly into the amniotic space usually produces uterine contractions within four hours, and the abortion is normally completed within 12 to 24 hours (vs. 24 to 36 hours or more for saline-induced abortions). In addition to the amniotic route, prostaglandins may be administered by multiple intramuscular injections or vaginal suppositories. Experience with prostaglandins administered by injection or vaginally to produce abortion is limited. Most providers of abortion services prefer prostaglandins over concentrated saline solutions when conducting amniocentesis (instillation) abortion.

Hysterotomy and Hysterectomy

Hysterotomy (an operation in which an incision is made in the uterus through which the fetal contents are removed) is a type of mini–cesarian section, is rarely used today as an abortion procedure, and is reserved for special cases. Hysterectomy involves removal of the uterus (and its contents in pregnancy) and is used as an abortion procedure only when other serious medical problems justify such a measure. Such justification is extremely rare.

THIRD TRIMESTER ABORTION (AFTER 24 WEEKS OF GESTATION)

Conditions under which a third trimester abortion is justified are extremely rare and limited by the legal system. A review of conditions under which third trimester abortions are typically legal and morally justifiable are included in the prior section of this chapter titled "Legal Status of Abortion in the U.S." Approximately 14,000 third trimester abortions are performed annually in the U.S.

ABORTION-INDUCED INTERFERENCE WITH SUBSEQUENT FERTILITY

There have been several nonconclusive reports from around the world that repeated abortions have decreased fertility and increased risk of premature birth, low birth weights, and other problems in subsequent pregnancies. Researchers in the U.S. and Great Britain have not found such trends when repeat abortions were legally acquired and complications did not develop. Subsequent fertility may be impaired if an infectious complication follows an abortion. If not promptly and effectively treated, pelvic inflammatory disease and tubal scarring can occur, thus ultimately affecting fertility. Risks of complications can be minimized by seeking an abortion in an appropriate medical facility.

EXPENSE OF ABORTIONS

Cost of an abortion is determined by (1) whether the procedure is performed in the first or second trimester, (2) whether it is performed in a nonhospital clinic or a hospital, and (3) whether it is performed near home or at a distance which necessitates costly travel. A 1984 national survey of the cost of a dilation and evacuation (D & E) at 14 weeks of gestation revealed that the average cost was

$740 if performed in a hospital and $358 if performed at a clinic. Amniocentesis (instillation) abortions during the second trimester cost an average of $940. Average charges in 1983 for all types of abortions performed at 10 weeks gestation where local anesthesia was employed were $194 (range $95 to $390) at abortion clinics, $213 (range $115 to $560) at other clinics, and $253 (range $75 to $650) in physician's offices. General anesthesia is offered by only 30 percent of abortion clinics and 17 percent of other clinics. General anesthesia in clinics will increase abortion costs by an average of approximately $150. General anesthesia during hospitalization will increase the cost of an abortion by several hundred dollars. Average costs of abortion services are increasing at a rate of 6 to 10 percent per year.

CONCLUSION

Pregnancy termination via abortion raises legal as well as moral, religious, ethical, and philosophical questions. There is no standard answer to the question . . . "Should I have an abortion?" Societal attitudes on the issue of abortion are varied. This chapter reviews logical steps to follow when considering an abortion and presents the various abortion procedures employed at various times during pregnancy so that full consideration can be given to matters concerning health.

22

Rational Approach to Feminine Hygiene

INTRODUCTION

Feminine hygiene products (douches, vaginal deodorant sprays, tampons, sanitary napkins, and thin pads) represent sales of over $1.5 billion per year. The American public appears to be obsessed with cleanliness and freedom from potentially offensive body odors. Use of feminine hygiene products is often rational, but all too frequently feminine hygiene products, particularly douches and vaginal deodorant sprays, are overvalued and misused. The focus of this chapter is upon the safe and appropriate use of feminine hygiene products with emphasis on feminine cleansing and deodorant products.

At one extreme we have "Madison Avenue" overpromoting these products, creating a demand where little or no demand previously existed, suggesting vague needs for the products, overstating value of the products, and being so successful in marketing that sales are setting records. At the other extreme are feminists who consider the marketing and sale of certain feminine hygiene products as a sexist exploitation of women. The appropriate approach to feminine hygiene is to be educated regarding risks and benefits associated with use of various products so you can make an informed decision about whether to purchase, and how to use a given product if purchased.

The appropriateness of using tampons, sanitary napkins, and thin pads is apparent. The primary questions of selection revolve around absorbency, aesthetics, comfort, cost, and risk of developing toxic shock syndrome if tampons are employed. Substantial controversy does exist, however, concerning the value of douches and feminine deodorant sprays. The prevailing medical opinion is that healthy vaginas are self-cleansing, and the external female genitalia may be cleaned and deodorized effectively with soap and water. Many physicians believe excessive douching presents a health risk because douching may disturb the normal environment of healthy vaginal tissue. If douches or deodorant sprays are utilized, they should be considered cosmetics unless they have been prescribed by a physician for a legitimate medical problem.

CONDITION (ENVIRONMENT) OF THE NORMAL VAGINA

Some discharge from the vagina is normal. The healthy vagina produces a secretion which cleanses and lubricates the vaginal tract and external genitals. A normal vaginal discharge is acidic, contains no pus, is free of blood, appears whitish or clear, is generally odorless, and does not normally produce irritation or itching. Volume and consistency of normal vaginal secretions will vary somewhat during the normal menstrual cycle. For a further review of the normal changes in vaginal secretions over a menstrual cycle see Chapter 6 (Other Contraceptive Methods).

Vaginal health is most dependent on good hygiene, the correct balance of pH (acidity or alkalinity), bacteria present, and hormonal activity. When the vaginal discharge causes vaginal irritation, itching, and/or burning; becomes offensively odorous; or discharge is excessive to the point of creating a need to utilize pads or change underwear frequently, something is wrong. If one or more of these conditions is present, you should contact your physician because these changes could be due to infection, hormonal changes, irritation, or other causes. The specific cause must be identified so appropriate treatment may be started.

One of the most frequent causes of excessive vaginal discharge, itching, burning, and pain of the female external genitals is the syndrome known as vaginitis (inflammation of vulvar and vaginal epithelium). Pain of vaginitis is due primarily to inflammation of the external genitalia; there are virtually no nerve endings within the vagina to perceive pain and inflammation. Odor may be associated with vaginitis, but odor alone does not indicate that vaginitis is present. Vaginal odor may also be due to bacterial decomposition of normal vaginal secretions left on the skin for excessively long periods between washing with soap and water. Other causes of vaginal odor include normal perspiration, presence of semen or old blood, infections, cervical cancer, or presence of foreign bodies (for example, a retained tampon or portion of a tampon, failure to remove diaphragm or contraceptive sponge at the recommended interval, or retention of a portion of a contraceptive sponge in the vaginal canal).

Estrogen is primarily responsible for controlling the thickness of the vaginal epithelium (lining). Epithelial cell height increases at puberty and decreases at menopause. The thicker the vaginal epithelium, the more healthy the vagina. In estrogen-deficient states (such as after menopause, during pregnancy, or during use of certain types of oral contraceptives) the vaginal epithelium may thin out and become more susceptible to infection and irritation.

Vaginal health also depends on the pH (acidity) of the vaginal area. For optimal vaginal health, the pH of the vaginal surface should be 3.5 to 5.0—that is, slightly acid. A shift in the pH toward alkalinity (pH greater than 7.0) may make the vagina more susceptible to infection. Menopause, pregnancy, and oral contraceptive use may decrease the acidity of vaginal tissue.

Numerous "friendly" bacteria inhabit the healthy vagina. These normal organisms include Döderlein's bacillus (a strain of lactobacillus), staphylococcal species, bacteroides, and streptococcal species. These organisms normally do no harm. Döderlein's bacillus is extremely useful because it metabolizes vaginal glycogen to lactic acid, which assists greatly in maintaining the normal acid pH of the vagina. The presence of glycogen is primarily controlled by estrogen. Without adequate estrogen and subsequent glycogen, the lactic acid levels and vaginal pH may increase toward alkalinity, thus increasing the risk of infection by "unfriendly" bacteria. Glycogen content in vaginal cells may be decreased after menopause, during pregnancy, or while using certain oral contraceptives.

THE MOST COMMON CAUSES OF VAGINITIS

Vaginitis may be caused by bacteria, fungi, protozoa, viruses, chemicals, or traumatic injury. Vaginitis in women of childbearing age (usually 15 to 44 years) is due primarily to infection. Infection of the vaginal area may be promoted by the following factors in this age group:

1. Suppression of normal bacteria of the vagina due to chronic use of broad spectrum antibiotics (for example, tetracycline or erythromycin) to treat acne or an infection. Suppression of normal bacteria allows abnormal

and "unfriendly" bacteria and fungi to grow and produce pain, burning, and itching.

2. Steroid therapy (including certain types of oral contraceptives) may decrease epithelial cell thickness and prevent the conversion of vaginal glycogen to lactic acid. A thinner, less acid vaginal surface increases the probability of infection. Certain oral contraceptives promote the development of vaginitis in a small percentage of users because the pill is progestin dominant, and overrides the protective value of estrogen.

3. Cancer of the female reproductive tract.

4. Pregnancy. Pregnancy results in a diminished protective effect from estrogen.

5. Diabetes.

6. Presence of a foreign body (for example, a tampon, diaphragm, contraceptive sponge, or fragment(s) of a tampon or contraceptive sponge).

Trichomonas vaginalis (a protozoan) and *Candida albicans* (a fungus) are the most common causes of vaginal infections in women of childbearing age. These agents are readily treatable with certain antibiotics. Chapter 15 presents, in detail, the symptoms of vaginitis due to *T. vaginalis* and treatment of that condition. Vaginitis due to *T. vaginalis* is transmitted primarily by sexual contact.

It may be very difficult for you to objectively and adequately distinguish abnormal from normal vaginal discharge. A physician should be seen if you feel the vaginal discharge is abnormal. A proper diagnosis must be made before treatment can be prescribed. Treatment with prescription drugs is usually quite effective. Self-treatment with douches and covering up odors with deodorant sprays can be a very unhealthy and ineffective practice.

ROLE OF DOUCHES AND VAGINAL DEODORANTS IN TREATING VAGINAL ITCHING, BURNING, EXCESSIVE DISCHARGE, AND VAGINAL ODOR

DOUCHES

Douches, available as liquids, liquid concentrates to be diluted in water, and powders to be dissolved in water, exert a cleansing effect by mechanically flooding the vaginal tract and washing away mucous secretions and accumulated debris. This mechanical flooding is perhaps the primary value of douching. Numerous active chemical ingredients are contained in douche liquids; some added ingredients are effective, but others are not. The typical ingredients added to douches are (1) antimicrobial agents (to suppress growth of bacteria), (2) counterirritants (to retard burning and itching), (3) astringents (to reduce inflammation), (4) proteolytics (to break down proteins in vaginal discharge and promote removal), (5) surfactants (to facilitate removal of vaginal secretions by promoting a thinning of the discharge), (6) substances affecting pH (to combat infection), and (7) various miscellaneous ingredients. Ingredients of douches, and their claimed activity, are included in Table 47.

The therapeutic value of most antimicrobials in douches utilized to treat vaginitis due to an infection is very questionable; there is general agreement that most antimicrobials in douches are ineffective. It is very difficult to objectively evaluate efficacy because most manufacturers do not list concentrations of ingredients. Typical "antimicrobial" ingredients include benzethonium and benzalkonium chlorides, boric acid, cetylpyridinium chloride, eucalyptol, menthol, oxyquinoline, povidone-iodine, sodium perborate, and thymol. Hexachlorophene- and phenol-containing douches are antimicrobial at adequate concentrations, but the FDA Advisory Panel on Over-the-Counter Contraceptive and Other Drug Products has judged these two products to be neither safe nor effective when used in douches.

With the exception of boric acid and povidone-iodine, you should consider all other antimicrobials in douches as lacking evidence of safety or effectiveness. Boric acid may be an effective antimicrobial in douche liquids in concentrations of five percent, particularly in the treatment of vaginitis caused by the fungus *C. albicans*. Treatment at this concentration requires physician supervision. Povidone-iodine (Betadine Douche®, Massengill Medicated Disposable Douche®, Femidine Douche®) may be an effective aid in managing vaginitis due to *C. albicans* or *T. vaginalis*. Local irritation or hypersensitivity reactions to antimicrobial ingredients may occur. If such reactions occur, you should discontinue douching and consult your physician.

Counterirritants are included in douches to aid in reducing the symptoms of burning and itching associated with vaginitis. There is insufficient evidence to substantiate the effectiveness of this group of chemicals, according to an expert FDA panel. Eucalyptol, menthol, methyl salicylate, and thymol may contribute to a soothing and refreshing feeling. Eucalyptol and methyl salicylate are aromatic and may mask vaginal odor.

Astringents are often included in douches to reduce inflammation. There is little proof of effectiveness at concentrations typically contained in douches. Many astringents become irritants in moderate to high concentrations. Astringent chemicals which may be contained in douches include alum, aloe vera, and zinc sulfate.

TABLE 47
TYPICAL INGREDIENTS OF VARIOUS DOUCHES

Agent	Activity
Acetic Acid	Alters pH
Aloe Vera (Stabilized)	Astringent
Alum	Astringent
Benzalkonium Chloride	Antimicrobial
Benzethonium Chloride	Antimicrobial
Benzocaine	Local Anesthetic
Boric Acid	Alters pH; Antimicrobial
Cetylpyridinium Chloride	Antiseptic; Antimicrobial
Citric Acid	Alters pH
Docusate Sodium	Helps Remove Vaginal Secretions
Eucalyptol	Antiseptic; Counterirritant; Deodorant
Lactic Acid	Alters pH
Menthol	Antiseptic; Counterirritant
Methyl Salicylate	Counterirritant; Deodorant
Nonoxynol-9	Helps Remove Vaginal Secretions
Octoxynol-9	Helps Remove Vaginal Secretions
Oxyquinoline	Antiseptic
Papain	Helps Remove Vaginal Secretions
Povidone-iodine	Antimicrobial
Sodium Bicarbonate	Alters pH
Sodium Perborate	Antiseptic; alters pH
Sodium Lauryl Sulfate	Helps Remove Vaginal Secretions
Thymol	Antiseptic; Counterirritant
Zinc Sulfate	Astringent

One proteolytic agent may be utilized in douche products—papain, which allegedly breaks down proteins in viscous vaginal discharge. This alleged value is highly theoretical, and papain may produce local allergic and inflammatory reactions.

Surfactants have been viewed somewhat favorably by the expert FDA panel evaluating vaginal products sold over-the-counter. These ingredients appear to facilitate spreading of the douche liquid over vaginal mucosa and folds and may assist in thinning vaginal discharge. Surfactant chemicals include docusate sodium, nonoxynol-9, octoxynol-9, and sodium lauryl sulfate.

Substances affecting pH include acetic acid, boric acid, citric acid, and lactic acid to increase acidity, and sodium perborate and sodium bicarbonate to increase alkalinity. If you need an acid douche, acetic acid (vinegar), as a solution of two tablespoonsful of white vinegar in one quart of water, may be as effective as any commercially available acid douche. Premixed disposable vinegar douches are also available commercially. Some individuals say that alkaline douches are more effective than acid douches for removing vaginal discharge, but there is little evidence to support this claim.

Miscellaneous ingredients in douche fluids include emollients, emulsifiers, fragrances, and numerous other chemicals. Most gynecologists agree that these ingredients have no therapeutic value.

In summary, the occasional use of douches to cleanse the vaginal canal may be appropriate. Self-diagnosing and self-treating vaginitis and other vaginal disorders by douching is a dangerous practice and is discouraged. If you have vaginal itching, burning, odor, and/or a heavy vaginal discharge, you should see your physician for a specific diagnosis. Douches of a particular type may be useful aids to treat a vaginal disorder, but only a physician will be able to determine when such use is appropriate for you and which product you should use.

RISKS ASSOCIATED WITH DOUCHING

There are numerous risks associated with indiscriminate and uninformed douching. Inappropriate douching may produce the following adverse events:

1. Direct irritation or allergic sensitivity from one or more of the ingredients.
2. Salpingitis (inflammation of fallopian tubes), endometritis (inflammation of the inner lining of the uterus), or pelvic inflammatory disease (see Chapter 14) if the douching is too vigorous.
3. Infection due to washing away of normal "friendly" bacteria and decreasing the acidity of the vaginal area.

4. Hemorrhage.
5. Local trauma.
6. Pregnancy if douching occurs sooner than six to eight hours after intercourse if a diaphragm, contraceptive sponge, or contraceptive jelly, cream, or foam was employed.
7. Pregnancy if douching is used as a contraceptive method. Douching is not a contraceptive. Sperm usually travel from the vagina into the cervix of the uterus within seconds to a few minutes after intercourse. Douching may propel viable sperm into the cervix of the uterus, thus increasing the probability of pregnancy.
8. Absorption of iodine from povidone-iodine may occur. If such a douche is used excessively during pregnancy, the absorbed iodine may lead to goiter, hypothyroidism, mental and/or physical retardation, and neurological disturbances in the developing fetus. Infrequent use of iodine-containing douches in pregnancy probably does not appear to harm a developing fetus.
9. Douching used to treat vaginal burning, itching, discharge, and/or odor will not generally treat the medical condition causing the symptoms. Furthermore, vaginal symptoms may be due to infections which cause gonorrhea, nongonococcal urethritis, and other serious medical disorders. Reliance on douching to treat symptoms may lead to costly delays in seeking appropriate medical diagnosis and treatment.

PROCEDURES TO BE EMPLOYED FOR PROPERLY USING A DOUCHE

Many complications of utilizing douches can be minimized or prevented if a few simple procedures are followed. These include the following:

1. A properly prepared and administered douche, used in the absence of vaginal symptoms, to cleanse the vaginal tract may be used once or twice weekly without significant risk of harm. Douching once or twice weekly is not required by most women, however.
2. Clean douching equipment before and after use, or use a prefilled disposable douche to avoid contamination.
3. Douches should never be instilled with excess pressure. If you use a douche bag, it should not be more than 24 inches above the hips.

4. Instill a douche lying down with your knees drawn up and hips raised (in a bathtub, for example).
5. Use lukewarm (not hot or cold) water to dilute douche solutions or powders.
6. Do not douche during pregnancy, except on the advice of your physician.
7. Do not douche if the cervical mucus (rhythm) method of contraception is employed. Douche liquid will interfere with evaluation of the mucus.
8. Do not rely on douching as a contraceptive.
9. Do not douche sooner than six to eight hours after intercourse if you use a diaphragm, contraceptive sponge, or contraceptive jelly, cream, or foam.
10. Do not use a douche 24 to 48 hours before a gynecological exam. The fluid may wash away cells that could be useful in diagnosis.
11. Discontinue use if burning, itching, or local inflammation develops or becomes worse.

VAGINAL DEODORANTS

Feminine hygiene deodorant sprays are available in mist or powder form, which are intended to be applied on the external genitalia to reduce or cover up objectionable odor. Their value is limited. They offer no proven advantage over soap and water. Soap and water remove the source of offensive odor; deodorant sprays only cover up odors for a short period of time.

The primary ingredient in vaginal deodorants is the fragrance, and many of the fragrances can cause local irritation and inflammation. Other ingredients include antimicrobials (see Table 47) and emollients (to soothe the skin). Aerosol sprays also contain a propellant (such as propane or isobutane) which is not dangerous unless the nozzle is held too close to the skin when applied.

Vaginal deodorant sprays have no therapeutic value; they should be considered cosmetics. If you have a persistent vaginal odor and/or vaginal burning, itching, or discharge, you should consult your physician, as the odor and other symptoms could be indicative of a serious medical disorder.

RISKS ASSOCIATED WITH USING VAGINAL DEODORANTS

There are risks associated with use of vaginal deodorants. The adverse effects induced by these products do not occur often, but occur too frequently to be ignored. The most common adverse effects reported to pharmacists, physicians, and the FDA are redness and itching of the vulva after application. Some severe cases of local irritation have occurred. Any number of ingredients could cause a local inflammatory or allergic reaction, depending on your susceptibility. Local inflammatory reactions may be compounded by wearing close-fitting and/or nonabsorbent undergarments, holding the nozzle too close to your body when you apply, or applying immediately after intercourse.

Use of vaginal deodorant sprays is controversial. Superiority of these products over soap and water utilized during a daily bath or shower has not been established. Removal of the source of offensive odor is logically more appropriate than covering it up for a few hours. Sales of these products are decreasing; this is believed to be reflective of a higher level of knowledge among consumers regarding the true value of vaginal deodorant sprays.

PROCEDURES TO BE EMPLOYED FOR PROPERLY APPLYING DEODORANTS TO THE VAGINAL AREA

Procedures for using vaginal deodorant sprays, which should minimize adverse effects, are included below:

1. Hold the spray at least eight inches from your vagina. If held too close, the spray may be too concentrated on a small area, may be forced into the vagina, or the propellant may "chill" the tissue.
2. Do not spread the labial folds before applying the spray, as this may allow entry of the spray into the vagina.
3. Avoid frequent (several times per day) application. Frequent application will increase the possibility of local irritation.
4. Do not use the spray prior to or immediately after intercourse.
5. Discontinue use of the spray if burning, itching, or local inflammation develops or becomes worse.
6. If you have a serious odor problem a few hours after bathing or applying a vaginal deodorant spray, you should see your physician.

TRENDS CONCERNING USE OF TAMPONS, SANITARY NAPKINS, AND PADS

Sanitary napkins have been available since the early 1900s, but their use declined dramatically after tampons were introduced. It is estimated that 70 percent of all menstruating women in America used tampons by 1980. The relationship between toxic shock syndrome (TSS) and tampon use (see Chapter 18) led to a precipitous drop in tampon use. The market share of tampons decreased from 70 percent to 55 percent during 1980. Although tampons have recaptured a significant share of this lost market, thin pads have been the real winner in feminine protection since 1980. The traditional and extremely bulky belted pads now account for less than 10 percent of the feminine protection market and should disappear from the market within a few years. Thin pads represent about 30 percent of feminine protection sales, and their market share is increasing.

American women are expressing a strong preference for feminine protection that is absorbent, convenient to use, and comfortable, and that poses little risk of contributing to the development of toxic shock syndrome (TSS). TSS associated with tampon use may have been more a factor of inappropriate consumer use than anything else. Since new guidelines have been developed for properly using tampons (see Chapter 18), the incidence of TSS has dropped dramatically. You should be very aware and mindful of the early warning signs of TSS if you use tampons. These signs and symptoms are presented in detail in Chapter 18. To avoid risks of TSS, many women now use both pads and tampons. The usual pattern is tampons by day and pad protection at night. This action is extremely wise and is encouraged.

Women desire total protection, so there has been an increase in use of multiple products over the past several years. For example, some users of tampons also use panty shields for added protection. The recently introduced breathable panty liners are certain to remain a popular item.

The adhesive backed thin pads, which were developed in the late 1970s and early 1980s, are replacing the more bulky pads. Thin pads offer varying degrees of absorbency, are often shaped like an hour glass and designed to fit the contour of the female body, and may be unscented or contain a deodorant. The key to success of thin pads is their superabsorbency and smaller size. The absorbency is as good as the traditional and bulkier maxipad, and the comfort index is higher.

23

Sexual Myths and Fallacies

INTRODUCTION

The subject of sexual response is of extreme interest to most people. Until the last two decades, however, human sexuality was not extensively studied, and open discussion of sexual themes rarely occurred. The sexual revolution of the 60s and 70s changed this. Its impact resulted in an explosion of information about virtually every aspect of sexual activity. Unfortunately, despite the proliferation of sex information, a great many sexual myths and fallacies persist. This chapter is intended to dispel some of the more prominent fictions that plague the sexual thinking of some men and women.

BACKGROUND

The first scientist to actually study and discuss sexuality in recent times was Sigmund Freud. His primary thesis was that much of human behavior was related to sex drive (libido).

The biologist Alfred Kinsey began to study sexual habits of men and women in the 1950s by developing structured interviews based on accepted scientific data collection methods. One of the major findings from Kinsey's research was that like many other forms of human activity, people were enjoying sex in a variety of forms.

Masters and Johnson were among the first to observe the physiological aspects of human sexual activity in a controlled setting. They were the first to analyze and categorize the various events of sexual response, dividing it into four phases: excitement, plateau, orgasm, and resolution.

Shere Hite used the questionnaire approach, eliciting responses from over three thousand women and seven thousand men. Her findings, published as *The Hite Report,* explored human feelings and understanding of sexual relationships. The report also reinforced much of the basic physiology associated with male and female orgasm.

Since the 1960s, sex research and therapeutic investigations of human sexual response has increased. Clinics that treat sexual impairment have sprung up across the U.S. Health professionals are becoming more aware of how important sexual health is to the general well-being of the individual. Many scientific journals are devoted to the reporting of sex research.

FACTORS THAT HAVE PERPETUATED SEXUAL MYTHS AND FALLACIES

Perhaps the basic difference between the sexual revolution of the last two decades and current trends in human sexuality can best be described as the desire for quantity in the 60s and 70s compared to the search for quality in sexual encounters seen developing in the 80s. An article in a popular women's magazine states "the headiness of the sixties soon vanished along with the last few remnants of sexual taboos." But have sexual taboos and myths really disappeared? A decade after the "sexual revolution," numerous myths and fallacies about sex remain.

Many states still have laws governing the types of sexual relations that may take place between consenting adults. Even though such moral conduct laws are seldom enforced, the fact that these archaic statutes still exist typifies the continued regimentation of societal attitudes about human sexual activity. Many parents inhibit sexual awareness as a result of their own lack of knowledge about sex, unfounded fears about telling their children about sex, or the influence of biases instilled in them during childhood. However, statistics do not bear out parental fears that increased sexual awareness and an environment for discussion of sex will push young people into sexual promiscuity.

Another reason myths about sexuality have persisted is the wealth of *mis*information that is presented in tabloids and the lay press. Probably the most guilty of these publications are several of the magazines and tabloids targeted to the woman reader. At the checkout stand of any grocery store the titles emblazoned across the displayed magazines or tabloids might include:

Sex: A Cure for Arthritis?
The Better Sex Diet

Titles such as these are designed purely to sell magazines, not to accurately and objectively inform the reader. Although these same publications may contain useful and accurate information from time to time, the average reader may have difficulty distinguishing fact and fallacy.

SOME COMMON MYTHS ABOUT FEMALE SEXUALITY

THE MYTH ABOUT "NICE GIRLS" AND "OTHER WOMEN"

Attitudes and beliefs about sexuality and sexual responses are shaped to a large extent by environment and childhood exposure. Distinctions have always been made between "nice girls" and "other women." Mothers have often suggested to daughters that they "get married, raise a family, and please their husband. Forget about sex, passion, and sensuality. Only nymphomaniacs and prostitutes revel in sexual activity." Many women were, and may still be, taught that:

- All men care about is your body.
- If you give them what they want, they won't respect you.
- Men will only use you.

This mentality has influenced the attitudes of some women toward men. With such a basis for male/female relationships, no wonder many women have feared sharing their true feelings about sex with men and vice versa.

In addition, sexual relationships for women hold the extra risk of childbearing. With today's contraceptive choices, there is less risk. With the development of the birth control pill, women experienced a sexual renaissance. The pill allows women the opportunity to separate sexual pleasure from reproduction and allows for a greater degree of sexual independence.

THE FEMALE ORGASM CONTROVERSY

During the late 1880s, Freud developed theories about female sexuality that shaped cultural attitudes for many years. Freud considered the clitoris a "masculine" organ—an inferior penis. The clitoris, when discovered by little girls, is often the focus of masturbation long before the vagina is found. Freud suggested that as a woman matures she stop her interest in the clitoris and focus pleasurable feelings to her vagina. Freud believed that orgasm resulting from clitoral stimulation was "immature," and that orgasm resulting from vaginal stimulation was "mature." He also stated that the sexually aroused female should be submissive during sexual intercourse. Errors arose in his theory because he did not adequately test his observations.

Karen Horney, a physician, challenged Freud's views on female sexuality as early as 1924. Horney acknowledged the role of culture on female sexual response. She believed female sexual response was largely influenced by the cultural belief that men were superior, and women's responses were shaped to fit that belief. The work of Margaret Mead, an American cultural anthropologist, suggests that the capacity for orgasm is a learned response, which a given culture may or may not help its women to develop.

So the debate over female orgasm raged. Since the "correct" way, according to Freud, to achieve "mature" orgasm was with vaginal stimulation, any woman who desired clitoral stimulation was, therefore, "immature." Thus, generations of women thought there was something wrong with them because they desired clitoral stimulation.

Masters and Johnson support the view that female orgasm involves the clitoris. They further believe that any perceived difference between orgasms is subjective because all female orgasms involve contact with the opening of the vagina, which generates stimulation of the clitoris. According to their research, women who report orgasm with repeated vaginal penetration may have learned to maximize clitoral stimulation during intercourse. Masters and Johnson found that female orgasm lasts about 4 to 12 seconds. It has since been determined that a woman is capable of having several different types of orgasm, each of which can occur with varying degrees of intensity. Furthermore, women do not have to have extended sessions of stimulation to reach orgasm.

A recently recognized element of female sexual response is continued or sequential orgasms, which may recur with restimulation to orgasm every few minutes. Researchers are finding that progressive, sequential orgasms with restimulation to orgasm every few minutes allows the individual to not only experience several orgasms, but also stay on an orgasmic plateau perhaps for hours.

In *The Hite Report,* some women reported that orgasm with vaginal penetration felt different from orgasm after clitoral stimulation. The most striking observation from the reports of these women is the variety of physical responses.

In 1980, the "source" of vaginal orgasm was reported to be the "G" Spot. The "G" or Grafenberg spot is named after Dr. Ernst Grafenberg, the first modern physician to describe it about thirty years ago. About two inches into the opening of the vagina, and in the top portion of the vaginal canal, the "G" spot is believed by some to be extremely sensitive to deep pressure, not soft touch as is the clitoris. When properly stimulated, the Grafenberg spot may swell and lead to orgasm in some women. With repeated stimulation of the "G" spot, some women may achieve multiple or sequential orgasms. Stimulation of both the clitoris and the "G" spot, alternatively or simultaneously, may bring on sequential orgasms.

MYTHS ABOUT FEMALE GENITALS

Women have natural secretions that appear as vaginal discharge and require no extraordinary cleansing practices. The amount, consistency, and color are variable. Most commonly, the vagina is clean and free from infection. It is unnecessary to use so-called "female deodorants" for vaginal cleanliness, and douching is unnecessary in the healthy female. Scented douches should be avoided because the perfumes included in these preparations may irritate the vaginal tissues. An abnormal discharge usually has a disagreeable odor and/ or unusual color, and may cause itching. It may be the result of infections such as candida (a fungus) or trichomonas (a protozoan). Any abnormal condition of the vagina should be evaluated medically and treated if necessary.

FEMALE SEXUAL DESIRE DURING MENSTRUATION

Many men are under the impression that women have no sexual desire during their menstrual period. *The Hite Report* surveyed 436 women about sexual drive during the menstrual cycle. An overwhelming majority (74 percent) reported an increase in sexual desire just before or during menstruation.

FEMALE SEXUAL ACTIVITY DURING PREGNANCY

There are few studies that provide factual data on sexual activity during pregnancy. Although there are an abundance of sexual taboos associated with pregnancy, few are based on biological or physiological fact and study.

Masters and Johnson found that sexual activity and behavior

varied in pregnant women. If nausea was present in the first trimester, then sexual activity was prone to decrease. Some women, however, reported an increase in libido. During the second trimester, they found that many women reported an increased interest in sex. However, by the third trimester almost all women reported a decrease in sexual interest and sexual activity.

Other studies have found that sexual activity decreased during all phases of pregnancy. The most common finding about sex during pregnancy is that there are no clear patterns of behavior other than a generally reduced frequency of sexual activity in the third trimester (last three months of pregnancy).

Why do many couples have sex less frequently during pregnancy? Most women feel uncomfortable during certain stages of pregnancy. Many women suffer from nausea early in pregnancy. Others suffer from fatigue, backache, and other complaints that could cause sexual desire to decrease. One of the most marked changes during pregnancy is breast tenderness. If a woman experiences significant discomfort of the breasts, she may have a decreased interest in sex.

Many couples fear damage related to penile thrusting. For example, they fear the membranes may rupture or bleeding may occur. A study of 260 healthy pregnant women revealed that this does not appear to be a threat. However, if substantial bleeding occurs, especially in the third trimester, it should be viewed as a serious symptom. It may indicate a condition called placenta previa, in which the placenta is positioned too low on the uterine wall. Bleeding is generally an indication not to have sexual intercourse.

Other couples fear that intercourse may cause infection. Intact uterine and placental membranes and a healthy cervix offer some protection against infection. However, intercourse is contraindicated in cases of ruptured membranes and a dilated cervix.

Orgasm may produce uterine contractions. This has probably been the most common reason why physicians recommend abstaining from intercourse during late pregnancy. Masters and Johnson reported no evidence to indicate fetal distress during orgasm. Intercourse late in pregnancy poses little direct danger to the fetus, unless there has been a previous history of premature labor or delivery. In this case, sexual intercourse should not occur in the third trimester.

FEMALE SEXUAL ACTIVITY AFTER LABOR AND DELIVERY

Most physicians recommend refraining from sexual intercourse for at least six weeks after delivery of a child. Sexual relations may be resumed sooner if there is no discomfort from an episiotomy, no persistent vaginal bleeding, and other physical problems are absent. If the woman had a cesarian section, sexual relations may be resumed sooner if no pressure is placed on the incision.

Many couples report little interest in sex for some time after birth. The woman may fear pain or feel that she is no longer attractive to her sexual partner. She may also suffer from postpartum depression, which may be due, in part, to hormonal changes. There is a period of adjustment after the birth of a child. There is also an increase in domestic activity, leading to preoccupation or fatigue, which may decrease sexual desire. The male partner may feel neglected or somewhat jealous of the time the mother spends with the child.

After the birth of a child, a temporary decrease of vaginal mucosal tissue may occur due to a decrease in estrogen levels, and this may account for some of the discomfort that women feel upon initially resuming sexual relations after delivery. If unresolved, this discomfort may lead to lack of interest in sex. This problem may be solved by the use of lubrication (such as K-Y Jelly®).

Nursing mothers may retain extra fat and feel unattractive. Their breasts may be sore from nursing. Particularly low estrogen levels in nursing mothers may cause breast and genital tenderness.

FEMALE SEXUAL ACTIVITY AFTER HYSTERECTOMY

The exact nature of female sexuality after hysterectomy is not well defined. The medical community is divided in their opinions. Hysterectomy may have great emotional impact. Women differ in how they perceive the surgery. Some see it as a symbol of aging or a loss of womanliness. It may cause depression, especially if associated with serious disease or malignancy. Other women may be glad to be free from menstruation, pain, or fear of pregnancy.

FEMALE SEXUAL ACTIVITY AFTER MENOPAUSE

For aging women, menopause is the most significant sign of sexual aging. The onset of menopause creates some psychological stress for almost all women. Some women grieve over the loss of the ability to bear children; others welcome the freedom from fear of pregnancy. Other women undergo episodes of depression.

Menopause occurs as the production of estrogen diminishes. The uterus and ovaries atrophy, the vagina is decreased in size, the entrance to the vagina becomes smaller, and the clitoris may reduce in size. In the absence of estrogen, lubrication of the vagina during sexual arousal decreases. This may result in dyspareunia (painful intercourse). Lubrication of the vagina may be accomplished by use of a lubricating material of personal preference. In some cases, estrogen replacement therapy may be initiated.

There is no evidence that sexual drive or capacity is decreased due to menopause. A reduction in clitoral size has never been correlated to reduction of responsiveness. About 60 percent of women continue to have intercourse at age 60. Masters and Johnson concluded that there is no age at which female sexual response automatically stops. In fact, they found the same clitoral responses in women over 40 that they found in younger women.

Many women report they enjoy sex more after 40 than when they were younger. Some reasons for this may be increasing independence, career success, financial security, dwindling family obligations, and a greater number of sexual experiences.

FEMALE SEXUAL FANTASIES

Many women fear they are abnormal because the only way orgasm is achieved is to fantasize during intercourse. To fantasize about sex during sexual intercourse seems to be a frequent and perfectly normal occurrence among women. Even though many women fantasize during sex, it seems to make some women uncomfortable. Most women feel they should be "turned on" entirely by their sexual partner. Should they fantasize, they may feel they are cheating themselves or their sexual partner.

The fantasies that women have may vary from mildly romantic scenes to acts that may be totally off limits in actuality. One woman in five reports fantasies in which she is forced to have sex against her will.

SOME COMMON MYTHS ABOUT MALE SEXUALITY

THE MYTH THAT MEN KNOW EVERYTHING ABOUT SEX

The man who knows all the right moves in every encounter is a mythical figure. What feels good to one woman may not feel good to another. Additionally, it is difficult for a man to know what a woman wants if she does not know herself. Although we tend to think of sex as natural and spontaneous, human sexuality is basically a learned phenomenon.

How do men and women learn about sex? Our culture and society do not assist us greatly in acquiring reliable information about sex. More permissive attitudes have not ended sexual misinformation. Some men and women have had understanding parents, teachers, or lovers that have taught or explained basic sexual technique.

MYTHS ABOUT MALE ORGASM

Many men and women believe that most males are capable of maintaining an erection for perhaps several minutes at best. This myth has stifled long, pleasurable sex for many couples and is probably based in past cultural attitudes. It is also widely held and practiced that once ejaculation has occurred, sexual activity is over for the male.

Many men may be surprised to learn they are capable of experiencing several orgasms in one lovemaking session. They are perhaps equally unaware that with proper training, exercise, and stimulation they can make love for more than an hour at a time.

MYTHS ABOUT MALE GENITALS

Penis size has nothing to do with whether or not a woman can achieve orgasm. Many men feel their penis is the wrong size, no matter what size it is, and that other penises are larger. Penis size is frequently mentioned in jokes. However, other than personal preference of the woman, penis size is relatively unimportant in bringing a woman to orgasm.

In the past, "premature ejaculation" referred to spontaneous male orgasm before or just at penetration of the vagina. Some use the term to denote male orgasm taking place during coitus, but prior to the woman experiencing orgasm. Nearly three-fourths of men in one study expressed concern over whether they continued intercourse long enough.

Thirty years ago Kinsey reported that 75 percent of men ejaculated within two minutes of beginning intercourse. Kinsey did not consider this to be premature ejaculation. The criteria of a good sexual performance have changed since then. Today the real test of good performance is the ability to satisfy one's partner. This may or may not include orgasm of the woman upon penetration. The woman may desire to be satisfied in other ways or may reach orgasm by other means of stimulation.

MALE PERCEPTIONS ABOUT SEXUAL INTERCOURSE

Many women believe that ejaculation and orgasm are the only reasons men enjoy sexual intercourse. Some men feel they are expressing their love through intercourse. Many men feel that having intercourse to orgasm with a woman is also giving her an orgasm and, therefore, love. Some men do not recognize that most women need more specific clitoral stimulation to achieve orgasm. Men are becoming increasingly aware that sex is more than just sexual intercourse and that sexual activity and orgasm may not necessarily involve just sexual intercourse in every instance.

Only three percent of men who answered the question "Why do you like intercourse?" mentioned orgasm. Only a few men mentioned the pleasure of the vagina on the penis. The most common reason men cited for wanting intercourse was the physical closeness, overall body contact, and the feeling of acceptance that sexual intercourse gave them. Another common reason men wanted sexual intercourse was that it allowed them to be more emotionally open with their partners. However, some women have scoffed at this idea, saying that it is easy for men to say orgasm is not important if it is always attained.

THE AGING MALE

Myths about man's decreased sexual ability in old age may have originated in China. The Chinese believed that a man's semen was limited and that he should only let himself reach orgasm infrequently. True gonadal failure is rarely due to age. Most erection and ejaculating difficulty in males over 40 is due to psychological, rather than physical, reasons. The male may become more concerned about performance as he gets older. Anxiety may assure performance failure. The man that fears aging may have more of a problem than those men who take the aging process in stride. The male may remain fertile to an advanced age. Men over 90 years of age have been reported to have fathered children.

The aging male experiencing erectile problems may be advised simply to vary the methods employed during lovemaking. An older male may only need more stimulation or longer stimulation. If the penis is pushed downward, erection may occur. Manipulation of the penis by the sexual partner may be required.

Even though male responsiveness may slow somewhat after age 40, this may be considered a blessing in disguise. Some women may consider him a better lover because the ejaculation reflex is not quite as fast as it once was. The man may learn to enjoy foreplay more.

MALE SEXUAL FANTASIES

Males, like females, may fantasize during sexual intercourse. This should not be viewed as pathological behavior if it contributes to more enjoyable sex for the male (and female) and the achievement of orgasm. Sexual fantasies that lead to behavior that is objectionable to, or abusive of, the female are abnormal and a cause for concern, however. Such a situation may require intervention by a professional counselor or therapist.

SOME OTHER MYTHS CONCERNING FEMALE/MALE SEXUALITY

THE MYTH ABOUT "EXCESSIVE" SEXUAL ACTIVITY

Some women fear that enjoyment of sex, or having sex too often, will lead to loss of control, mental disorders, epileptic seizures, heart attacks, irresponsible behavior, or even ridicule from their partner. As they approach the orgasmic stage of sexual excitement, they may "turn off" because they are afraid. A relatively high incidence of sexual activity is not associated with any medical disorder. In fact, the more the body is stimulated sexually, the easier it is to achieve orgasm. A low level of sexual activity makes it more difficult to maintain sexual function in later years. Frequent sex in the early and middle adult years is an important factor in whether or not an individual is capable of having sex after age 60.

MYTHS ABOUT MASTURBATION

Western culture often frowns on masturbation as a debased or evil sexual activity. Old wives' tales had masturbation associated with acne, insanity, blindness, and numerous diseases. Until recent times, anyone who masturbated was subject to admonitions of impending doom from continuing the practice. However, there is no evidence that masturbation causes any illnesses or physical deformity.

Masturbation has served as a method to learn about the body and orgasmic potential. Sex therapists recommend masturbation as a learning tool for some women who have difficulty in attaining orgasm. Most women who masturbate state that they enjoy it physically, but not psychologically. Many males and females masturbate as a substitute for sexual activity when a partner is not available. Still others masturbate purely for the pleasure.

"APHRODISIACS"

"Aphrodisiacs" are substances that supposedly enhance sexual desire. Throughout history man has searched for foods and drugs that would increase sexual desire and performance. Substances reported to possess these qualities are numerous, even today. Proof that any substance is a true "aphrodisiac" is lacking, however.

Many legendary "aphrodisiac" foods originated in countries such as China and India where good nutrition among the general population was rare. Many of the so-called "aphrodisiac" foods contain protein and nutrients which were probably lacking in most diets in these countries. If a person improved the nutritional content of the diet with these foods, it would follow that sexual appetite might increase as a result of improved general health.

For the Greeks, it was onions, eggs, honey, seafood, and snails. The Dutch gynecologist, Theodoor Van deVelde, recommended venison, eggs, milk, rice, beets, carrots, and turnips (stewed in milk sauce). Peruvian Indians recommended cocoa and chocolate for men. Publications such as *The Better Sex Diet* cite balanced nutrition as a contributing factor to better lovemaking.

Unsolicited mail and sexually explicit magazines, such as *Playboy, Penthouse, Hustler, Gallery,* and many others, may contain advertisements for so-called nutritional "aphrodisiacs." Some ads feature mega or super vitamins that are supposed to make men more virile, featuring key phrases like "men's tonic," or "make her want you more." The messages insidiously refer to certain vitamins and minerals, such as iron, zinc, and vitamin E, capitalizing on sensational articles purporting these substances to have special sexual enhancing powers. Other ads are directed at the female with claims that their product will make her a more sensuous or total woman.

Perhaps the most insulting of all ads for "aphrodisiacs" are those for spurious remedies. Federal law prohibits advertising using unsupportable claims. Makers of these remedies navigate federal regulatory waters by inserting the word *spurious* into their ads. Some readers are not aware that spurious means fictitious, false, or unsupported. Ads for bogus sex potions use phrases such as "dynamic placebo capsule." Should these remedies enhance sexual prowess, it would not be due to their chemical properties because any placebo is, by definition, an inert or inactive substance.

Amyl Nitrite

In the 1970s amyl nitrite became a "social drug" in North America and Western Europe. Amyl nitrite is a relaxer of smooth muscles, such as those found in the intestines and colon. For this reason, it is especially favored by male homosexuals to aid rectal intercourse. It has been reported to prolong and intensify orgasm. There have been no formal clinical trials of amyl nitrite as an "aphrodisiac." Large doses may cause cardiovascular collapse and sudden death. Chronic exposure to nitrites may result in physical dependence, with blood vessel spasm when the drug is withdrawn.

In the United States, the sale of amyl nitrite requires a prescription, but preparations containing butyl or isobutyl nitrite can be purchased in sex shops. Many of these preparations contain toxic impurities, depending upon the manufacturing process used.

Ginseng

Ginseng, the root of which has been prized in the Orient for centuries, has traditionally been hailed as a cure for everything from headache to sexual inadequacy. In 1733 the first shipload of American ginseng was sent to China. The root was used in teas, elixirs, and tonics for almost any abnormal condition and to prevent almost every disease. During the next 250 years, there was a very lucrative market for American ginseng in the Orient. American ginseng became scarce, and its scarcity only heightened its demand. In 1976 over 329,000 pounds of ginseng were exported from the United States where dealers were paying diggers $90 per pound. In 1978 an international trade commission placed ginseng, or *Panax quinquefolius,* under control as an endangered species. Tight regulations and continued scarcity has enabled ginseng to command the current price of $200 a pound. Marathon County, Wisconsin, produces 90 percent of the entire American crop, with a market value of roughly $25 million annually.

The high demand for ginseng is difficult to explain, however. There has been very little research showing it to be safe and effective for the treatment of any medical disorder, including sexual impairment. Nor has ginseng been shown superior to placebo (inert substance) for increasing sexual desire or performance.

Yet, what about the numerous men and women who report enhanced sexual performance after ingesting ginseng? In a report in the April 13, 1979, issue of the *Journal of the American Medical Association,* 133 ginseng users were studied. Of these, only nine reported increased sexual performance. However, 47 persons experienced diarrhea, 33 had skin eruptions, 65 experienced sleeplessness, and 22 had episodes of hypertension. Other reported adverse effects include depression, hypotension, and amenorrhea. In 1978 the *British Medical Journal* reported that six women developed swollen, tender breasts after chronic ingestion of ginseng. This effect may be due to the small amount of estrogen-like chemicals present in ginseng root. There have also been isolated reports of vaginal bleeding in postmenopausal women who consumed ginseng.

It seems there may be some minor enhancement of sexual feelings in a small number of persons who take ginseng because of its hormonal content or its placebo effect. However, very serious side effects occur in a far greater number of persons who take ginseng. Long-term ingestion of ginseng is not recommended.

Marijuana

Many persons have reported they enjoy sex more under the influence of marijuana. Most scientists who have studied this drug believe that occasional marijuana use immediately prior to sexual activity only removes social inhibitions that may prevent some people from enjoying sex more.

Marijuana alters time perception and causes a perceived sense of pleasure. Actually, long-term use of marijuana is associated with a decrease in levels of hormones that contribute to sexual desire. With chronic use of marijuana, it would be possible to believe that sexual prowess is increasing when it is actually decreasing.

Spanish Fly

Spanish fly is probably one of the most well-known of the "traditional" aphrodisiacs. It is another name for the drug cantharidin, obtained from iridescent beetles found in southern France and Spain. This drug is a very harsh irritant and can be very corrosive to tissue. When swallowed in liquid form it burns the mucous membranes from the mouth to the intestines. It can cause dilation of genital blood vessels, causing erection of the penis or engorgement of the labia. Men may experience priapism, an often uncomfortable condition in which there is prolonged failure of an erection to subside in the absence of sexual stimulation. A large dose of Spanish fly can be dangerous or even life-threatening and has no aphrodisiac properties.

Yohimbine

Yohimbine is actually undergoing scientific testing as a potential aphrodisiac. In the 1970s, several research grants were awarded to scientists to study drugs with potential for use in treating sexual dysfunction. Laboratory experiments with both male and female rats have revealed that injections of yohimbine may cause sexual arousal. The precise mechanism by which yohimbine affects sexual function in rats is not clear. It is not known if yohimbine will work in humans, as it appears to work in rats, or if it is safe to use in humans.

CONCLUSION

Perpetuation of sexual myths and fallacies and failure to allow dissemination of accurate, objective information on human sexuality and sexual health due to societal attitudes may have serious negative consequences. Confusion, misinformation, or lack of information may impair social and marital relations, create psychological difficulties, or produce physical harm. This chapter reviews some of the more common sexual myths and fallacies and presents factual information in an attempt to minimize risk and maximize understanding of human sexuality.

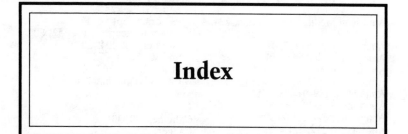

Index

A

Abortion
  amniocentesis, 359–61
  controversy, 352–54
  cost, 362–63
  death, 361
  definition, 347–48
  and fertility, 362
  history, 350*t*, 351–52
  and IUD, 52, 54, 55
  legal status, 349–51
  methods, 357–62
  preparation, 355–56
  public funding of, 355
  services, 354–55
  teenage, 73
  tubal sterilization, 148
  and ultrasound, 340
Abortion, spontaneous. *See*
    Miscarriage
Acetaminophen, 47–48, 143, 210–11,
    244, 302–03
Acne, 32, 167, 171–72
Acquired Immune Deficiency
    Syndrome. *See* AIDS
Acyclovir, 206–08, 210
Addison's disease, 323
Adrenal glands, 319
A-Gen 53®, 179
Aging, 326
AIDS
  cause, 219
  and children, 218, 230–31
  condom, 72, 228

controversies about, 230–31
cost, 231
and death, 218
definition, 216–17*t*
and fungal infections, 224, 225
and herpes, 205, 217, 225
history, 215–16
and immune system, 219–22
and pneumonia, 217, 225
prevention, 227–29
Public Health Service and, 218,
    223, 224, 228
risk factors, 226–27
symptoms, 224–25
testing for, 223–24
treatment, 229–30
AIDS-Related Complex, 216, 224–25
Alcohol, 273, 323, 326, 330
Allergy
  to diaphragm, 85, 90
  to douches, 370
  to oral contraceptives, 32
  to penicillin, 244
  to sperm, 74
  to spermicide, 85, 96, 105
  to vaginal deodorants, 373
Alpha-interferon, 230
Amenorrhea
  and hormonal implants, 171
  and IUD, 50
  and oral contraceptives, 21
  and post-oral contraceptives, 36
  and pregnancy detection, 335,
    342
  and sexual dysfunction, 322

American Board of Obstetrics and
   Gynecology, 157
American Medical Association, 224,
   387
Aminocaproic acid, 330
Ammonium chloride, 301
Amniocentesis, 357, 359–61
Amoxicillin, 189–91, 285, 286
Ampicillin, 189–91, 285, 286
Amyl nitrate, 330, 386–87
Analgesics. *See* Painkillers
Androgens, 319, 321
Anemia, 47, 224, 240
Anesthesia, 151, 152, 211
Aneurysm, 239
Ansamycin, 230
Antibiotics, 189–92, 261–64, 265,
   313, 315, 366–67
Antihistamines, 303
Antihypertensive drugs, 326–28
Antinausea drugs, 329
Antipregnancy vaccine, 177–78
Antivertigo drugs, 329
Antiviral drugs, 230
Aphrodisiacs, 386–89
Appetite suppressants, 329
Arthritis, 187, 196, 325
Ascheim-Zondek pregnancy test,
   334
Azidothymidine (AZT), 230

B
Baclofen, 329
"Band-aid" sterilization. *See*
   Laparoscopy
Bartholin's glands, 9
Basal body temperature, 119–22
Bateman, Thomas, 195
Benztropine, 330
Better Sex Diet, The, 386
Birth control. *See* Contraception
Birth defects, 35–36, 57, 105, 145,
   273, 344, 357
Blood, 54, 145, 227, 229
Blood pressure
   and oral contraceptives, 26, 29,
      30, 31
   and sexual dysfunction, 323
   and toxic shock syndrome, 308,
      311, 312–13
Boric acid, 368
Boston Collaborative Study, 31, 32
Breast cancer, 34, 324

Breastfeeding
   and AIDS, 228
   as contraceptive, 135
   and contraceptive use, 52, 80
   and herpes, 204, 207
   and vaginitis, 273
Breasts, 9, 296, 302, 320
Burkitt's lymphoma, 226

C
Caffeine, 299, 301
Cancer
   and contraceptives, 34–35, 57,
      97
   and DES, 134
   and herpes, 204–05
   and injectable progestin, 164,
      166
   and sexual dysfunction, 324,
      330–31
   and vaginitis, 272, 367
Candida albicans, 246, 268, 271, 367
Cardiovascular disorders
   and injectable progestin, 167
   and oral contraceptives, 26, 29–
      31
   and sexual dysfunction, 322–23
   and syphilis, 239
   and toxic shock syndrome, 312
   see also Clots; Strokes
Castration, 138, 147
Catholic Church. *See* Roman
   Catholic Church
Cefoxitin, 262–63
Ceftriaxone, 190–92, 285
Centers for Disease Control, 217,
   262, 273, 308
Cephalosporin, 189–91, 241
Cerebral lymphoma, 226
Cervical cancer, 34–35, 56, 72, 91,
   204–05
Cervical cap, 80–81, 111–12, 158–64
Cervical mucus, 122–26, 164–65
Cervix
   described, 8
   and gonorrhea, 186, 187, 189
   and herpes, 200–01
   and IUD, 49, 54
   and syphilis, 237
   see also Cervical cap; Pelvic
      inflammatory disease
Chanchroid, 203
Chancre, 234, 237–38

Chicken pox, 195–96
Childbirth
    contraception after, 57, 74, 85
    and gonorrhea, 185
    sexual activity after, 380–81
    teenage, 73
    tubal sterilization after, 148
Children
    and AIDS, 218, 230–31
    and *chlamydia trachomatis,* 250
    and gonorrhea, 185, 187
    and herpes, 203–04, 210
    and syphilis, 240, 243
    and toxic shock syndrome, 307
    see also Teenagers
Chlamydia trachomatis, 49, 189,
        191, 203, 248, 250, 265, 284
Chlorinated sugars, 177
Cholesterol, 26, 28, 30
Chronic lymphadenopathy
        syndrome, 224
Cinnamedrine, 303
Clindamycin, 264
Clitoris, 9, 317–18, 377–79, 381–82,
        284
Clofibrate, 331
Clomiphene, 345
Clotrimazole vaginal tablets, 272
Clots, 15, 26, 30–31, 167, 224
Cocaine, 330
Codeine, 329
Coitus interruptus, 129–30
Cold sores, 195–96
Colpotomy, 138, 148, 149t, 152
Combination pill, 15–18, 20–22, 26
Comstock Act, 77
Condoms
    acceptance, 74–77, 81
    advantages, 66–74
    and AIDS, 72, 228
    characteristics, 61t
    for disease prevention, 60, 68–
        73, 184, 192, 228, 244
    FDA regulation, 60
    history, 59–60
    and IUD, 58
    and pelvic inflammatory
        disease, 265
    and multiple sex-partners, 73
    and spermicides, 66, 101
    teenagers and, 73, 77
    types, 60–66
Condylomata lata, 238

Contact lens, 29, 33
Contraception
    barrier, 79–98
    breastfeeding, 135
    condoms, 59–78
    douche, 131–32
    experimental, 158–80
    failure, 1, 67, 83
    IUD, 39–58, 134–35, 357
    oral, 15–38
    postcoital, 132–35, 357–58
    rhythm method, 115–29
    spermicidal, 99–114
    withdrawal, 129–30
Copper-containing IUDs, 42–45, 53,
        55, 56, 134–35
Copper-7®, 43, 44, 55
Coronary artery disease, 145
Corynebacterium genetalium, 246
Cowper's glands, 11
Crabs. *See* Pubic lice
Crotamiton, 278
CS-85, 230
Culdoscopy, 138, 148, 149t, 152
Cushing's syndrome, 323
Cyclobenzaprine, 329
Cystitis, 90
Cytomegalovirus, 217, 225

D
Dalkon Shield®, 40, 41
Death
    and abortion, 361
    and AIDS, 218
    and hepatitis B, 280
    and oral contraceptives, 26, 29
    during sexual activity, 323
    and syphilis, 235, 239, 240, 241
    and toxic shock syndrome, 313
    and tubal sterilization, 155
Depo-Provera®, 164–68
Depression (mental)
    and hormonal implants, 172
    with menopause, 381
    and oral contraceptives, 29, 32–
        33
    postpartum, 381
    and premenstrual syndrome,
        296, 300, 301–02
DES (diethylstilbestrol), 132–34, 357
Diabetes, 28, 30, 55, 145, 323, 367

Diaphragm
advantages, 79–80, 83
care of, 90
characteristics, 81–82
disadvantages, 80, 90–91
for disease prevention, 80, 91, 184
and douches, 372
fit, 83–85
history, 80–81
insertion and removal, 85–90
and lactation, 80
and pelvic inflammatory disease, 265
rate of use, 81
and spermicides, 111–12
and toxic shock syndrome, 90–91, 309
types, 82
and urinary tract infections, 85
and vaginitis, 366, 377
Diethylpropion, 329
Diethylstilbestrol. See DES
Dilation and evacuation (D&E), 359
Dimenhydrinate, 329
Diphenhydramine, 329
Disopyramide, 331
Diuretics. See Fluid retention
DMSO (dimethysulfoxide), 208–09
Döderlein's bacillus, 267, 366
Dopamine, 313
Douches
as contraceptives, 131–32, 371
and diaphragm, 89
and gonorrhea, 192
ingredients, 367–70
and IUD, 57
proper use, 371–72
risks and safety, 368–70
and syphilis, 244
and toxic shock syndrome, 309
Doxycycline, 262–64
Droegemueller, William, 261
Drug interactions, 37t, 38, 54
Drugs. See specific kinds and names
Dumas cap, 159, 160
Dysmenorrhea, 47
Dyspareunia, 321, 325, 382

E
Ears, 239, 240–41
Ectopic pregnancy
defined, 7
and DES, 134
detection, 340, 344, 345
and IUD, 46, 47, 48, 50–51, 53, 55, 172
and oral contraceptives, 35
and pelvic inflammatory disease, 259, 260
symptoms, 50
and tubal sterilization, 156
Ejaculation, 10, 11, 73–74, 130, 318
Encephalitis, 205, 225
Endometrium, 8, 12, 34, 45, 54, 166, 370
Endorphins, 297
Enzyme immunoassay (EIA), 339
Ephedrine, 303
Epididymis, 10, 146, 185, 187, 284–86
Epididymo-orchitis, 284–86
Epstein-Barr virus, 196
Erythromycin, 189–91, 242, 243, 250, 251, 252–53t, 264
Escherichia coli, 286
Estradiol, 19
Estrogen
and cardiovascular complications, 26, 167
in female reproduction, 6, 7t, 9
and IUD, 45
and oral contraceptives, 15, 19, 22–23
and premenstrual syndrome, 297, 302
as postcoital contraceptive, 132
synthetic, 22
Eyes, 198, 208, 225, 238–40
see also Contact lens; Glaucoma; Ophthalmia neonatorum

F
Fallopian tubes, 7–12, 147–56, 163, 186
see also Pelvic inflammatory disease
Fallopius, 59
Fantasies, sex, 382, 384–85
Female reproductive system, 6–9, 11–12
Feminine hygiene products, 364–74
Fenfluramine, 329

Fertility, 36, 46, 52–53, 165, 166, 362
see also Infertility; Ovulation;
    Sterilization
Food and Drug Administration
    (FDA)
  and cervical cap, 159
  and condoms, 60
  and contraceptive sponge, 97
  and douches, 368, 370
  and oral contraceptives, 15, 34
  and spermicides, 101
  and toxic shock syndrome, 311
  and vaginal deodorants, 373
Freud, Sigmund, 375, 377–78
Friedman, M. H., 334
Fulguration, 153
Fungal infections, 205, 224, 225

G
Gall bladder disease, 31–32
Gamma-interferon, 230
Gastrointestines, 29, 225, 261, 312
Genital herpes. *See* Herpes
Genitourinary tract infections. *See*
    Urinary tract infections
Gentamicin, 264
Gestational age, 348
Ginseng, 387–88
Glaucoma, 240
Glycogen, 366
Gonadotrophin, 321
Gonorrhea
  antibiotic resistance, 192
  causes, 184
  complications, 187–89
  diagnosis, 189
  and diaphragm use, 91
  history, 183
  in-home test, 189
  nicknames, 183
  and nongonococcal urethritis,
    246–47
  and pelvic inflammatory
    disease, 2, 265
  "ping-pong effect," 192
  prevalence, 183–84
  prevention, 192
  and Skene's glands, 9
  and spermicide use, 113
  spread, 184–85
  symptoms, 185–87
  teenage, 73

  treatment, 189–92
  types, 185–87
Gossypol, 175, 176–77
Grafenberg, Ernst, 379
"G" spot, 379
Gummas (granulomas), 239, 240, 241
Gynecomastia, 320, 329, 330

H
Headache, 32, 133, 146, 167, 174,
    202, 238, 239, 244, 297, 302
Hematoma, 146
Hemagglutination assay, 338–39
Hepatitis B, 238, 279–81
Hernia, 145, 155
Heroin, 329
Herpes
  and AIDS, 205, 217, 225
  complications, 203
  and condom use, 68, 72
  death, 204, 205, 210
  and diaphragm use, 91
  history, 194–95
  neonatal, 210
  and pregnancy, 203–04
  preventative drugs, 211–12
  psychological effects, 212–13
  quack remedies, 211–12
  sexual dysfunction, 325
  and spermicide use, 113
  spread, 196–98
  symptoms, 200–03
  and toxic shock syndrome, 309
  treatment, 205–11
  types, 195–96, 198–200
Herpitex, 212
Hippocrates, 183, 333
Hite, Shere. *See Hite Report, The*
Hite Report, The, 376, 378, 379
Hodgkin's disease, 226
Hormonal implants, 168–72
Hormones. *See* names
Horney, Karen, 378
HP-23, 230
HTLV-III virus. *See* AIDS
Human chorionic gonadotrophin
    (HCG), 177, 334–46
Hyde Amendment, 355
Hydrochlorothiazide, 301
Hydromorphone, 329
Hydroxyzine, 329
Hyperprolactinemia, 323–24
Hypertension. *See* Blood pressure

Hypoglycemia, 297, 299
Hypo-ovarianism, 324
Hypothyroidism, 324, 371
Hysterectomy, 138–39, 157, 362, 381
Hysterotomy, 362

I
Ibuprophen, 211, 302
Idoxuridine, 208–09
Immunological assay, 334, 338
Implantation, 7, 12, 165
Inderal®, 179–80
Indomethacin, 302
Infertility, 74, 176–77, 189, 259–60, 261, 286
Injectable progestin. *See* Progestin, injectable
Interferons, 209–10
Interleukin-2, 230
Intracervical devices, 179
   see also Cervical cap
Intrauterine device. *See* IUD
IUD (intrauterine device)
   bleeding, 45, 46–47, 55
   cancer link, 56
   characteristics, 43–44
   complications, 45–53, 57
   cost, 57
   effectiveness, 45, 46t, 57
   fertility after using, 46, 52–53
   and gonorrhea, 184
   and herpes, 195
   history, 39–40
   insertion and removal, 55
   and miscarriage, 46, 51–52, 56, 57
   myths about, 56–58
   and oral contraceptives, 18
   postcoital, 132, 134–35, 357
   rate of use, 40
   types, 39–43
   and vaginal discharge, 51
   see also Pelvic inflammatory disease

J
Jaundice, 32, 240, 280

K
Kaposi's sarcoma, 217, 222, 225, 230
Keratitis, 240

Kidney problems, 238, 312
Kinsey, Alfred, 375–76, 383

L
Labia, 9, 237, 317
Lactation. *See* Breastfeeding
Laminaria digitala, 358, 360
Laparoscopy, 138, 148, 149t, 151, 154
Laparotomy, 138, 148, 149t, 150, 154
   see also Minilapotomy
Levodopa, 330
Levonorgestrel, 168, 169, 170, 174
Libido, 177, 319, 321, 375
Librium, 300
Lindane, 278, 279, 283
Lippes Loop®, 40, 41
Lithium carbonate, 330
Liver, 31, 247, 279, 280, 312
LSO-1, 212
Luteinizing hormone, 20, 117, 127, 164, 176, 178, 321, 345
Lymph glands, 200, 238, 240
Lymphoblastic lymphoma, 226
Lysine tablets, 212

M
Macrophages, 221
Magnesium, 308, 310
Malathion, 283, 284
Male contraceptives, experimental, 175–76
Male Reproductive System, 9–10
Marijuana, 330, 388
Masters and Johnson, 376, 378, 379–80, 382
Masturbation, 385
Mead, Margaret, 378
Meclizine, 329
Medicated IUDs, 41–43
Medroxyprogesterone. *See* Depo-Provera®
Mefenamic acid, 302
Melanoma, 35
Meningitis, 187, 205, 225, 238, 239
Menopause, 118, 326, 381–82
Menstrual cycle
   condom use during, 74
   described, 6–7, 12
   diaphragm use during, 80

and ectopic pregnancy, 50, 56
and gonorrhea, 186
and herpes, 203
and hormonal implants, 171
and IUD, 47, 48, 50, 53–54, 57
and oral contraception, 19, 36
and rhythm method, 116–27
and sexual dysfunction, 322, 329
and *trichomonas vaginalis,* 269
and vaginal rings, 174
see also Premenstrual syndrome
Menstrual extraction, 357
Meperidine, 329
Mercury-containing spermicides,
    100
Methadone, 329, 345
Metronidazole, 73, 264, 271–74, 331
Mifepristone (RU 486), 357
Minilaparotomy, 138, 148, 149*t,* 151,
    152, 154
Minipill, 15–18, 20–22, 51
Miscarriage
    and IUD, 46, 51–52, 56, 57
    and oral contraceptives, 35
    prevention, 340, 344–45
    rate, 347
    see also Stillbirth
Monoclonal antibodies, 127
Monoclonal antibody assays, 339
Mononucleosis, 196, 225
"Morning after" pill. *See* DES
Mucus. *See* Cervical mucus
Multiple sclerosis, 325
Muscle relaxants, 329
Muscular dystrophy, 325

N
Naprosyn, 302
Narcotics, 329–30, 388
Nasal sprays, contraceptive, 178
Neisser, Albert, 183
Neisseria gonorrhoeae, 183, 184,
    187, 189, 191, 192, 284–85,
    287
Neurosyphilis, 239, 242
Nongonococcal urethritis, 246–53*t*
Norgestrel, 175
Norplant® system, 169–70, 171, 172

O
Obesity, 154–55
Oligospermia, 320

Ophthalmia neonatorum, 286–89
Oral contraceptives
    action mechanism, 19–20
    and birth defects, 35–36, 57
    cancer link, 34–35
    cost, 18
    death from, 29
    dose, 21–22
    effectiveness, 18, 57
    experimental, 175–77
    hormonal balance, 25*t*
    and injectable progestins, 164
    pharmacologic effects, 24*t*
    and premenstrual syndrome, 300
    and rheumatoid arthritis, 36
    and sexually transmitted
        diseases, 36
    side effects, 28–33
    types, 15–18, 22–23
    usage rates, 18
    and vaginitis, 367
Orgasm, 317–18, 321–22, 278–79,
    383
Orphenadrine, 329
Ovarian cancer, 34
Ovaries, 6, 12, 163
Ovulation, 7, 12, 27, 36, 116–27,
    164, 167, 174
Oxycodone, 329
Oxytocin, 360

P
Painkillers, 47–48, 143, 151, 210–11,
    244, 302–03, 360
Pamabron, 301
Papilloma virus, 91
PAP smear, 35, 53, 55, 205
Parkinson's disease, 325, 330
Pelvic inflammatory disease
    and abortion, 362
    causes, 256–57
    and *chlamydia,* 265
    complications, 259–60
    and condoms, 70, 265
    and contraceptive sponge, 80,
        265
    and diaphragm, 80, 91, 265
    and douches, 370
    and gonorrhea, 186–89, 265
    and injectable progestin, 165
    and IUD, 46–50, 53, 54, 55, 56,
        262, 265

Pelvic inflammatory disease *(cont.)*
  and oral contraceptives, 36–37,
    265
  prevention, 264–65
  risk factors, 256*t*
  and sexual dysfunction, 319,
    324–25
  symptoms, 257–59
  treatment, 260–64
  and tubal scarring, 259, 261
Penicillin, 189–92, 233, 241–44, 251,
    252–53*t*, 288
Penis
  and condoms, 59–78
  described, 11
  and herpes, 200–01
  priapism, 320
  and sexual response, 317–18
  size, 383
  and syphilis, 237
Perforation, uterine, 48, 49, 55
Peritonitis, 261
Permethrin, 279
Pharylyngeal gonorrhea, 185
Phentermine, 329
Phenylmercuric acetate, 100
Pituitary gland, 20
Pituitary tumors, 35
Placenta, 12
Pneumonia, 217, 225, 250
Postcoital contraception, 132–35,
    357–58
  see also Abortion
Povidone-iodine, 210, 368, 371
Prednisone, 281
Pregnancy
  and AIDS, 227
  and cervical cap, 164
  and diaphragm, 80
  and douches, 371, 372
  and epididymitis, 286
  and herpes, 194, 204, 207
  and IUD, 49, 53, 54, 56
  and metronidazole, 272
  and narcotics, 329
  sexual activity during, 379–80
  and spermicides, 105
  and syphilis, 234, 237, 240, 243
  symptoms, 335
  and vaginitis, 269, 272–73, 367
  see also Childbirth
Pregnancy detection
  A–Z test, 334, 337

  current methods, 336–39
  false pregnancy, 345
  history, 333–34
  in-home kits, 341–43
  limitations, 345–46
  ultrasound, 340
  urine test, 334, 336
Premenstrual syndrome (PMS)
  awareness of, 3, 298
  causes, 297
  complications, 298
  definition, 294–95
  and depression, 296, 300, 301–
    02
  and drug therapy, 299–306
  economic implications, 294
  as legal defense, 298
  and menstrual chart, 298
  and oral contraceptives, 300
  painkillers, 302–03
  psychoactive drugs, 300
  symptoms, 294–97
  treatment, 297–99, 301–02
Prentif cap, 159, 160, 162
Priapism, 320
Probenecid, 189–91, 242, 285
Proctitis, 249
Prodrome, 200
Progestasert®, 42–47, 50–51, 54, 55,
    172
Progesterone
  and abortion, 358
  in female reproduction, 6, 7*t*, 9
  and IUD, 51
  and oral contraceptives, 19
  and premenstrual syndrome,
    297, 298, 300
  and rhythm method, 116–117,
    119
Progestin, 15
Progestin implants. *See* Hormonal
    implants
Progestin, injectable, 164–68
Progestin-releasing IUDs, 172
Progestogen, 132
Prolactin, 297, 302, 321
Prolactinomas, 35
Propranolol, 179–80
Prostaglandins, 297, 302
Prostate gland, 10–11, 185, 269, 317
Pseudomonas aeruginosa, 286
Psychoactive drugs, 328, 345
Pubic lice, 281–83

Pubic Health Service, U.S., 72, 218, 223, 224, 228
Pyrethrins, 283, 284
Pyridoxine. *See* Vitamin B.
Pyrilamine maleate, 303

Q
Quinestrol, 175

R
Rabbit test, 334
Reproductive system. *See* Female reproductive system; Male reproductive system
Rheumatoid arthritis, 37–38
Rhythm method
  advantages, 128
  biological basis, 116–17
  calendar, 117–18
  cervical mucus, 122–26
  disadvantages, 129
  and douches, 372
  effectiveness, 128
  in-home ovulation test, 127
  sympto-thermal, 127
  thermal, 119–22
Ribavirin, 230
Rifampin, 250, 251, 251–53*t*
Robins Co., A. H., 40
Roe vs. *Wade,* 348, 349, 350, 352
Roman Catholic Church, 116, 128, 353

S
Saf-T-Coil®, 40–41
Saline abortion, 360–61
Saliva, 198, 279, 280
Salpingitis, 257, 259–60
Sanitary napkins, 373–74
Scabies, 275–79
Searle Co., G. D., 42–43
Seminal vesicles, 10, 269, 317
Septic arthritis, 187
Sex therapy, 332
Sexual activity
  and AIDS, 219, 225, 226, 227–29
  and cervical cancer, 35
  and epididymitis, 284
  and gonorrhea, 185, 192
  and hepatitis B, 279, 281
  and herpes, 196, 213

  after menopause, 326, 381–82
  myths about frequent, 385
  and pubic lice, 282
  and scabies, 277
  and syphilis, 234, 237, 244
  and toxic shock syndrome, 309
Sexual dysfunction, 319–32
Sexual fantasies, 382, 384–85
Sexual myths and fallacies, 375–89
Sexual response, 317–19
Sexually transmitted diseases
  and cervical cap, 163
  and condoms, 68–73
  and contraceptive sponge, 80
  and diaphragm, 80
  and IUD, 56
  and oral contraceptives, 36–37
  prevention, 1
  and spermicides, 113
  see also specific disease names
Shingles, 195–96
Sickle-cell disease, 165
Silastic®, 168–69, 172
Silver nitrate solution, 287, 288, 289
Skene's glands, 9, 269
Skin disorders
  and gonorrhea, 187
  and herpes, 196, 198, 200–03
  and pubic lice, 282
  and syphilis, 234, 237, 238, 244
  and toxic shock syndrome, 312
  see also Kaposi's sarcoma; Melanoma; Scabies
Smoking, 28, 29–30, 31
Spanish fly, 388
Spectinomycin, 190–92, 285
Sperm, 10, 11–12
  Allergy to, 74
  enzyme inhibitors, 179
  granuloma, 144, 146
  IUD and, 44–45
  reduced count, 320
Spermicides
  allergy to, 85, 96, 105
  and cervical cap, 160, 163
  characteristics, 100, 104*t*
  with condoms, 70, 110
  and contraceptive sponge, 91, 92, 96, 97, 98
  and diaphragm, 83, 87, 91, 110–12
  disease prevention, 70, 91, 113
  and douches, 372

Spermicides *(cont.)*
  effectiveness, 105–12
  and gonorrhea, 192
  history, 99–100
  limitations, 114
  safety, 101, 105
  and syphilis, 244
  and toxic shock syndrome, 91
  types, 100–01, 102–03*t*
  use procedure, 108–09
Spinal cord injury, 325
Sponge, contraceptive
  advantages, 79–80
  characteristics, 93–94
  disadvantages, 80
  and douches, 372
  effectiveness, 96
  FDA approval, 97
  insertion and removal, 94–95
  and lactation, 80
  rate of use, 97–98
  side effects, 96–97
  and vaginitis, 366, 367
Spontaneous abortion. *See*
    Miscarriage
Staphylococcus aureus, 91, 97, 308,
    310, 313, 314
Sterilization, 136–41
  see also specific procedures
Steroid drugs, 281, 313, 367
Stillbirth, 35, 52, 57
Strokes, 30–31, 323
Suction curettage, 358–59
Sulfamethoxazole-trimethoprim,
    192, 286
Sulfur ointments, 279
Sunlight, 32, 35, 202, 203
Supreme Court, U.S., 77, 348, 349,
    350, 352
Suramin, 230
Surfactants, 100, 101
Sympathomimetic amines, 303
Syphilis
  acquired, 234
  causes, 235
  and children, 240, 243
  complications, 237–41
  and condom use, 60, 244
  congenital, 234, 240
  and death, 235, 239, 240, 241
  and gonorrhea, 184
  and herpes, 203
  history, 233
  latent, 239, 244
  and pregnancy, 234, 237, 240,
    243
  prevalence, 233–34
  prevention, 244
  stages, 234–35, 237–39, 244
  symptoms, 237–41
  transmission, 235–37
  treatment, 241–44
  treponema pallidum, 235–37,
    238, 239, 241, 242, 244

T
Tampons, 57, 308–12, 314–15, 366,
    367, 373–74
Tatum-T®, 43, 44, 55
Teenagers
  births and abortions, 73
  condom use, 73, 77
  gonorrhea, 73
  minor-consent law, 254
  nongonococcal urethritis, 247
  pregnancy detection, 346
  rhythm method use, 118
  sex education, 1–2
  syphilis, 240
  withdrawal method, 129
Temperature, body, 119–20
Teratogenicity, 272
Testicles, 10, 145, 146, 284
Testicular cancer, 324
Testosterone
  in contraceptive nasal spray, 178
  described, 10
  and long-acting hormones, 176
  and sexual dysfunction, 319–20,
    330
  and sexual response, 318
Tetracycline, 189–92, 242, 285
Thromboembolic disorders. *See*
    Clots
T lymphocytes, 221–22
Today® contraceptive sponge, 92–98
Toxic shock syndrome
  awareness of, 3
  and blood pressure, 308, 311,
    312–13
  causes, 308
  and children, 307
  and contraceptive sponge, 97,
    309

and death, 313
definition, 307–08
and diaphragm, 90–91, 309
and herpes, 309
nonmenstrual, 309
prevention, 314–15
symptoms, 311–12
and tampons, 308–12, 314–15, 365, 373–74
treatment, 312–13
Toxoplasma, 217
Treponema pallidum. See Syphilis
Trichomonas vaginalis
and cancer, 272
causes, 267–68
and condoms, 73
defined, 267
and lactation, 273
location, 268–69
and pregnancy, 272–73
side effects, 273
and spermicides, 113
transmission, 266
treatment, 270–74
Trifluridine, 209
Triglycerides, 28, 30
Trihexyphenidyl, 330
Triphasic pill, 15, 18, 22
Tubal litigation, 152–53
Tubal pregnancy. *See* Ectopic pregnancy
Tubal sterilization, 138, 147–56
2, 4 toluenediamine (4, 4-TDA), 97

U
Ulene, Art, 3
Ultrasound, 340
Umbilical cord, 12
Ureaplasma urealyticum, 246, 248
Urea-prostaglandin abortion, 361
Urethra, 9, 185, 187, 189, 269, 270, 317–18
Urethritis, 90, 259
see also Nongonococcal urethritis
Urinary tract infections, 84, 90, 121, 325
Uterine
bleeding, 46–47, 50, 52
cancer, 56
perforation, 48, 49, 55

Uterus, 6, 7, 8, 12, 54, 138–39, 247, 336

V
Vaccine
anti-AIDS, 229
antipregnancy, 177–78
antisyphilis, 243
Vagina
chemical balance, 267, 365–66
described, 7, 11, 12
lubrication, 322
and sexual response, 317–18
Vaginal deodorants, 262, 372–73
Vaginal rings, 172, 173*f.,* 174
Vaginismus, 322
Vaginitis
causes, 366–67
and cervical cap, 162
and condom, 73
described, 365–66
and diaphragm, 90
and IUD, 46, 49, 51
and spermicide, 113
treatment, 367–73
and vaginal rings, 174
see also Candida albicans; Trichomonas vaginalis
Valium, 300
Van de Velde, Theodoor, 386
Varicose veins, 28
Vas deferens, 10, 138, 141–43, 269, 317
Vasectomy, 138, 141–47
VD Hotline, 254
Vidarabine, 209, 210
Vimule cap, 159–60, 162
Vitamin B_6, 33, 297, 301–02
Vitamin C, 37, 212
VLI Corporation, 97
Vulva, 9, 237
Vulvovaginal gonorrhea, 185

W
Walnut Creek Drug Study, 28, 32
Weight gain, 166, 171, 335
see also Appetite suppressants; Obesity
White blood cells, 44, 257
Withdrawal, 129–30

World Health Organization (WHO),
140, 179

X
X-ray examination, 44

Y
Yohimbine, 388
Youngs, Merle, 60

Z
Zinc, 212